# OCULAR ACCOMMODATION, CONVERGENCE, & FIXATION DISPARITY

## Clinical Testing, Theory, & Analysis

### Third Edition

**David A. Goss, O.D., Ph.D., FAAO, FCOVD-A**

Professor of Optometry, Indiana University,
Bloomington, IN

Optometric Extension Program Foundation Press

The OEP Foundation, founded in 1928, is an international non-profit organization
dedicated to continuing education and research for the advancement of human prog-
ress through education in behavioral vision care.

OEP Foundation, Inc.
1921 E. Carnegie Ave., Suite 3-L
Santa Ana, CA 92705
www.oep.org

Managing editor: Sally Marshall Corngold
Cover design: Kathleen Patterson

Library of Congress Cataloging-in-Publication Data

Goss, David A., 1948-

Ocular accommodation, convergence & fixation disparity : clinical testing, theory &
analysis / David A. Goss. -- 3rd ed.

    p. ; cm.

Rev. ed. of: Ocular accommodation, convergence, and fixation disparity / David A.
Goss. 2nd ed. c1995.

Includes bibliographical references and index.

ISBN 978-0-929780-24-5

1. Eye--Accommodation and refraction. I. Goss, David A., 1948- Ocular accommodation, convergence, and fixation disparity. II. Optometric Extension Program
Foundation. III. Title. IV. Title: Ocular accommodation, convergence, and fixation
disparity.

[DNLM: 1. Accommodation, Ocular. 2. Convergence, Ocular. 3. Vision Disor-
ders--diagnosis. 4. Vision Disparity. WW 109 G677oa 2009]

RE925.G67 2009

617.7'55--dc22

2009015107

The opinions expressed in this book do not necessarily reflect the policies or philosophy of the Optometric Extension Program Foundation. The Optometric Extension Program Foundation does not endorse any specific assessment or treatment methodology.
The contents are intended for information purposes only and are not to be substituted
for professional advice from readers' health care providers.

\*\*\*\*\*\*\*\*\*\*\*\*\*\*\*\*\*\*\*\*\*\*\*\*\*\*\*\*\*\*\*\*\*\*\*\*\*\*\*\*

Optometry is the health care profession specifically licensed by state law to prescribe lenses, optical devices and procedures to improve human vision. Optometry
has advanced vision therapy as a unique treatment modality for the development
and remediation of the visual process. Effective vision therapy requires extensive
understanding of:the effects of lenses (including prisms, filters and occluders)
  •   the variety of responses to the changes produced by lenses
  •   the various physiological aspects of the visual process
  •   the pervasive nature of the visual process in human behavior
As a consequence, effective vision therapy requires the supervision, direction
and active involvement of the optometrist.

\*\*\*\*\*\*\*\*\*\*\*\*\*\*\*\*\*\*\*\*\*\*\*\*\*\*\*\*\*\*\*\*\*\*\*\*\*\*\*\*

**To my Dad, Arthur Goss,
my best mathematics teacher**

# Epigraph

Plotting data on coordinates or graph paper is for many of us the simplest possible way to grasp a trend or gain a clear picture of the interrelationship of two or more variables.

Henry W Hofstetter

He who is theoretic as well as practical is therefore doubly armed: able not only to prove the propriety of his design but equally so to carry it into execution.

Vitruvius

For when the one great scorer comes
To write against your name,
He'll write not that you won or lost,
But how you played the game.

Grantland Rice

# Contents

Preface     vii

1. Introduction     1

2. Dissociated Phorias and Introduction to ACA Ratios     10
   and Binocular Vision Syndromes

3. Blur, Break, Recovery, and Amplitude Findings     24
   and the Zone of Clear Single Binocular Vision

4. Effects of High Lag of Accommodation and Proximal     36
   Convergence on the Zone of Clear Single
   Binocular Vision

5. Definitions of Terms     42

6. Simple Guidelines for Evaluating the Stress     49
   on Fusional Vergence

7. Dissociated Phoria, Fusional Vergence, and     61
   Relative Accommodation Test Norms

8. Accommodative Facility and Vergence Facility     70

9. Introduction to Fixation Disparity     81

10. Clinical Application of Fixation Disparity     88

11. Diagnosis and Prescription Guidelines in Vergence     107
    Disorders

12. Presbyopia     136

13. Nonpresbyopic Accommodative Disorders     151

14. Introduction to Vision Therapy for Accommodation     171
    and Vergence Disorders

15. Vertical Imbalances     187

16. Additional Considerations and Concepts in     192
    Case Analysis

17. Other Systems of Case Analysis     215

18. Oculomotor Dysfunction     228

19. Historical and Biographical Notes     232

20. Appendix A. Answers to Selected Practice Problems          253

21. Appendix B. Equipment Sources                              265

22. Appendix C. Glossary and Acronyms                          266

23. Appendix D. Phorometry Test Procedures                     273

24. Index                                                      277

# Preface

This manual is an introduction to the collection, organization, and analysis of clinical optometric data used in the diagnosis and management of accommodation and vergence disorders. The purposes of this edition remain the same as the purposes of the first and second editions: to help students learn basic concepts of clinical evaluation of accommodation and convergence, and to provide the fundamentals for a systematic analysis of nonstrabismic binocular vision problems and accommodative disorders.

The primary intended audience of this edition, like the previous ones, is first and second year optometry students. This edition will help students acquire a basic understanding of concepts of accommodation and vergence analysis, and have some confidence in their initial encounters with patients with nonstrabismic binocular vision problems. Mastery of the concepts in this book also will help prepare students for any of the various books available on vision therapy techniques, advanced aspects of accommodation and vergence, and diagnosis and management of strabismus aimed mainly toward third and fourth year optometry students and established practitioners. This book could serve as a review for third and fourth year optometry students. It also might be of some interest to ophthalmology residents or to vision scientists who seek information on clinical evaluation of accommodation and convergence. The summaries of normative values for various tests may be of use to even experienced practitioners.

Accommodation and vergence disorders are among the most common clinical conditions the optometrist encounters. Accommodation and vergence problems can cause significant ocular discomfort and can adversely affect educational, recreational and occupational performance. It is essential, therefore, that the optometrist conduct comprehensive testing of accommodation and vergence, and have a systematic approach to the analysis of those test findings. The analysis approach presented in this book is essentially a normative analysis system, in which particular patterns of abnormal test findings are diagnostic of corresponding accommodation and vergence disorders. Treatment regimens can then be planned based on the disorder present.

As in previous editions, initial chapters present important background concepts necessary to an understanding of accommodation and vergence disorders. Additional information on testing procedures has been included in the beginning chapters in this edition. The coverage of norms for common accommodation and vergence tests in chapter 7 has been expanded from the previous edition. Chapter 8 is a new chapter devoted to accommodative facility and vergence facility testing. Chapters 9 and 10 discuss fixation disparity. Then chapter 11 synthesizes that material to give a systematic method for evaluating non-strabismic vergence disorders. Chapter 12 deals with presbyopia. Chapter 13 has expanded coverage of the clinical evaluation of accommodation in nonpresbyopes. Chapter 14 provides a brief introduction to some of the common training procedures used in vision therapy. New to this edition, in chapter 14, is a sampling of the results of studies on the effectiveness of vision therapy for accommodation and vergence disorders. Chapter 15 deals with vertical imbalances. Chapters 16 and 17 present some additional considerations, concepts, and analysis systems for understanding and evaluating accommodation and convergence function on a clinical basis. Chapter 18, a brief introduction to oculomotor dysfunction, is a new chapter. Oculomotor dysfunction is abnormal saccadic or pursuit eye movement function. Such disorders technically do not fall within the topics described by the title of this book. However, oculomotor dysfunction is included here because it can produce symptoms similar to the symptoms associated with accommodation and vergence disorders. Also new to this edition is chapter 19, which presents biographical sketches of some of the persons who made important contributions to the knowledge and care of accommodation and vergence disorders. Two appendices have been added, a glossary and a series of tables summarizing phorometry testing procedures. The definitions in the glossary are usually worded somewhat differently from definitions in the chapters so that readers not understanding definitions when reading the chapters can potentially see if a definition in the glossary makes the meaning more clear.

The framework used for the teaching of many of the concepts in this book is a graphical display of accommodation and convergence data. I have found this to be an excellent teaching tool for conveying concepts of accommodation and vergence analysis. The insights that students gain by plotting accommodation and convergence graphs help them achieve a better understanding of accommodation and convergence relationships and clinical analysis. It helps to show the interrelations of different tests and why various tests are grouped together in the normative analysis of examination data. It is also an excellent way of assessing the pattern and consistency of phoria, fusional vergence, and relative accommodation findings. The plotting of examination findings in clinical practice can be valuable for that reason, but the principles presented in this book can guide the practitioner in the diagnosis and management of accommodation and vergence disorders, whether or not a formal plot of the data is completed.

In 1980, when I joined the faculty of the Northeastern State University College of Optometry in Oklahoma, I was assigned to teach a course on "graphical analysis." The manuscript for the first edition of this book, published in 1986, developed from hand-outs prepared for that course. At that time another required course was a course in OEP case analysis. Students were then expected to integrate and apply concepts from the two courses when they had patient encounters supervised by faculty. In today's crowded optometric curricula, there is no longer the luxury of having separate courses on particular systems of case analysis. Trends in accommodation and convergence case analysis over the last few decades include integration of concepts from different case analysis systems, increased application of various testing methods previously considered to be auxiliary tests, and increased emphasis on normative analysis.

Many of the revisions in this book were prompted by those changing trends. The basic outline for this edition is similar to that of the second edition, but all chapters have undergone revision and much new material has been added. Practice problems have been revised, and there are many new practice problems. A major change from the second edition to this one is the addition of numerous tables summarizing the means and standard deviations for common accommodation and vergence tests from published studies. By studying these tables the reader can gain an appreciation for the expected or normal findings for accommodation and vergence tests.

I thank former students for their kind comments concerning the ease of reading and the usefulness of earlier editions of this book. These comments have helped motivate me to continue to improve and update this book. I thank Dr. Doug Penisten for his encouragement and suggestions, Dr. Scott Cooper for interesting email discussions, and Dr. David Grisham for suggestions for revisions. And I have benefited throughout my career from the influence of Dr. Henry Hofstetter (1914-2002), who was an outstanding mentor during my years as a graduate student and for many years thereafter. His emphasis on the power of a graph as a tool for examining data is one of the most important lessons I learned from him. I thank former students Drs. Jaimie Kruger and Rana Zargar for work that served as a first draft of Appendix D. Several persons helped locate historical material, supply biographical information, provide photographs, and answer historical questions for chapter 19, including Drs. Charles Letocha, Richard Keeler and Piers Percival, Linda Draper of the International Library, Archives, and Museum of Optometry in St. Louis, and Doug Freeman and Cris Coffey of the Indiana University Optometry Library. I also thank staffs of libraries and archives at Pacific University, University of Waterloo School of Optometry, and the College of Physicians of Philadelphia for providing biographical information and photographs. Lastly, I appreciate the efforts of Robert Williams and Sally Corngold of the Optometric Extension Program in the production of this book.

A book reviewer for the magazine Science once observed "three principal motivations behind writing a scientific book: to unify questions, solutions, advancements, and discussion on a particular topic; to summarize one's lifetime work; and to have fun." (Tsonis AA. Science 1998;280:1210) That observation applies to this book. I have attempted to weave together useful classical clinical concepts, evolving conventional wisdoms, and recent research results in this book. My professional lifetime work has been largely teaching and research on the topics in this book and on refractive errors and optometric history. And it can be fun trying to explain concepts in a clear concise manner; I hope that has been achieved to some small measure.

David A. Goss, O.D., Ph.D.

Sae here content I quat the pen,
Until my Muse return again.

David Sillar
(Sillar D. Poems. Kilmarnock, Scotland: John Wilson, 1789: 236)

# Chapter 1
# Introduction

**A**ccommodative disorders and non-strabismic binocular vision problems are very common eye and vision conditions. Only refractive conditions are more common. The consequences of accommodation and vergence problems range from minor nuisance to significant discomfort to interference with optimal school, recreational, or occupational performance. To detect and properly diagnose accommodation and vergence disorders it is important to have a comprehensive battery of accommodation and vergence tests as well as a systematic method of analysis of the results of those tests.

Two components of such a systematic analysis are (1) the comparison of a patient's test findings to normal or average values and (2) assessment of the overall pattern of the patient's test findings to recognize a case type. For the first component, statistical studies have determined normative values for accommodation and vergence tests.[1] For the second component, one expects certain clusters of test findings to be outside of normal ranges in particular case types. In addition, an x,y coordinate plot of accommodation and vergence test results can help to identify patterns and internal consistency of test findings and to evaluate accommodation and vergence relationships.

## ACCOMMODATIVE STIMULUS AND CONVERGENCE STIMULUS
In most tests in a clinical vision examination we know the accommodation and convergence stimulus values, but we usually do not measure the actual accommodative response and convergence response. We know the accommodative stimulus from the combination of the test distance and the lens power in relation to the subjective refraction. We know the convergence stimulus from the test distance and the power of any prisms through which the patient views.

If we assume that the patient's ametropia is exactly corrected, the stimulus to accommodation in diopters is the reciprocal of the target distance from the spectacle plane in meters. For units other than meters, we can use the following formula:

$$\text{Accommodative stimulus in diopters} = \frac{\text{Number of units in a meter}}{\text{Measured units from the spectacle plane}}$$

The stimulus to accommodation for an object 40 cm from the spectacle plane would be: Accommodative stimulus in diopters = 100/40 = 2.50 D

When we calculate the stimulus to accommodation for various selected test distances, we get the results shown in Table 1.1.

The convergence stimulus is a measure of how much the eyes must converge from parallelism to fixate a given object binocularly. One prism diopter of convergence is a movement of the lines of sight equal to 1 cm as measured at a distance of 1 meter from the base line. (The base line in this context is the line connecting the centers of rotation of the two eyes) For fixation of a near-point target the lines of sight of the eyes must move in from parallelism a distance equal to the interpupillary distance (PD). Therefore, one way to calculate the amount of convergence stimulus is to divide the PD in centimeters by the distance from the object of regard to the base line in meters. We will use the symbol d for the distance from the object of regard to the base line. Figure 1.1 shows an example of convergence for an object 40 cm from the spectacle plane of a person with a 64 mm PD. We usually make the assumption that the spectacle plane is 2.7 cm from the base line. The convergence stimulus would be:

$$\text{Convergence stimulus} = \frac{\text{PD (in cm)}}{d \text{ (in m)}} = \frac{6.4 \text{ cm}}{0.427 \text{ m}} = 15\Delta$$

For the more convenient use of common units for the measurement of PD (mm) and test distance (cm), we can calculate the convergence stimulus in prism diopters with the following formula:

$$\text{Convergence stimulus} = \frac{10 \text{ X PD (in mm)}}{d \text{ (in cm)}}$$

The formula using test distance from the object of regard to the spectacle plane is thus:

$$\text{Convergence stimulus} = \frac{10 \text{ X PD (in mm)}}{\text{test distance (in cm)} + 2.7 \text{ cm}}$$

So if a person with a PD of 64 mm views an object 40 cm from the spectacle plane, the convergence stimulus in prism diopters is:

Convergence stimulus = (10 X 64) / (40 + 2.7) = 15$\Delta$

Table 1.2 shows the calculated convergence stimuli for various test distances for one individual with a PD of 60 mm and another with a PD of 64 mm.

## THE ACCOMMODATION AND CONVERGENCE GRAPH

The x,y coordinate plot of accommodation and vergence is a method of graphing clinical accommodation and vergence test findings to determine the zone in which a given individual has clear single binocular vision and then to relate that to accommodation and vergence stimuli.[2] We will also use the graph as a means of learning about the interrelationships of accommodation and vergence, the effects of lenses and prisms on accommodation and vergence, and other fundamental clinical concepts. The graph makes it possible to readily evaluate accommodation and convergence relationships. It also makes the interdependence of various test findings obvious. Other potential uses of a graphical display of clinical data are to assess the internal consistency of the data for a given individual and to assist in determining a case type.

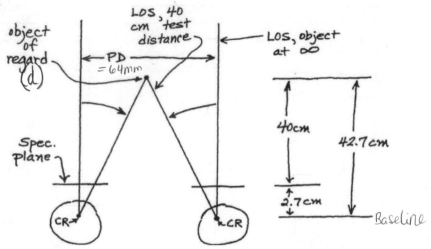

*Figure 1.1. Illustration of the concept of calculating convergence stimulus in prism diopters. In this example, interpupillary distance (PD) is 64 mm. The spectacle plane is 2.7 cm from the base line, the line connecting the centers of rotation (CR) of the two eyes. The lines of sight (LOS) of the two eyes rotate in from parallelism to fixate the object of regard at 40 cm from the spectacle plane.*

| Table 1.1. | |
|---|---|
| Dioptric accommodative stimulus for selected test distances with the patient viewing through their sub-jective refraction to best visual acuity (BVA). (For convenience in graphing and calculations, the accommodative stimulus for 6 m is often assumed to be 0) | |

| Test distance | Accommodative stimulus |
|---|---|
| 6 m | $\frac{1}{6m}=$ 0.17 D |
| 4 m | $1/4m$ 0.25 D |
| 1 m | $\frac{1}{1m}$ 1.00 D |
| 50 cm | $\frac{100}{50cm}=$ 2.00 D |
| 40 cm | $\frac{100}{40cm}=$ 2.50 D |
| 33.3 cm | $\frac{100}{33.3cm}=$ 3.00 D |
| 25 cm | $\frac{100}{25cm}=$ 4.00 D |
| 20 cm | $\frac{100}{20cm}$ 5.00 D |
| 16.7 cm | $\frac{100}{16.7}=$ 6.00 D |
| 14.3 cm | $\frac{100}{14.3cm}$ 7.00 D |
| 12.5 cm | $\frac{100}{12.5cm}$ 8.00 D |
| 11.1 cm | $\frac{100}{11.1cm}$ 9.00 D |
| 10 cm | $\frac{100}{10cm}$ 10.00 D |

Many graphical representations have been used through the years.[2-7] The earliest dates to Donders in the middle of the 19th century.[8] The one that we will use was developed through the pioneering efforts of Glenn Fry and Henry Hofstetter.[2,9-12] Test findings are plotted on a graph like the one in Figure 1.2.

3

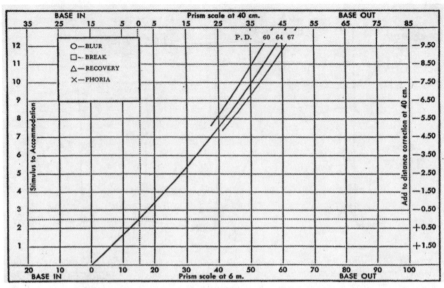

*Figure 1.2. The graph used to plot optometric findings. Convergence stimulus values are on the x-axis. Accommodative stimulus values are on the y-axis. The box toward the upper left hand corner shows the symbols used for plotting blur, break, recovery, and dissociated phoria findings.*

**Table 1.2.**

Convergence stimulus in prism diopters for various test distances for individuals with interpupillary distances of 60 mm and 64 mm. Test distance is the distance from the test object to the spectacle plane. (For convenience in graphing and calculations, the convergence stimulus for 6 m is often assumed to be 0)

| Test distance | Convergence stimulus 60 mm PD | Convergence stimulus 64 mm PD |
|---|---|---|
| 6 m | 1.0 | 1.1 |
| 4 m | 1.5 | 1.6 |
| 1 m | 5.8 | 6.2 |
| 50 cm | 11.4 | 12.1 |
| 40 cm | 14.1 | 15.0 |
| 33.3 cm | 16.7 | 17.8 |
| 25 cm | 21.7 | 23.1 |
| 20 cm | 26.4 | 28.2 |
| 16.7 cm | 30.9 | 33.0 |
| 14.3 cm | 35.3 | 37.7 |
| 12.5 cm | 39.5 | 42.1 |
| 11.1 cm | 43.5 | 46.4 |
| 10 cm | 47.2 | 50.4 |

The graph that we will study in the first few chapters of this book displays the results of dissociated phoria, fusional vergence range, relative accommodation, amplitude of accommodation, and convergence amplitude testing. Interpretation of other important tests, such as fixation disparity, dynamic retinoscopy, and accommodative facility will be discussed in later chapters.

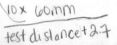

4

The graph has convergence stimulus in prism diopters on the x-axis, and accommodative stimulus in diopters on the y-axis (Figure 1.2). The line drawn obliquely up and to the right on the graph starting from the (0,0) point is the demand line. The demand line indicates the accommodation and convergence stimulus levels for various distances when patients view through lenses equal in power to their refractive errors.

To draw in the demand line, we would simply plot a point at the stimulus to accommodation and convergence stimulus for the various test distances for which we made such determinations (Tables 1.1 and 1.2). Since convergence stimulus is different for different PDs, there is more than one demand line. However, this becomes important only for very close test distances. For instance, Table 1.2 shows that the convergence stimuli for these two PDs are only 0.9Δ apart for a 40 cm test distance. This is why demand lines for three different PDs are shown only at the very top of Figure 1.2. For intermediate and further distances, a demand line for only a 64 mm PD is shown, since 64 mm is close to the population mean for PD in adults.

By convention, the formula for accommodative stimulus takes into account the distance of the test object from the spectacle plane, whereas the formula for convergence stimulus uses the distance of the test object from the base line. As a result, the demand line is nonlinear.

## EFFECTS OF LENSES AND PRISMS ON ACCOMMODATIVE STIMULUS AND CONVERGENCE STIMULUS

Stimulus to accommodation can be altered by changing testing distance or lens power. Variations in lens power are considered in relation to the patient's maximum plus subjective refraction to best visual acuity (BVA). Lens powers which are more plus than the BVA are said to be plus adds, and lens powers which are more minus power than the BVA are referred to as minus adds. For example, lenses which are 1.00 D more plus or less minus than the BVA would be considered to represent a +1.00 D add. Plus adds reduce the accommodative stimulus, and minus adds increase the accommodative stimulus.

Plus and minus adds change accommodative stimulus but not convergence stimulus. To take an example, let's say a patient with a 64 mm PD views an object at 40 cm through a +1.00 D add. The convergence stimulus would be:

$$(10 \times 64) / (40 + 2.7) = 15\Delta$$

The accommodative stimulus would be 1.00 D less than the dioptric stimulus for the 40 cm distance through the BVA:

$$(100 / 40) - 1.00 = 1.50 \text{ D}$$

Or, if a patient with a 64 mm PD views an object at 40 cm through a -1.00 D add, the convergence stimulus would be 15Δ, and the accommodative stimulus would be 1.00 D greater than the dioptric accommodative stimulus through the BVA:

$$(100 / 40) + 1.00 = 3.50 \text{ D}$$

Similarly, convergence stimulus can be altered by changing distance or adding prisms. As we have already seen, closer distances represent greater convergence stimuli. Base-out prisms increase the convergence stimulus without changing accommodative stimulus. Base-in prisms decrease the convergence stimulus without changing the accommodative stimulus. For a patient with a 64 mm PD viewing an object at 40 cm through the BVA and 6Δ base-out prism, the accommodative stimulus would be 2.50 D, and the convergence stimulus would be:

$$[(10 \times 64) / (40 + 2.7)] + 6 = 21\Delta$$

If a patient with a 64 mm PD viewed an object at 40 cm through the BVA and 6Δ base-in prism, the accommodative stimulus would be 2.50 D, and the convergence stimulus would be:

$$[(10 \times 64) / (40 + 2.7)] - 6 = 9\Delta$$

## SCALES ON THE GRAPH

The convergence stimulus is plotted on the x-axis of the accommodation and convergence graph. A convergence stimulus of 0 represents the situation in which the lines of sight of the two eyes are parallel to each other, as when they are binocularly fixating an object at infinity. Clinically, distance testing often is at 6 meters or at 4 meters. The assumption is often made that this distance represents optical infinity, so the convergence stimulus (as well as the accommodative stimulus) for 6 m or 4 m is assumed to be zero. The base-out values on the x-axis indicate the number of prism diopters of vergence from parallelism. Convergence can be stimulated by either moving the target in or adding base-out prism.

The scales on the bottom of the graph (for convergence) and on the left-hand side of the graph (for accommodation) are absolute scales, and are all that would be necessary for plotting of test results. But there is also a convergence scale at the top of the graph for convenience in plotting near-point findings taken at 40 cm from the spectacle plane since this is the most common testing distance for near testing. In Table 1.2 the convergence stimulus for 40 cm for a person with a 64 mm PD is 15Δ. Therefore, 0 on the top scale is lined up with 15 on the bottom (absolute) scale. If a patient views an object at 40 cm through a 25Δ base-out prism, the total convergence stimulus is 40Δ. So 40 on the bottom scale lines up with 25 on the top scale.

The scale on the left side of the graph is an absolute scale for stimulus to accommodation in diopters. There is also a scale on the right side of the graph; like the convergence scale on the top of the graph, this scale is designed for convenience in the use of a 40 cm testing distance. Since 40 cm represents a 2.50 D stimulus to accommodation, 2.50 D on the left-hand scale is at the same place on the y-axis as 0 is on the right-hand scale. The numbers on the right-hand scale give the add powers that would result in the accommodative stimuli at the corresponding position on the left-hand scale for a patient viewing an object at 40 cm. If a patient views an object at 40 cm through a +1.50 D add, the accommodative stimulus is 1.00 D. So 1.00 D on the left-hand scale lines up with +1.50 D on the right-hand scale.

The upper and right-hand scales are for use with a 40 cm test distance only. For any distance, the effect of lens adds on the stimulus to accommodation is represented by moving up from the demand line point for the test distance for minus adds and moving down from the demand line point for plus adds. Changes in convergence stimulus induced by prism are represented by horizontal movement from the demand line point for the test distance: to the left for base-in prism because it decreases convergence stimulus and to the right for base-out prism because it increases convergence stimulus.

## TESTS PLOTTED AND SYMBOLS USED

Tests typically plotted on the accommodation and convergence graph are dissociated phorias, fusional vergence ranges (base-in and base-out to blur, break, and recovery), relative accommodation (plus to blur and minus to blur), amplitude of accommodation, and near point of convergence. The dissociated phorias and fusional vergence ranges are usually done at distance and at 40 cm and the relative accommodation tests are usually done at 40 cm, but it is possible to perform these tests at other distances and graph the results.

Some clinicians suggest that tests should be done in the following order: (1) a free-posture test (theoretically no stimulation or inhibition), (2) an inhibitory test, and (3) a stimulatory test. According to this thinking, the dissociated phoria would be tested before fusional vergence tests, and base-in fusional vergence ranges would be tested before base-out fusional vergence ranges. Base-out testing yields a greater fusional after-effect or vergence adaptation than does base-in.[13-15] Similarly, for relative accommodation testing, many clinicians recommend doing the plus to blur test before the minus to blur test.

## PREVALENCE OF ACCOMMODATION AND VERGENCE DISORDERS

Accommodation and vergence disorders are very common clinical conditions. For example, Hokoda[16] found that of 119 patients 35 years of age and younger seen in a municipal workers' optometry clinic in New York during a six month period of time, 21% had symptomatic accommodation and/or vergence dysfunctions. Accommodative disorders were found in 16.8% of patients, symptomatic esophoria in 5.9%, and convergence insufficiency in 4.2%. Scheiman et al[17] reported on the prevalence of eye and vision conditions in 6 to 18 year old patients seen in the clinic at the Pennsylvania College of Optometry. Nonstrabismic binocular vision problems were seen in 16.3% of patients and accommodative disorders in 6.5%. In Spain, Porcar and Martinez-Palomera[18] found 32% of 65 university students with an average age of 22 years to have accommodation and/or vergence disorders.

## REFERENCES

1. Jackson TW, Goss DA. Variation and correlation of standard clinical phoropter tests of phorias, vergence ranges, and relative accommodation in a sample of school-age children. J Am Optom Assoc 1991;62:540-547.

2. Hofstetter HW. Graphical analysis. In: Schor CM, Ciuffreda KJ, eds. Vergence Eye Movements: Basic and Clinical Aspects. Boston: Butterworth-Heinemann, 1983:439-464.

3. Hofstetter HW. The graphical analysis of clinical optometric findings. In: Transactions of the International Ophthalmic Optical Congress 1961. London: Lockwood, 1962:456-460.

4. Hofstetter HW. Optometric contributions in accommodation and convergence studies. Am Optom Assoc J 1954;25:431-439.

5. Borish IM. Clinical Refraction, 3rd ed. Boston: Butterworth-Heinemann, 1970:875-894.

6. Daum KM, Rutstein RP, Houston G IV, Clore KA, Corliss DA. Evaluation of a new criterion of binocularity. Optom Vis Sci 1989;66:218-228.

7. Goss DA. Pratt system of clinical analysis of accommodation and convergence. Optom Vis Sci 1989;66:805-806.

8. Donders FC. Moore WD, trans. On the Anomalies of Accommodation and Refraction of the Eye. London: New Sydenham Society, 1864:110-126.

9. Fry GA. Fundamental variables in the relationship between accommodation and convergence. Optom Weekly 1943;34:153-155, 183-185.

10. Hofstetter HW. The zone of clear single binocular vision. Am J Optom Arch Am Acad Optom 1945;22:301-333, 361-384.

11. Fry GA. Basic concepts underlying graphical analysis. In: Schor CM, Ciuffreda KJ, eds. Vergence Eye Movements: Basic and Clinical Aspects. Boston: Butterworth-Heinemann, 1983:403-437.

12. Michaels DD. Visual Optics and Refraction: A Clinical Approach, 3rd ed. St. Louis: Mosby, 1985:380-391.

13. Alpern M. The after effect of lateral duction testing on subsequent phoria measurements. Am J Optom Arch Am Acad Optom 1946;23:442-446.

14. Rosenfield M, Ciuffreda KJ, Ong E, Super S. Vergence adaptation and the order of clinical vergence range testing. Optom Vis Sci 1995;72:219-223.

15. Goss DA. Effect of test sequence on fusional vergence ranges. New Eng J Optom 1995;47:39-42.

16. Hokoda SC. General binocular dysfunction in an urban optometry clinic. J Am Optom Assoc 1985;56:560-562.

17. Scheiman M, Gallaway M, Coulter R, Reinstein F, Ciner E, Herzberg C, Parisi M. Prevalence of vision and ocular disease conditions in a clinical pediatric population. J Am Optom Assoc 1996;67:193-202.

18. Porcar E, Martinez-Palomera A. Prevalence of general binocular dysfunctions in a population of university students. Optom Vis Sci 1997;74:111-113.

## PRACTICE PROBLEMS

1. Calculate the dioptric accommodative stimulus for the following testing distances and lens adds:

   (a) 55 cm, BVA _____

   (b) 45 cm, +1.00 D add _____

   (c) 40 cm, +1.50 D add _____

   (d) 40 cm, -2.00 D add _____

   (e) 36 cm, BVA _____

   (f) 36 cm, +1.25 D add _____

   (g) 33.3 cm, +1.00 D add _____

2. Calculate the convergence stimulus for each of the following test distances and prism powers:

(a) 64 mm PD, 40 cm, 4Δ base-out _____

(b) 64 mm PD, 33.3 cm, 6Δ base-in _____

(c) 60 mm PD, 40 cm, 8Δ base-in _____

(d) 60 mm PD, 33.3 cm, 9Δ base-out _____

3. On the figure below, plot the demand line for an individual with a PD of 70 mm. (Do the necessary calculations) Where is the most deviation from the demand line for a person with a PD of 64 mm?

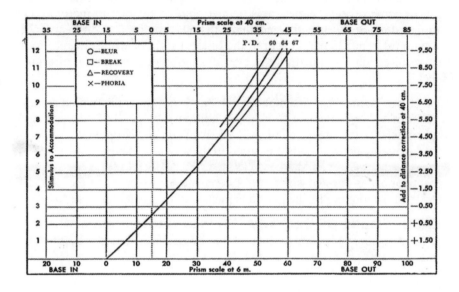

# Chapter 2
# Dissociated Phorias and Introduction to ACA Ratios and Binocular Vision Syndromes

In the Dictionary of Visual Science and Related Clinical Terms, dissociated phoria is defined as "the direction or orientation of one eye, its line of sight, or some other reference axis or meridian, in relation to the other eye, manifested in the absence of an adequate fusion stimulus, and variously specified with reference to parallelism of the lines of sight or with reference to the relative directions assumed by the eyes during binocular fixation of a given object."[1]

In other words, the dissociated phoria indicates the amount by which the lines of sight of the eyes deviate from the condition in which both lines of sight would intersect the object of regard, when fusion is disrupted. By definition, the dissociated phoria is measured in the absence of binocular fusion. In exophoria the lines of sight are divergent with respect to the object of regard. In esophoria the lines of sight are convergent with respect to the object of regard. Most commonly, the phoria is measured in prism diopters ($\Delta$).

## MEASUREMENT OF DISSOCIATED PHORIAS
The word dissociated refers to the fact that binocular fusion is prevented; that is, the eyes are dissociated.[2] The methods by which the non-fused condition of dissociated phoria testing can be achieved can be classified into four categories:

1. exclusion, such as in the cover test;
2. diplopia or displacement, such as in the von Graefe technique;
3. distortion, such as in the Maddox rod test and the modified Thorington test;
4. nonfusable or independent objects, such as those present on some stereoscope phoria cards or the Maddox wing test.

On the cover test, vision in one eye is excluded because it is covered. On the von Graefe test for lateral phorias, a vertical prism over one eye optically displaces the object of regard to induce diplopia.[3] On the Maddox rod test, the Maddox rod distorts the image reaching one eye, so that there is typically a white spot seen by one eye and a red line seen by the other eye. A Maddox rod is also used in the performance of the modified Thorington test.[3] On some stereoscope cards and on the Maddox wing test, an arrow is seen by one eye and a scale is seen by the other eye.

Dissociated phoria tests also involve some method for determining the magnitude of the phoria is measured. Different dissociated phoria tests use either

*Base direction is determined by the direction the eye moves.*

prisms or scales to determine the magnitude of the phoria. On the alternating cover test, prism can be increased (such as with a prism bar) until the movement of the eyes is neutralized; the power of the neutralizing prism is the amount of the dissociated phoria. On the von Graefe test, the rotary prisms on the phoropter are adjusted until the two charts are aligned (aligned vertically for a lateral phoria and aligned horizontally for a vertical phoria). Base-in prism is necessary for vertical alignment in exophoria, and base-out prism is needed for vertical alignment in esophoria. The amount of the prism for alignment is the amount of the dissociated phoria. On the Maddox rod test, prism is added until the red line runs through the white light. On the modified Thorington test and the Maddox wing test, there are scales to indicate the magnitude of the phoria. On the modified Thorington, the patient reports the point on the scale where the red line from the Maddox rod crosses. On the Maddox wing test and on some stereoscope card tests, the patient reports the point on a numbered scale to which an arrow points.

## PROCEDURES FOR THE VON GRAEFE TEST

Because the von Graefe dissociated phoria test and the modified Thorington dissociated phoria test are commonly used tests, the procedures for conducting them will be discussed. The von Graefe test is performed with the rotary prisms in the phoropter.[3,4] The distance lateral phoria is performed with the patient viewing through the subjective refraction to best visual acuity (BVA). The phoropter is set at the patient's distance PD. The target viewed by the patient is a vertical row of letters or a single letter. The letter(s) used should be one line above the patient's best visual acuity. The steps in performing the distance lateral phoria are as follows:

1. The rotary prism over the right eye is set at $12\Delta$ base-in and the rotary prism over the left eye is set at $6\Delta$ base-up. The patient's eyes should be closed or occluded when the prisms are being set up. The BU prism is the dissociating prism and the lateral prism is the measuring prism.

2. The patient should be asked if he or she sees two letters (or lines of letters). The expected answer is yes. Possible reasons for the patient not seeing two are misalignment of the phoropter, inadvertent occlusion of one eye, or deep suppression. It may also be necessary in some cases to increase the power of the BU dissociating prism. Sometimes the examiner must alternately occlude the two eyes so that the patient can locate the two images.

3. If the patient sees two, then the examiner should ask if the top letter (or line) is to the right or to the left of the bottom one. If to the left, the amount of base-in prism over the right eye should be increased.

4. If the top letter (or line) is to the right of the bottom one, instruct the patient to look at the lower letter(s) and keep the letter(s) clear. Inform the patient that the top letter (or line) will be moved and that he or she should say "now" when the top letter (or line) is lined up directly above the bottom one in a straight line.

5. Reduce the amount of base-in prism by about 2Δ per second. Observe the amount of prism when the patient says "now." (Continue into base-out prism if necessary)

6. Continue moving the prism past the alignment point without stopping. Now tell the patient to again say "now" when the targets are aligned and reverse the direction of movement of the prism. Again note the amount of prism when the patient says "now."

7. If the two values are within 3Δ of each other, record the average. If not, repeat the test and average the two closest values.

The vertical phoria can be performed next without changing the lenses or PD in the phoropter. The target viewed by the patient is a horizontal row of letters or a single letter. The letter(s) used should be one line above the patient's best visual acuity. The steps for the distance vertical von Graefe phoria are as follows:

1. The rotary prism over the right eye is set at 12Δ base-in and the rotary prism over the left eye is set at 6Δ base-up. The patient's eyes should be closed or occluded when the prisms are being set up. The BI prism is the dissociating prism and the vertical prism is the measuring prism.

2. The patient should be asked if he or she sees two letters (or lines of letters). The expected answer is yes. Possible reasons for the patient not seeing two are misalignment of the phoropter, inadvertent occlusion of one eye, the amount of base-in prism not being great enough to break fusion, or deep suppression.

3. If the patient sees two, then the examiner should ask if the top letter (or line) is to the right or to the left of the bottom one.

4. If to the right, instruct the patient to look at the letter (or line) to the right. Inform the patient that the letter (or line) on the left will be moved and that he should say "now" when the two are lined up side by side at the same height.

5. Reduce the amount of base-up prism by about 2Δ per second. Observe the amount of prism when the patient says "now." (Continue into base-down prism if necessary)

6. Continue moving the prism past the alignment point without stopping. Now tell the patient to again say "now" when the targets are aligned and reverse the direction of movement of the prism. Again note the amount of prism when the patient says "now."

7. If the two values are within 2Δ of each other, record the average. If not, repeat the test and average the two closest values.

For the near lateral von Graefe phoria, the phoropter is set at the near PD. The target is a line or block of small letters (20/20 or 20/30) on a nearpoint card. The card should be placed at 40 cm on the phoropter reading rod, and good illumination should be directed toward the card. Once those adjustments have been made, the steps in performing the test are the same as for the distance lateral phoria.

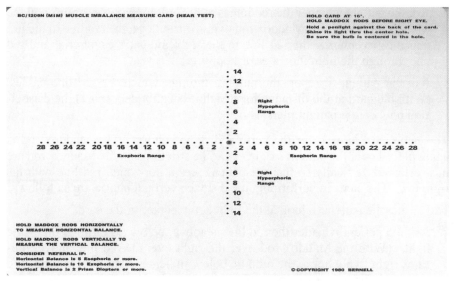

*Figure 2.1. The near Muscle Imbalance Measure card, a modified Thorington test card calibrated for use at 40 cm.*

The same target and PD can be used for the near vertical von Graefe phoria. The steps for the near vertical phoria are the same as for the distance vertical phoria.

It should be noted that an instruction to keep the letter(s) clear was part of the instructions to the patient for the distance and near lateral phorias. This is important in order to control accommodation. Such an instruction is not necessary for the vertical phoria because changes in accommodation will not affect the vertical phoria.

## PROCEDURES FOR THE MODIFIED THORINGTON TEST

The modified Thorington test requires a special test card with a calibrated scale and a hole in the card at the zero point. Commercially available cards are the Muscle Imbalance Measure cards, one calibrated for use at 10 feet and the other for use at 40 cm. A picture of the near card is shown in Figure 2.1. To use either the distance card or the near card, the examiner holds a penlight against the back of the card and shines the light through the center hole toward the patient. A Maddox rod is placed over the patient's right eye. The cards can be used either with or without a phoropter.

To do the distance lateral phoria, patients view through their BVA lenses either in the phoropter or in a trial frame. The striations on the Maddox rod are oriented horizontally so that the patient sees a vertical red line with his right eye. The steps in performing the distance lateral phoria are as follows:

1. Instruct the patient to keep the numbers on the card clear (to control accommodation).

2. Instruct the patient to next look at the light at the center of the card.

3. Ask the patient whether the red line is to the left, to the right, or through the white light. (With the Maddox rod over the right eye, the red line to the left indicates exophoria, the red line to the right indicates esophoria, and red line through the light indicates orthophoria)

4. Ask the patient to report the number through which the red line passes. (With the card at the distance for which it is calibrated, this is the dissociated phoria in prism diopters)

The same card is used for the vertical distance phoria. The Maddox rod is again placed over the patient's right eye. The striations on the Maddox rod are now oriented vertically so that the patient sees a horizontal red line with his right eye. The steps in performing the distance vertical phoria are as follows:

1. Instruct the patient to look at the light at the center of the card.

2. Ask the patient whether the red line is above, below, or through the white light. (With the Maddox rod over the right eye, the red line above indicates right hypophoria, the red line below indicates right hyperphoria, and through indicates zero vertical phoria)

3. Ask the patient to report the number through which the red line passes. (With the card at 10 feet, this is the vertical dissociated phoria in prism diopters)

The procedures for the near phorias are the same as for the distance phorias except that the near card is used and the card is held at the distance for which it is calibrated. It is important for the patient to keep the numbers clear on the near lateral phoria just as with the distance lateral phoria to control accommodation. The near card is calibrated to give the phoria in prism diopters when the card is 40 cm from the patient.

## PLOTTING DISSOCIATED PHORIAS ON THE GRAPH
To plot phorias on the accommodation and convergence graph, follow these steps:

1. Find the point on the demand line corresponding to the test distance. Perhaps the easiest way is to determine where the level of accommodative stimulus for that test distance falls on the demand line.

2. If the lenses in place during the phoria test differ from the distance subjective refraction, move straight up one space for each diopter of minus or straight down one space for each diopter of plus. (This is done because the addition of minus lenses over the subjective refraction increases the stimulus to accommodation, and the addition of plus lenses reduces it.)

3. Move one space to the right for each 10Δ of esophoria or one space to the left for each 10Δ of exophoria.

4. Mark this point with an X.

5. Connect the X symbols with straight-line segments. The single best-fit line for all the X symbols is called the phoria line.[5,6]

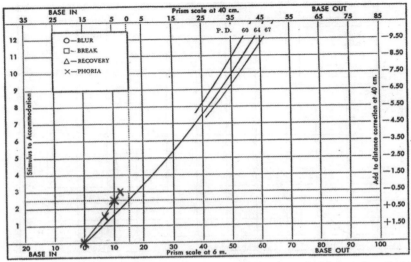

Figure 2.2. As an example of the graphing of phorias and the drawing of the phoria line, the following findings are plotted on the graph:

6 m through the subjective refraction to best visual acuity (BVA): ortho
40 cm through the BVA: 5Δ exo  2·5D
40 cm through a +1.00 D add: 8Δ exo  2·50D
33.3 cm through the BVA: 6Δ exo  3·00D

Figures 2.2 and 2.3 show examples of phoria plotting. The phoria line should approximate a straight line. If one phoria is way off a straight line through the other points, the validity of that finding should be doubted. In phoria testing, the greatest single source of error is inadequate control of accommodation. To avoid this problem, the examiner should use close to the smallest letters that the patient can see clearly and should instruct the patient to keep the letters clear. Another tactic is to ask the patient to read (aloud) the nonmoving letters forward and backward while the measuring prism is being adjusted.

## TYPES OF CONVERGENCE

It is useful to conceive of convergence as being divided into four types: tonic, proximal, accommodative, and fusional.[7] Tonic convergence represents the physiologic position of rest. The distance phoria with the subjective refraction in place is taken to be a measure of tonic convergence. Proximal convergence is convergence that occurs because of the awareness of nearness of the target in near-point testing. Accommodative convergence occurs with a change in accommodation as part of the neurological link of accommodation and convergence.[8,9] Fusional convergence is the convergence that responds to maintain singleness of the object of regard. This classification of the types of convergence is known as the Maddox classification; definitions are summarized in Table 2.1.

In the measurement of a nearpoint phoria, fusional convergence is eliminated by dissociation. The amount of tonic convergence is known from the distance phoria. The amount of convergence that occurs in going from distance to the near-point testing distance is due to accommodative convergence and proximal

15

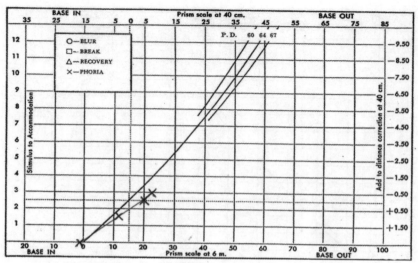

*Figure 2.3. Plotting of phorias. This graph was created using data from an individual with the following phorias:*

    *6 m through the BVA: 1Δ exo*
    *40 cm through the BVA: 5Δ eso*
    *33.3 cm through the BVA: 6Δ eso*
    *40 cm through a +1.00 D add: 3Δ exo*

| Table 2.1. | | |
|---|---|---|
| Definitions of the Maddox components of convergence | | |
| Tonic convergence | Convergence at the physiological position of rest of the eyes; vergence position during distance fixation under unfused conditions and with no accommodation occurring | |
| Accom-modative convergence | Convergence due to the neurological link of accommodation and convergence and occurring as a result of the stimulation of accommodation | |
| Proximal convergence | Convergence due to an awareness of nearness | |
| Fusional convergence | Convergence occurring in response to retinal disparity in order to maintain binocular fusion | |

convergence. Accommodative convergence also can be induced by altering lens power while maintaining a constant testing distance.

## ACA RATIOS

The ratio of accommodative convergence (AC) to the change in stimulus to accommodation (A) is known as the stimulus ACA ratio. (ACA can also be written as AC/A) The ratio of accommodative convergence to the change in accommodative response is the response ACA ratio. Because accommodative response measurements usually are not measured simultaneously with the phoria measurement in clinical practice, the clinically measured ACA ratios are almost always stimulus ACA ratios. The ACA ratio is the foundation for various aspects of clinical decision making.

# CALCULATION OF STIMULUS ACA RATIOS

A general formula for the stimulus ACA ratio is:

$$\text{Stimulus ACA ratio} = \frac{\text{Accommodative convergence (in } \Delta)}{\text{Change in accommodative stimulus (in D)}}$$

The formula can be adapted for use with changes in stimulus to accommodation induced by either a change in testing distance or a change in lens power. The accommodative stimulus is changed by a change in test distance when two phorias are performed through the subjective refraction, one at distance and one at some near-point distance, In that case, the ACA formula becomes:

$$\text{Stimulus ACA ratio} = \frac{\text{Convergence stimulus of near target - distance phoria } + \text{ near phoria}}{\text{Accommodative stimulus of near target}}$$

The stimulus ACA ratio determined with this formula is called the calculated ACA ratio. In emmetropia or corrected ametropia, the convergence stimulus and the accommodative stimulus of the distance target are assumed to be 0. An esophoria is a plus value in the formula, because it represents a convergent posture in relation to the object of regard; an exophoria is a minus value in the formula, because it represents a divergent posture in relation to the object of regard.

Let's look at an example with this formula. A person with a 64 mm PD has a dissociated phoria at 6 m of $1\Delta$ eso and a phoria at 40 cm of $4\Delta$ exo. Both phorias are taken through the subjective refraction to best visual acuity. What is the stimulus ACA ratio?

$$\text{Stimulus Calculated ACA ratio} = \frac{15 - 1 + (-4)}{2.50 \text{ D}} = 4\Delta/D$$

The stimulus ACA ratio also can be determined by two phorias taken at the same distance but with different lenses using the following formula:

$$\text{Stimulus ACA ratio} = \frac{\text{phoria \#1 - phoria \#2}}{\text{stimulus to accommodation \#1 - stimulus to accommodation \#2}}$$

For example, if a patient has a 40 cm phoria of $3\Delta$ eso through a -1.00 add and a 40 cm phoria of $2\Delta$ exo through a + 1.00 add, the stimulus ACA ratio is calculated as follows:

$$\text{Stimulus ACA ratio} = \frac{3 - (-2)}{3.50 - 1.50} = 2.5\Delta/D$$

The same formula can be used with the gradient test to determine the stimulus ACA ratio. In the gradient test, usually two phorias are performed at 40 cm, one through the subjective refraction and one through a +1.00 D add. The

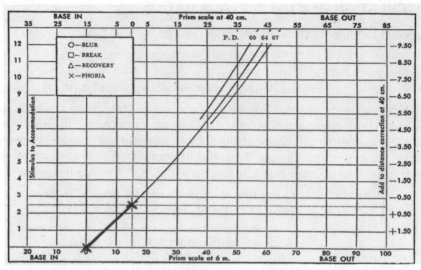

*Figure 2.4. The phoria line falls on the demand line for an individual with ortho at both 6 m and 40 cm (both phorias through the subjective refraction to best visual acuity). If this person has a 64 mm PD, the stimulus calculated ACA ratio is 6Δ/D.*

### Table 2.2.
Phoria findings characteristic of Duane's binocular vision syndromes. (More complete information on diagnosis of these conditions will be given in chapter 11)

|  | Distance phoria | Near phoria | ACA ratio |
|---|---|---|---|
| Convergence insufficiency | Approximately ortho | High exo | Low |
| Convergence excess | Approximately ortho | Eso | High |
| Divergence insufficiency | Eso | Low exo or approximately ortho | Low |
| Divergence excess | High exo | Low exo or approximately ortho | High |

stimulus ACA ratio determined in this way is called the gradient ACA ratio. For example, if the phorias are 3Δ exo through the BVA and 9Δ exo through a +1.00 D add, the ACA ratio will be:

$$\text{Stimulus Gradient ACA ratio} = \frac{-3-(-9)}{1} = 6\Delta/D$$

The stimulus calculated ACA ratio and the stimulus gradient ACA ratio which have just been presented are the ACA ratios which are used clinically most of the time. Stimulus ACA ratios also can be estimated from the graph. Because convergence is on the x-axis and stimulus to accommodation is on the y-axis, the stimulus ACA ratio is the inverse of the slope of the phoria line. If the phoria line is parallel to the demand line, the ratio is 6Δ/D. (This is strictly true only for persons with 64 mm PDs, but it is a good approximation for all patients) A simple example of a stimulus ACA ratio of 6Δ/D is given in Figure

18

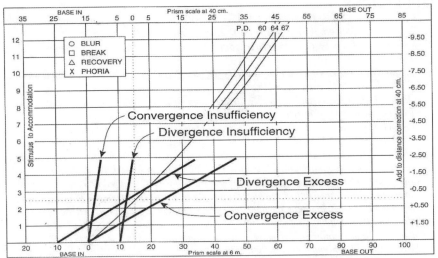

*Figure 2.5. Examples of phoria lines representing Duane's four binocular vision syndromes. Although the examples represent four different individuals, they are plotted together here for illustrative purposes.*

2.4. If the phoria line is tipped more toward the abscissa (lesser slope), the ratio is greater than 6; if it is tipped less (greater slope), the ratio is less than 6.

The ACA ratio is expressed here as a single number rather than as a ratio for simplicity, because the denominator is always expressed as 1. Thus, 6Δ/D is equivalent to 6Δ:1D.

## BINOCULAR VISION SYNDROMES

Duane described four types of binocular vision syndromes: convergence insufficiency, convergence excess, divergence insufficiency, and divergence excess.[10,11] These syndromes have been defined in somewhat different ways by different authors. A clinically useful description of the syndromes based on the phoria findings characteristic of each is given in Table 2.2. The phoria lines typical of each are shown in Figure 2.5. Convergence insufficiency and divergence insufficiency are characterized by low stimulus ACA ratios; convergence excess and divergence excess are characterized by high stimulus ACA ratios. The normal range for distance phorias according to Morgan is ortho to 2Δ exo, and the normal range for near phorias is ortho to 6Δ exo.

In convergence insufficiency, the distance phoria is normal and the near phoria is high exo. In convergence excess, the distance phoria is normal and the near phoria is eso. In divergence insufficiency, the distance phoria is eso and the near phoria is normal. In divergence excess, the distance phoria is high exo and the near phoria is normal. These phoria findings can be used to make a tentative diagnosis, and then the pattern of other test findings can be examined to confirm the diagnosis or suggest another one. Diagnosis and management of these syndromes will be discussed in more detail in chapter 11.

# REFERENCES

1. Hofstetter HW, Griffin JR, Berman MS, Everson RW. Dictionary of Visual Science and Related Clinical Terms, 5th ed. Boston: Butterworth-Heinemann, 2000:387.

2. Grosvenor T. Primary Care Optometry, 5th ed. St. Louis: Butterworth Heinemann Elsevier, 2007:224-227.

3. Carlson NB, Kurtz D. Clinical Procedures for Ocular Examination, 3rd ed. New York: McGraw-Hill, 2004:164-169,176-181,208-213.

4. Saladin JJ. Phorometry and stereopsis. In: Benjamin WJ, ed. Borish's Clinical Refraction, 2nd ed. St. Louis: Butterworth Heinemann Elsevier, 2006:899-960.

5. Pitts DG, Hofstetter HW. Demand-line graphing of the zone of clear single binocular vision. Am Optom Assoc J 1959:31:51-55.

6. Hofstetter HW. The graphical analysis of clinical optometric findings. In: Transactions of the International Ophthalmic Optical Congress 1961. London: Lockwood, 1962:456-460.

7. Morgan MW. The Maddox analysis of vergence. In: Schor CM, Ciuffreda KJ, eds. Vergence Eye Movements: Basic and Clinical Aspects. Boston: Butterworth-Heinemann, 1983:15-21.

8. Ciuffreda KJ. Accommodation, the pupil, and presbyopia. In: Benjamin WJ, ed. Borish's Clinical Refraction. Philadelphia: Saunders, 1998:77-120.

9. Schor CM. Neural control of eye movements. In: Kaufman PL, Alm A, eds. Adler's Physiology of the Eye, 10th ed. St. Louis: Mosby, 2003:830-858.

10. Scheiman M, Wick B. Clinical Management of Binocular Vision: Heterophoric, Accommodative, and Eye Movement Disorders, 2nd ed. Philadelphia: Lippincott Williams & Wilkins, 2002:73-78.

11. Griffin JR, Grisham JD. Binocular Anomalies: Diagnosis and Vision Therapy, 4th ed. Amsterdam: Butterworth-Heinemann, 2002:92-96.

## OTHER SUGGESTED READING

Daum KM. Heterophoria and heterotropia. In: Eskridge JB, Amos JF, Bartlett JD, eds. Clinical Procedures in Optometry. Philadelphia: Lippincott, 1991:72-90.

Grosvenor T. Primary Care Optometry, 5th ed. St. Louis: Butterworth Heinemann Elsevier, 2007:235-336.

## PRACTICE PROBLEMS

1. For the patients with the following test findings, plot the phorias, draw the phoria lines, and determine the calculated and gradient ACA ratios. Findings were taken with the subjective refraction to best visual acuity lenses in place unless otherwise noted.

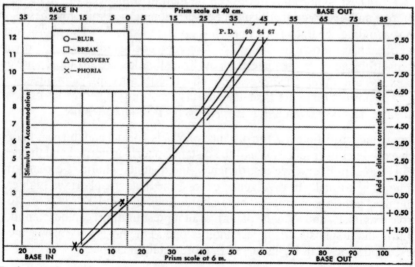

Patient AK: 64 mm PD; 6 m phoria, 2 exo; 40 cm phoria, 2 exo.

Left exo
Right ESO

up or down for add

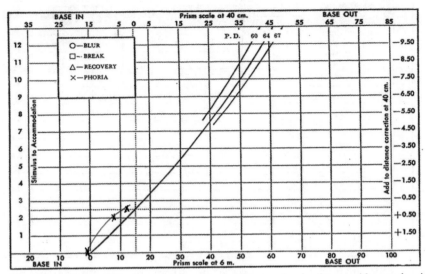

Patient ED: 64 mm PD; 6 m phoria, 1 exo; 40 cm phoria, 3 exo; 40 cm phoria / +1.00 D add, 7 exo.    +1.00D - go down

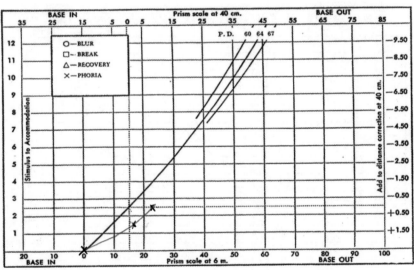

Patient DB: 64 mm PD; 6 m phoria, ortho; 40 cm phoria, 8 eso; 40 cm phoria / +1.00 D add, 1 eso.

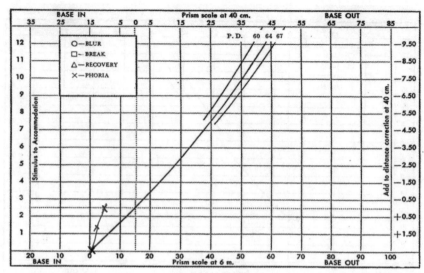

Patient SR:  64 mm PD; 6 m phoria, ortho; 40 cm phoria, 10 exo; 40 cm phoria / +1.00 D add, 11 exo.

Phoria line not tilted much = low ACA

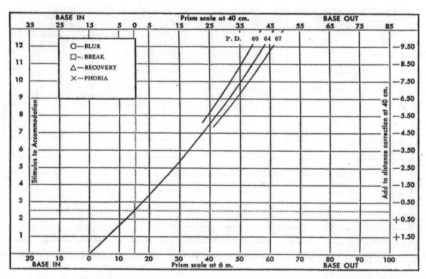

Patient LP:  60 mm PD; 6 m phoria, 1 exo; 33.3 cm phoria, 2 exo.

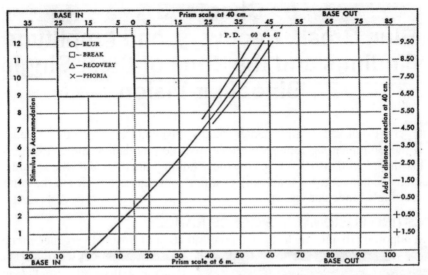

Patient TC:  63 mm PD; 4 m phoria, 2 exo; 40 cm phoria, 6 exo; 40 cm phoria / +1.00 D add, 9 exo.

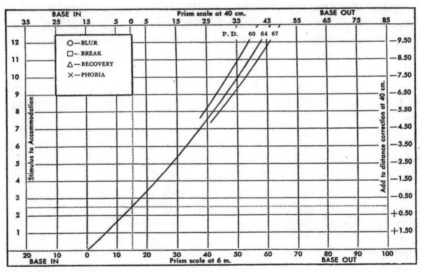

Patient BE:  67 mm PD; 4 m phoria, 2 eso; 40 cm phoria, 4 eso; 40 cm phoria / +1.00 D add, 1 exo.

# Chapter 3
# Blur, Break, Recovery, and Amplitude Findings and the Zone of Clear Single Binocular Vision

Tests discussed in this chapter include fusional vergence ranges, relative accommodation, and amplitudes of accommodation and convergence. This chapter will also describe how these findings are plotted on the accommodation and convergence graph and examine some characteristics of the zone of clear single binocular vision.

## TESTING FUSIONAL VERGENCE RANGES

An important diagnostic test is the determination of fusional vergence ranges.[1] Fusional vergence is stimulated by prism. Base-in prism causes divergence, and base-out prism causes convergence. During a fusional vergence test, base-in prism is increased gradually until the patient reports a blur and then diplopia (break). Then the prism is decreased until the patient is able to regain single vision (recovery). This is repeated with base-out prism. The patient is instructed to report when letters blur, then break into two, and then come back into one again. Prisms are placed in front of each eye when using the phoropter rotary prisms, and the prisms are increased in power equally in front of the two eyes. Prism power is slowly and smoothly increased at a speed of about $1\Delta$ per second over each eye. When the break is reached, prism power is increased slightly further and then reduced until the recovery is reached. Prism adjustment is stopped after the recovery to record the results, rather than stopping prism movement after the blur or break. The total amount of prism over the two eyes is recorded. Some patients do not report a blur before the break.

Prism power can alternatively be varied with a prism bar outside the phoropter. The prism bar is held over one eye and the power is increased from one level to the next after a pause of about two seconds on each power. As with rotary prisms, patients are asked to report when they see a blur, two (break), and one (recovery). A break without a blur is more likely on prism bar vergence testing than on rotary prism testing.

Fusional vergence ranges are determined with distance fixation and with nearpoint fixation, using letters near the patient's best visual acuity as the test target. Blur, break, and recovery are recorded in that order, with slashes between the values. So, for example, a blur of 10, break of 20, and recovery of 12 would be recorded 10/20/12. Some patients do not have a recovery until passing zero and going into the opposite base direction. So, for example, if on a base-in fusional vergence test, recovery does not occur by the time prism has been reduced to zero, the examiner should continue into base-out prism until the patient reports seeing one again. In such cases, the recovery is recorded as a negative number. Normal values for fusional vergence ranges will be discussed later in chapter 7.

## PLOTTING BASE-IN AND BASE-OUT FINDINGS ON THE GRAPH

The base-in and base-out to blur, break, and recovery findings are plotted on the accommodation and convergence graph in the same manner as for phorias but with different symbols. Use the following steps to plot fusional vergence findings:

1. Find the point on the demand line for the given testing distance.

2. Go straight up one space for each diopter of minus added to the distance subjective refraction or go straight down one space for each diopter of plus over the subjective.

3. Move to the right one space for each 10 D of base-out or to the left one space for each 10 D of base-in.

4. Mark blurs with circles, breaks with squares, and recoveries with triangles.[2]

## TESTING RELATIVE ACCOMMODATION

In relative accommodation testing, lens power is increased binocularly in 0.25 D steps until the patient reports the first blur that cannot be cleared.[3] Most commonly, the patient is viewing reduced 20/20 letters at 40 cm from the spectacle plane. When plus power is increased to blur, the test is called the plus to blur test. It is also called the negative relative accommodation (NRA) test because plus decreases accommodation. Another name for the minus to blur test is the positive relative accommodation (PRA) test because minus increases accommodation. For non-presbyopic patients, the starting point for NRA and PRA tests is usually the subjective refraction to best visual acuity (BVA). Normal values for the NRA and PRA in non-presbyopic patients are discussed later in chapter 7.

## PLOTTING PLUS TO BLUR AND MINUS TO BLUR FINDINGS

Relative accommodation findings can be plotted on the accommodation and convergence graph and the plotted points can be connected as follows:

1. Find the point on the demand line corresponding to the testing distance.

2. If the test was performed through prisms (not usually done), move to the right or left appropriately.

3. Move straight up one space for each diopter of minus added to the distance subjective correction or straight down one space for each diopter of plus added to the distance subjective correction. (If the test was started with lenses added to the subjective, include the difference in power from the subjective when moving up or down.)

4. Use a circle to mark the point at which a blur occurs. If a break occurs without a blur, use a square to mark the point.

5. Connect the distance and near base-in to blur (or the base-in to break without blur) findings. This line will also usually connect with the minus-to-blur findings. (If the minus-to-blur finding falls on the amplitude of accommodation line, which is described in the next section, it is not necessary to connect the base-in finding with the minus to blur) Similarly connect distance and near base-out to blur (or the base-out to break without blur) findings. The base-out line will connect with the plus-to-blur finding if the plus-to-blur does not fall on the bottom of the graph (in other words, connect the base-out findings with the NRA if the NRA is less than 2.50 D for a 40cm test distance).

6. If breaks beyond blurs are also plotted, the breaks in the base-in direction can be connected with line segments to show the divergence limits and all the breaks in the base-out direction to show the convergence limits, although this is not commonly done. Similarly the base-in and base-out recovery points can optionally be connected to enclose the fusion recovery range at the various accommodative stimulus levels.[2]

## AMPLITUDE OF ACCOMMODATION

Amplitude of accommodation usually is measured by means of the push-up or near point of accommodation test, in which a target is brought closer and closer to the patient until the best visual acuity letters appear blurred to the patient. The stopping point is the first blur that cannot be cleared.[3] This test generally is done with the patient wearing correction for his or her ametropia or, for the presbyope, with some added plus. The near point of accommodation test is typically performed as a preliminary test. If it is subsequently found on the subjective refraction that the correction worn during the near point of accommodation test is not the same as the subjective refraction, an adjustment in the calculated amplitude of accommodation should be made. This is because uncorrected hyperopia will increase the amount of accommodation needed for any test distance and uncorrected myopia will decrease the amount of accommodation required for any test distance.

The near point of accommodation distance is converted into diopters of stimulus to accommodation, with any amount of plus over the subjective refraction worn during the test subtracted or any minus over the subjective refraction added. For example, if a near point of accommodation of 10 cm is obtained with unaided vision and the patient is subsequently found to be a 1.00 D hyperope, the amplitude of accommodation is 1/0.1m + 1.00 D = 11.00 D. The one diopter was added because a 1 D hyperope will be accommodating 1 D at infinity when unaided. Similarly, if a near point of accommodation is measured to be 10 cm for a patient while wearing a habitual prescription of -1.50 D sph OU and the subjective refraction is later found to be -2.25 D sph OU, the amplitude of accommodation is 1/0.1 m - 0.75D = 9.25D.

A formula that incorporates the difference in the power of the lenses through which the patient was tested (L) and the patient's distance subjective refraction (RE for refractive error) and that uses centimeters as the unit for near point of accommodation (NPA) is as follows:

$$\text{Amplitude of accommodation (in D)} = \frac{100}{\text{NPA (in cm)}} + (\text{RE} - \text{L})$$

The amplitude of accommodation can be plotted on the accommodation and convergence graph by drawing a horizontal line across the graph, starting at the stimulus to accommodation level equal to the amplitude of accommodation. This line demarcates the top of the zone of clear single binocular vision (ZCSBV) on the graph. Amplitude of accommodation varies with patient age. The expected values for amplitude of accommodation will be discussed later.

## NEARPOINT OF CONVERGENCE TEST

A simple and very useful test is the near point of convergence (NPC) test. To determine the NPC, a small object is brought toward the patient until the patient reports diplopia or until one eye swings out or fails to converge further as the object is brought nearer.[4] That is the break point and the distance from the patient's spectacle plane is measured. Then the target is moved away from the patient until the patient again reports single vision or the examiner observes movement of one eye to regain binocular fixation. That is the recovery point and again the distance from the target to the spectacle plane is measured. Some clinicians prefer to use a letter target so that accommodation is controlled during the test, while other clinicians use a penlight for fixation. Using children and young adults as subjects, Adler et al[5] found that a pencil tip, a fingertip, and a target with a single letter yielded NPC measurements that did not vary significantly. They did find that using a penlight resulted in more remote NPC break and recovery when compared to pencil tip and fingertip.

Different authorities give varying cut-off values for separating normal from reduced performance on the NPC test. The results of three studies on the NPC test are summarized in Table 3.1. Based on the results of their study, Hayes et al[6] suggested that a cut-off of 6 cm for the break best distinguished between symptomatic and asymptomatic children. Jiménez et al[7] agreed with a cut-off of 6 cm for the break and recommended a cut-off of 12 cm for the recovery for children. Looking at data from young adults, Scheiman et al[8] recommended cut-offs of 5 cm for the break and 7 cm for the recovery. Based on scores on a quality of life survey for 5 to 10 year old children, Maples and Hoenes[9] also recommended a cut-off of 5 cm for the NPC break. Chen et al[10] reported the NPC to be significantly closer in children five years of age and younger than in children seven to ten years of age when colored pictures were used as targets.

## CONVERGENCE AMPLITUDE

Convergence amplitude is determined from the NPC test and the formula for convergence stimulus. The distance of this point from the spectacle plane is measured; this distance can then be added to 2.7 cm to obtain the value d in the following formula:

$$\text{Convergence stimulus (in } \Delta) = \frac{10 \times \text{PD (in mm)}}{\text{d (in cm)}}$$

**Table 3.1.**
Findings of four studies on nearpoint of convergence test results.

| Study | Subjects | Target | Break: Mean + SD | Recovery: Mean + SD |
|-------|----------|--------|------------------|---------------------|
| Hayes et al[6] | Kindergarten (N=100)<br>3rd grade (N=89)<br>6th grade (N=108) | letters<br>letters<br>letters | 3.3 + 2.6<br>4.1 + 2.4<br>4.3 + 3.4 | 7.6 + 4.8<br>8.7 + 4.2<br>7.2 + 3.9 |
| Jiménez et al[7] | 6 to 12 years of age (N=1016) | penlight | 5.2 + 4.4 | 11.4 + 7.2 |
| Scheiman et al[8] | 22 to 37 years of age; normal binocular vision (N=175) | letters<br>penlight | 2.5 + 1.7<br>2.1 + 1.9 | 4.4 + 2.7<br>3.7 + 2.9 |
| Maples and Hoenes[9] | 6 years old (N=132)<br>7 years old (N=162)<br>8 years old (N=164)<br>9 years old (N=63) | reflective sphere<br>reflective sphere<br>reflective sphere<br>reflective sphere | 2.6 + 2.7<br>3.1 + 6.1<br>2.7 + 3.3<br>3.3 + 4.2 | |

For example, an individual with a 58 mm PD and a 6 cm NPC will have a convergence amplitude of

$$\frac{10 \times 58 \text{ mm}}{6 \text{ cm} + 2.7 \text{ cm}} = 66.7\Delta$$

A person with a 64 mm PD and a 7 cm NPC will have a convergence amplitude of

$$\frac{10 \times 64 \text{ mm}}{7 \text{ cm} + 2.7 \text{ cm}} = 66.0\Delta$$

To mark convergence amplitude on the graph, find the value of the convergence amplitude on the base-out side of the distance prism scale and draw a vertical line through that point. Alternatively, a vertical line can be drawn through the point on the demand line corresponding to the NPC. In most instances, however, as in the two examples, the convergence amplitude will exceed the maximum demand line value provided for on the standard graph.

## ZONE OF CLEAR SINGLE BINOCULAR VISION
After plotting the results of tests described in this and the previous chapters, the accommodation and convergence graph is ready for completion. The base-out to blur value or base-out to break without blur findings should be connected with the point of intersection of the convergence and accommodative ampli-tude lines. In the absence of either of the two amplitude lines, the trend of the base-out to blur limits should be continued as a dashed line obliquely up and to the right until it reaches the other amplitude line. In principle, the positive fusional convergence border and the convergence and accommodative ampli-tude lines have a common intersection. Similarly, the base-out to break beyond the blur values can be extended to the point of intersection of the conver-gence and accommodative amplitude lines. The trends of the phorias and the base-in blurs, breaks, and recoveries can all be extended obliquely upward as dashed lines to the accommodative amplitude line at slopes approximating

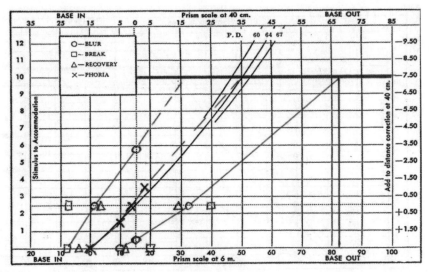

*Figure 3.1. A completed graph. The area inside the blur point lines, the amplitude of accommodation line, and the x-axis is the zone of clear binocular vision. The numerical findings are given in the table below; all the findings were taken through the subjective refraction unless other wise noted.*

| | Phoria | Base-in | Base-out | Plus to blur | Minus to blur |
|---|---|---|---|---|---|
| 6 m | Ortho | X/8/4 | 10/20/12 | | |
| 40 cm | 1 exo | 14/22/12 | 17/25/14 | +2.00 | -3.25 |
| 40 cm +1.00 D add | 5 exo | | | | |
| 40 cm -1.00 D add | 3 eso | | | | |

Amplitude of accommodation, 10 D; NPC, 5 cm; PD, 63 mm.

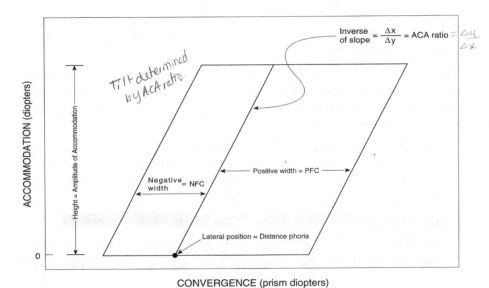

CONVERGENCE (prism diopters)

*Figure 3.2. The five geometrical properties of the ZCSBV and their clinical correlates.*

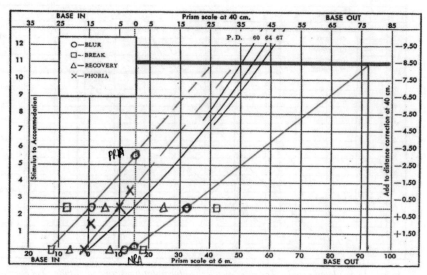

*Figure 3.3. A graph with a possibly erroneous finding (the 40 cm phoria with a +1.00 D add). The test findings presented in the following table were taken through the subjective refraction unless otherwise noted.*

|  | Phoria | Base-in | Base-out | Plus to blur | Minus to blur |
|---|---|---|---|---|---|
| 6 m | 1 exo | X/12/7 | 12/18/8 |  |  |
| 40 cm | 5 exo | 14/23/10 | 17/27/10 | +2.25 | -3.00 |
| 40 cm +1.00 D add | 14 exo |  |  |  |  |
| 40 cm -1.00 D add | 2 exo |  |  |  |  |

Amplitude of accommodation, 11 D; NPC, 4 cm; PD, 63 mm.

their respective line-segment slopes at the lower accommodative levels. In other words, interpolation is indicated by solid line segments, and extrapolation is indicated by dashed lines.

The zone of clear single binocular vision (ZCSBV) is the area within the blur lines, the amplitude lines, and the base line on the bottom of the graph through zero stimulus to accommodation. Figures 3.1 and 3.2 provide examples of completed graphs.

The ZCSBV represents the area in which the patient can see clearly and singly. It predicts how the patient will respond to different viewing distances, lenses, and prisms. To better understand the nature of the ZCSBV, we can relate five of its geometric properties to clinical correlates:

1. The lateral position of the graph corresponds to the distance phoria.

2. The height of the zone corresponds to the amplitude of accommodation.

3. The correlate of the slope of the zone is the reciprocal of the stimulus ACA ratio.

4. The positive width corresponds to positive fusional convergence, the lateral distance from the phoria line to the base-out boundary.

5. The negative width represents negative fusional convergence, the lateral distance from the phoria line to the base-in boundary.[11-13]

The five geometric properties of the ZCSBV are illustrated in Figure 3.2. If we do not consider for the moment variability in lateral position, slope, height, and widths of the ZCSBV; we can describe its general form as follows:

1. The phoria line is expected to approximate a straight line.

2. The line formed by the base-in to blur (or base-in to break if no blur is obtained) and minus-to-blur findings is expected to be parallel to the phoria line. It should be approximately straight.

3. The line connecting the base-out to blur (or base-out to break if no blur is obtained) and the plus-to-blur findings also should be approximately straight and parallel to the phoria line. NRA

4. The ZCSBV should approximate a parallelogram with the phoria line making it a double parallelogram.

5. Because of accommodative convergence, phoria and blur lines should tilt toward the right.

One of the uses of a plot of the ZCSBV is that it can give the examiner an idea of the internal consistency of the findings for a given patient. The findings for a given patient are likely to be consistent with each other if the pattern of the ZCSBV conforms to the expected configuration outlined in the five points above. If a given finding departs significantly from placement in the double parallelogram arrangement of the ZCSBV, it may indicate procedural error during the performance of that test. Such findings are easy to identify if tests are done with a number of lens and test distance combinations. Figure 3.3 provides an example of the detection of erroneous test results.

One common deviation from the expected graph form, which is not considered due to error but rather due to normal variation, may occur with an individual who exhibits a large amount of proximal convergence.[14] In this case the ZCSBV will appear to fan out. That is, the lateral distance from the base-in and minus to blur line to the base-out and plus to blur line will appear to increase as the stimulus to accommodation level increases. Proximal convergence and its effect on the appearance of the ZCSBV will be discussed in more detail in the next chapter.

A second clinical use of the ZCSBV is to assist in the recognition of case types. Differences in the lateral position, tilt, and width of the ZCSBV can help in the identification of a particular vergence disorder case type.

## REFERENCES

1. *Daum KM. Vergence amplitude. In: Eskridge JB, Amos JF, Bartlett JD, eds. Clinical Procedures in Optometry. Philadelphia: Lippincott, 1991:91-98.*

2. Pitts DG, Hofstetter HW. Demand-line graphing of the zone of clear single binocular vision. Am Optom Assoc J. 1959;31:51-55.

3. Grosvenor T. Primary Care Optometry, 5th ed. St. Louis: Butterworth Heinemann Elsevier, 2007:227-234.

4. London R. Near point of convergence. In: Eskridge JB, Amos JF, Bartlett JD, eds. Clinical Procedures in Optometry. Philadelphia: Lippincott, 1991:66-68.

5. Adler PM, Cregg M, Viollier A-J, Woodhouse JM. Influence of target type and RAF rule on the measurement of near point of convergence. Ophthal Physiol Opt 2007;27:22-30.

6. Hayes GJ, Cohen BE, Rouse MW, DeLand PN. Normative values for the nearpoint of convergence of elementary schoolchildren. Optom Vis Sci 1998;75:506-512.

7. Jiménez R, Pérez MA, García JA, González MD. Statistical normal values of visual parameters that characterize binocular function in children. Ophthal Physiol Opt 2004;24:528-542.

8. Scheiman M, Gallaway M, Frantz KA, Peters RJ, Hatch S, Cuff M, Mitchell GL. Nearpoint of convergence: Test procedure, target selection, and normative data. Optom Vis Sci 2003;80:214-225.

9. Maples WC, Hoenes R. Near point of convergence norms measured in elementary school children. Optom Vis Sci 2007;84:224-228.

10. Chen AH, O'Leary DJ, Howell ER. Near visual function in young children. Part I.: near point of convergence. Part II: amplitude of accommodation. Part III: Near heterophoria. Ophthal Physiol Opt 2000;20:185-198.

11. Fry GA. Fundamental variables in the relationship between accommodation and convergence. Optom Weekly 1943;34:153- 155, 183-185.

12. Hofstetter HW. The zone of clear single binocular vision. Am J Optom Arch Am Acad Optom 1945;22:301-333, 361-384.

13. Hofstetter HW. Graphical analysis. In: Schor CM, Ciuffreda KJ, eds. Vergence Eye Movements: Basic and Clinical Aspects. Boston: Butterworth-Heinemann, 1983:439-464.

14. Hofstetter HW. The relationship of proximal convergence to fusional and accommodative convergence. Am J Optom Arch Am Acad Optom. 1951;28:300-308.

## OTHER SUGGESTED READING

Carlson NB, Kurtz D. Clinical Procedures for Ocular Examination, 3rd ed. New York: McGraw-Hill, 2004:162-193.

Saladin JJ. Phorometry and stereopsis. In: Benjamin WJ, ed. Borish's Clinical Refraction, 2nd ed. St. Louis: Butterworth Heinemann Elsevier, 2006:899-960.

## PRACTICE PROBLEMS

1. Graph the test findings for the following cases. All findings are taken with the subjective refraction in place unless otherwise indicated. For each patient, draw in the boundaries of the ZCSBV, determine whether there are any inconsistent findings, and determine the stimulus calculated ACA ratio and the stimulus gradient ACA ratio.

2. What is the amplitude of accommodation in each of the following cases:

   (a) Near point of accommodation with habitual Rx: 10 cm; habitual Rx: plano sph OU;
   Subjective refraction: +2.00 D sph OU.
   (b) Near point of accommodation with habitual Rx: 8 cm; habitual Rx: -1.00 D sph
   OU; Subjective refraction: -2.50 D sph OU.

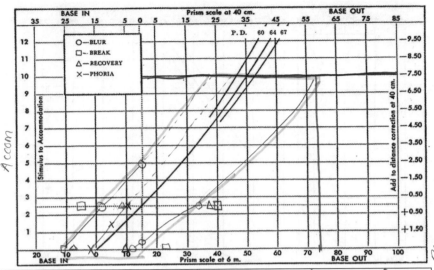

Handwritten annotations: "Accom" (left side), "converg" (below graph), "normal ACA ratio / demandline / is 1/1 to", "zone of clear single bino vision. (ZCSBV)"

| Patient AR | | | | | |
|---|---|---|---|---|---|
| | Phoria X | Base-in | Base-out | Plus to blur | Minus to blur |
| 6 m | 2 exo | X/11/8 | 12/22/10 | | |
| 40 cm | 4 exo | 14/20/7 | 19/25/22 | +2.00 | -2.50 |
| 40 cm +1.00 D add | 8 exo | | | | |

Near point of accommodation, 10 cm; NPC, 6 cm; PD, 64 mm.

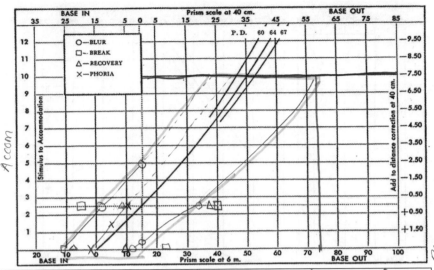

| Patient BP | | | | | |
|---|---|---|---|---|---|
| | Phoria | Base-in | Base-out | Plus to blur | Minus to blur |
| 6 m | 2 exo | X/9/5 | 10/18/6 | | |
| 40 cm | 2 eso | 9/15/4 | 23/30/16 | +2.25 | -1.50 |
| 40 cm +1.00 D add | 3 exo | | | | |

Near point of accommodation, 8 cm; NPC, 4 cm; PD, 62 mm.

(12.5D)

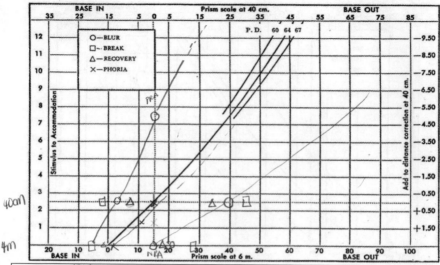

40cm

4m

Patient DT  EXO                                                                                           ESO

|  | Phoria | Base-in | Base-out | Plus to blur | Minus to blur |
|---|---|---|---|---|---|
| 4 m | 2 eso | X/5/2 | 21/28/18 |  |  |
| 40 cm | Ortho | 12/18/8 | 25/30/20 | +2.50 | -5.00 |
| 40 cm +1.00 D add | 4 exo |  |  |  |  |

Near point of accommodation, 9 cm; NPC, 3 cm; PD, 64 mm.

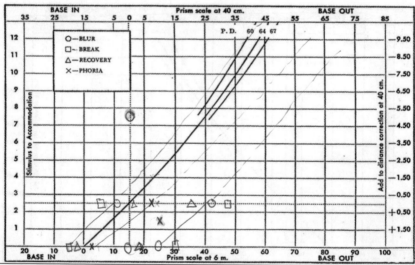

Patient GL

|  | Phoria | Base-in | Base-out | Plus to blur | Minus to blur |
|---|---|---|---|---|---|
| 6 m | 3 eso | X/4/2 | 25/30/18 |  |  |
| 40 cm | 8 eso | 4/10/-2 | 27/32/20 | +2.50 | -5.00 |
| 40 cm +1.00 D add | 10 eso |  |  |  |  |

Near point of accommodation, 7 cm; NPC, 2 cm; PD, 60 mm

(14.3Δ)

PRA + Gradient does not fit in

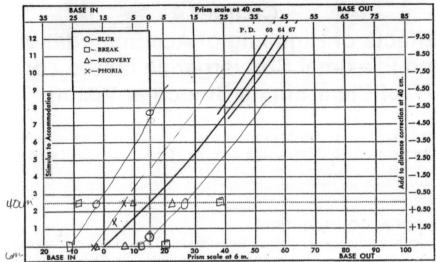

| Patient DK | | | | | |
|---|---|---|---|---|---|
| | **Phoria** | **Base-in** | **Base-out** | **Plus to blur** | **Minus to blur** |
| 4 m | 4 exo | X/12/4 | 12/20/6 | | |
| 40 cm | 8 exo | 18/24/6 | 12/24/8 | +2.00 | -5.25 |
| 40 cm +1.00 D add | 12 exo | | | | |

Near point of accommodation, 10 cm; NPC, 9 cm; PD, 64 mm.

# Chapter 4
# Effects of High Lag of Accommodation and Proximal Convergence on the Zone of Clear Single Binocular Vision

In Chapter 3 we saw that the expected shape of the zone of clear single binocular vision (ZCSBV) is a parallelogram. With the inclusion of the phoria line it becomes a double parallelogram. Two common causes of departure from this expected form are an abnormally high lag of accommodation and proximal convergence.

## LAG OF ACCOMMODATION

Clinically we try to assure that the accommodative response will be approximately equal to the accommodative stimulus by instructing the patient to keep the test letters clear during testing procedures such as dissociated phoria tests. Because of the depth of focus, the accommodative response does not have to exactly equal the stimulus to accommodation for clear vision. For example, if the depth of focus is 1.00 D and the patient is wearing the correction for ametropia, the accommodative response can vary from approximately 2.00 D to approximately 3.00 D while target clarity is retained at 40 cm. For most individuals the accommodative response tends to be less than the stimulus to accommodation; this is referred to as the lag of accommodation. The term lag of accommodation was coined by Sheard.[1]

The ACA ratio that would most closely describe the physiologic interaction of accommodative convergence and accommodation would be the ratio of the amount of accommodative convergence to the corresponding change in accommodative response. This is called the response ACA ratio and it can be determined if accommodative response is measured by an optometer or a retinoscopic arrangement. During clinical testing, we know the accommodative stimulus from the test distance and the test lenses used, but we usually do not measure the accommodative response. As a result, the ACA ratio derived clinically usually is the ratio of the amount of accommodative convergence to the corresponding change in stimulus to accommodation (stimulus ACA ratio).

The stimulus calculated ACA ratio will not equal the response calculated ACA ratio if there is a lag of accommodation during the near phoria test (accommodative stimulus and accommodative response would both theoretically be zero during the distance phoria test because accommodation should be relaxed when viewing through the maximum plus subjective refraction to best visual acuity). The stimulus gradient ACA ratio will not equal the response gradient ACA ratio if the lag of accommodation changes from one dissociated phoria test to the next. The lag of accommodation can be minimized during dissociated phoria testing by requiring patients to view letters close to their best visual acuity and instructing them to keep the letters clear. In fact, the single

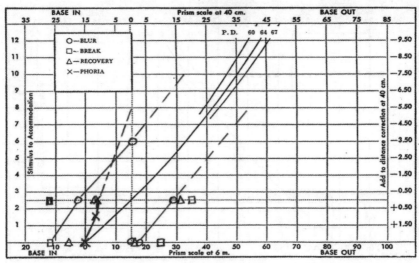

Figure 4.1. The findings in the following table are plotted in the graph. The phoria line is not parallel to the base-in and base-out blur lines. The ACA ratio is thus evidently higher than the phoria line would indicate. The case type typified by this set of findings has been called pseudoconvergence insufficiency. Test findings were taken with the patient viewing through the subjective refraction to best visual acuity unless otherwise noted.

|  | Phoria | Base-in | Base-out | Plus to blur | Minus to blur |
|---|---|---|---|---|---|
| 6 m | Ortho | X/12/6 | 18/24/16 |  |  |
| 40 cm | 11 exo | 18/28/12 | 14/20/16 | +2.50 | -3.50 |
| 40 cm +1.00 D add | 12 exo |  |  |  |  |

most common source of error in clinically measured phorias and ACA ratios is the failure to include this requirement. It is important to control accommodation on any dissociated phoria measurement, whether it be by alternating cover test, von Graefe test, or other test.

A lag of accommodation that shows a sizable increase with an increase in accommodative stimulus will result in a phoria line that is tipped less toward the right (thus indicating a lower stimulus ACA ratio) than are the base-in and base-out limit lines. If there is a large lag of accommodation at the higher stimulus to accommodation, calculation of the stimulus ACA ratio will yield a significantly lower value than the response ACA ratio. An example is provided in Figure 4.1. Because the accommodative response is low, there is less accommodative convergence occurring than if the accommodative response had more closely approximated the accommodative stimulus. That results in a more divergent dissociated phoria than if the accommodative response had been normal. The near phoria is more exo than it would be if the phoria line were parallel with the left and right sides of the ZCSBV. Cases with findings similar to those in Figure 4.1 even though an instruction is made to keep the letters clear during phoria testing, have been called pseudo convergence insufficiency or false convergence insufficiency.[2,3] In pseudo convergence insufficiency the high exophoria is secondary to an accommodative problem, so

37

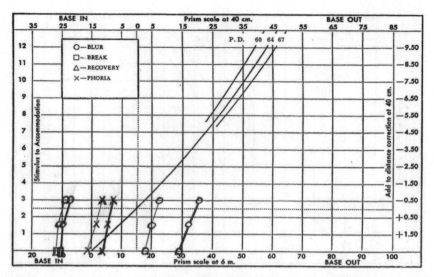

Figure 4.2. To demonstrate proximal convergence, base-in and base-out limits and phorias were taken at 6 m (thin lines) and 33 cm (heavy lines) with various adds over the subjective refraction to best visual acuity. The data are given in the following table.

| | Phoria | Base-in limit | Base-out limit |
|---|---|---|---|
| 6 m | 1 exo | 12 | 18 |
| 6 m -1.50 D add | 2 eso | 11 | 20 |
| 6 m -3.00 D add | 4 eso | 9 | 22 |
| 33 cm | 10 exo | 25 | 18 |
| 33 cm +1.50 D add | 12 exo | 27 | 14 |
| 33 cm +3.00 D add | 14 exo | 28 | 12 |

Amplitude of accommodation, 10 D; NPC, 5 cm; PD, 63 mm.

treatments can include plus adds and/or vision therapy to improve accommodative function.[2-5]

## PROXIMAL CONVERGENCE

Proximal convergence is convergence caused by awareness of nearness of a target.[6] Individuals who exhibit a great deal of proximal convergence have a characteristic alteration in the ZCSBV: the zone appears to fan out; that is, it is wider at the higher stimulus to accommodation. This is due to the fact that the base-out findings are affected the most by proximal convergence and the base-in findings are affected the least, with the phorias falling somewhere in between.[7] One way to demonstrate this is to obtain one set of findings at distance with different minus adds over the subjective refraction and another set of findings at near-point with plus adds over the subjective refraction. The two sets of data will thus have used the same levels of stimulus of accommodation but different test distances.

If the subject in this experiment happens to show proximal convergence, results similar to those shown in Figures 4.2 and 4.3 may be obtained. In Figure 4.2 the lines connecting points for 6 m test distance findings are separate from the

38

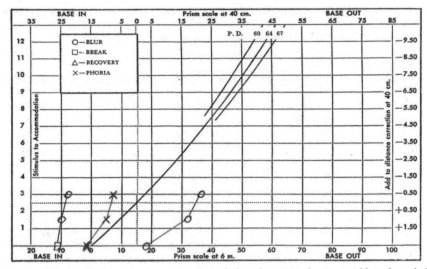

*Figure 4.3. Plot of the findings taken at 6 m through the subjective refraction, at 33 cm through the subjective refraction, and at 33 cm through a +1.50 D add from the example in Figure 4.2. Note that the zone fans out, a characteristic configuration for an individual who exhibits a typical amount of proximal convergence.*

lines connecting 33 cm findings. In Figure 4.3, lines connect the points that more closely represent a typical clinical routine. In the same figure the base-in and base-out boundaries of the ZCSBV fan out.

In Figure 4.2, the two base-out lines are separated more than the two phoria lines, which in turn are separated more than the two base-in findings. This agrees with the hierarchy mentioned earlier for the findings most affected by proximal convergence. Hofstetter[7] found that for a group of 21 young adult subjects in an experiment similar to the one shown in Figures 4.2 and 4.3, the average amounts of displacement of the base-in, phoria, and base-out lines were 1.5 Δ, 2.6 Δ, and 7.6 Δ, respectively.

One possible explanation for differing amounts of proximal convergence on the base-out, phoria, and base-in lines is that perception of distance changes as prism power is added under binocular conditions. As base-out prism power is increased, the target seems to get smaller and closer. As base-in prism power is increased, the target seems to get larger and farther away. This is often called the SILO effect, with SI standing for smaller and (closer) in with convergence and the LO standing for larger and (farther) out with divergence. The observation that proximal convergence is greater under conditions of binocular fusion than under unfused conditions[8] would suggest that the effect of proximal convergence would be greater on fusional vergence ranges than on dissociated phorias.

## REFERENCES

1. Sheard C. Dynamic skiametry and methods of testing the accommodation and convergence of the eyes. In: The Sheard Volume-Selected Writings in Visual and Ophthalmic Optics. Philadelphia: Chilton, 1957:125-230 (originally published as a monograph in 1920).

2. Grosvenor TP. *Primary Care Optometry*, 5th ed. St. Louis: Butterworth Heinemann Elsevier, 2007:263-64.

3. Richman JE, Cron MT. *Guide to Vision Therapy*. South Bend, IN: Bernell Corp, 1987:17-18.

4. Heath GG. The use of graphic analysis in visual training. *Am J Optom Arch Am Acad Optom* 1959;36:337-50.

5. Mazow ML, France TD, Finkelman S, et al. Acute accommodative and convergence insufficiency. *Trans Am Ophthalmol Soc* 1989;87:158-73.

6. Hofstetter HW. The proximal factor in accommodation and convergence. *Am J Optom Arch Am Acad Optom* 1942;19:67-76.

7. Hofstetter HW. The relationship of proximal convergence to fusional and accommodative convergence. *Am J Optom Arch Am Acad Optom* 1951;28: 300-08.

8. Wick B. Clinical factors in proximal vergence. *Am J Optom Physiol Opt* 1985; 62:1-18.

## OTHER SUGGESTED READING

Ciuffreda KJ. Accommodation, the pupil, and presbyopia. In: Benjamin WJ, ed. *Borish's Clinical Refraction*, 2nd ed. St. Louis: Butterworth Heinemann Elsevier, 2006:93-144 *(see especially pages 99-101)*.

Hokoda SC, Ciuffreda KJ. Theoretical and clinical importance of proximal vergence and accommodation. In: Schor CM, Ciuffreda KJ, eds. *Vergence Eye Movements: Basic and Clinical Aspects*. Boston: Butterworth-Heinemann, 1983: 75-97 *(see especially pages 90-92)*.

## PRACTICE PROBLEMS

1. Which would you expect to be higher in a person exhibiting considerable proximal convergence: the gradient ACA ratio or the calculated ACA ratio? Explain.

2. Why is the stimulus calculated ACA ratio less than the response calculated ACA ratio in a patient with a high lag of accommodation?

3. Plot the findings on the next page for a patient diagnosed as having pseudo convergence insufficiency. Tests were taken through the subjective refraction to best visual acuity unless otherwise noted. Note that the phoria line does not tilt to the right as much as the base-in and base-out lines.

4. Plot the phorias and vergence range blurs on the next page. Tests were done through different lens powers at 6 m and then different lens powers at 40 cm to demonstrate the effect of proximal convergence. Connect the 6 m points with one color and the 40 cm points with a second color. Which line (phoria, base-in, or base-out) shifts the most and which shifts the least from 6m to 40 cm? Now take a third color to connect the points taken through the BVA. Which line drawn with the third color tilts the most to the right and which the least?

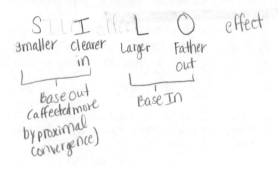

## Question 3.

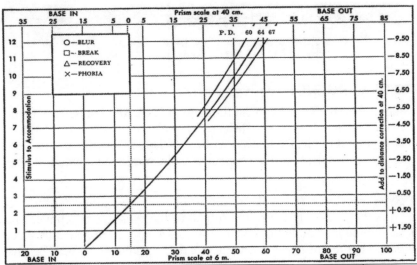

|  | Phoria | Base-in | Base-out | Plus to blur | Minus to blur |
|---|---|---|---|---|---|
| 6 m | 1 exo | X/10/4 | 12/18/8 |  |  |
| 40 cm | 10 exo | 12/20/8 | 14/20/8 | +2.00 | -2.25 |
| 40 cm +1.00 D add | 11 exo |  |  |  |  |

## Question 4.

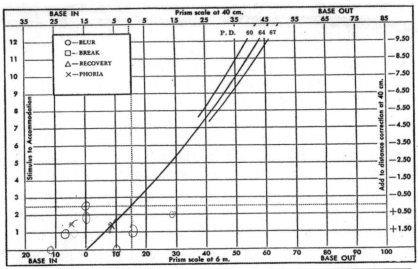

|  | Phoria | Base-in blur | Base-out blur |
|---|---|---|---|
| 6 m / BVA | 1 exo | 11 (break) | 10 |
| 6 m / -1.00 D add | 3 eso | 7 | 14 |
| 6 m / -2.00 D add | 8 eso |  |  |
| 40 cm / BVA | 2 exo | 15 | 14 |
| 40 cm / +1.00 D add | 6 exo | 19 | 8 |
| 40 cm / +2.00 D add | 10 exo |  |  |

# Chapter 5
# Definitions of Terms

## TYPES OF VERGENCE

To aid in theoretical and clinical thinking, it is useful to classify vergence eye movements into types. The early classification scheme of Maddox[1-3] provides a helpful clinical framework. In the Maddox classification scheme vergence eye movements are described as tonic, accommodative, proximal, and fusional.

Tonic convergence represents the result of tonus in the extraocular muscles; that is, it is the physiologic position of rest of the eyes. Tonic convergence can be said to be the amount of convergence of the eyes when no stimulus to convergence is present and the accommodative stimulus is zero. The position of the eyes under these conditions is the combination of tonic convergence and the anatomic position of rest of the eyes. The clinical correlate of this position is the distance phoria through the subjective refraction. Thus, the distance phoria is said to represent tonic convergence. Accommodative convergence is convergence that occurs as part of the synkinesis of convergence and accommodation. The ACA ratio is the accommodative convergence in prism diopters per diopter of accommodation. Proximal convergence is convergence caused by the awareness of nearness of a given object of fixation. Fusional convergence is convergence which serves to maintain fusion of the two retinal images. Disparity vergence often is used as a synonym for fusional convergence because the effective stimulus for these movements is retinal disparity.[4-6] The definitions of the Maddox components of convergence were summarized earlier in Table 2.1.

Maddox's writings were based on clinical experience rather than controlled experimentation.[3] Maddox's concepts are an oversimplification of the neurophysiology of vergence eye movements, but the Maddox classification is a useful construct that aids in understanding clinical analysis of convergence.

The above terms describing the Maddox classification of vergence have been defined earlier. They appear here for review as a background for the terms to be discussed next.

## TERMS USED TO DESCRIBE FUSIONAL VERGENCE EFFORT AND CAPABILITY

Fusional vergence is of particular interest because strain on fusional vergence can cause eyestrain or ocular discomfort. A number of terms are used to describe the amount of fusional vergence the patient can exert and the amount of fusional vergence the patient uses to maintain single vision. To illustrate what these terms mean, Figure 5.1 shows the positions of the lines of sight during various tests. DT represents the position of the lines of sight when viewing an infinitely distant object binocularly. DT for the left eye is thus

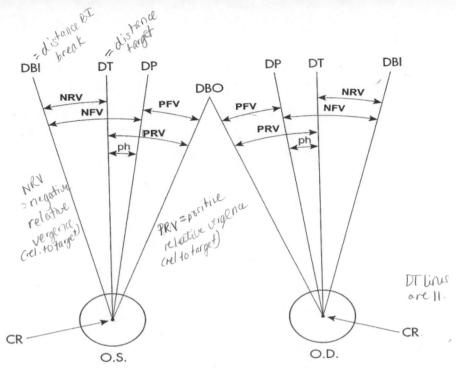

Handwritten annotations in figure:
- = distance BI break (pointing to DBI)
- = distance target (pointing to DT)
- NRV = negative relative vergence (rel. to target)
- PRV = positive relative vergence (rel. to target)
- DT lines are ll.

*Figure 5.1. Positions of the lines of sight of the eyes during various tests for a patient with esophoria at distance. CR, center of rotation; DBI, position at distance base-in break; DT, position if target is fused at infinity (parallelism of the lines of sight); DP, distance phoria position; DBO, position at distance base-out blur; ph, dissociated phoria. See text for explanations of NRV, PRV, NFV, and PFV.*

parallel with DT for the right eye. DP represents the position of the lines of sight during the dissociated phoria test. This patient has an esophoria because DP is convergent with respect to DT. The angle between DT and DP is the amount of the dissociated phoria. DBI shows the position of the lines of sight at the break on the distance base-in fusional vergence range test, and DBO represents the distance base-out blur.

When the distance dissociated phoria test is done, tonic convergence is in play. From there fusional vergence can be exerted in a positive direction (lines of sight rotating in toward each other) or a negative direction (lines of sight moving out away from each other). DBO and DBI represent the limits of these excursions, respectively. Negative fusional vergence (NFV) is the angle between DP and DBI. Positive fusional vergence (PFV) is the angle between DP and DBO. These values represent the maximum fusional vergence capabilities of the patient. Positive relative vergence (PRV) is the angle between DT and DBO. Because DT represents the position of the lines of sight with no prism, PRV is equal to the amount of prism added to reach the base-out limit. Negative relative vergence (NRV) is the angle between DT and DBI. The NRV and the PRV are the base-in and base-out limits, respectively, as read from the prism used for fusional vergence range testing. (The base-in and base-out limits are the blur findings with increasing prism or the break findings if no blur occurs)

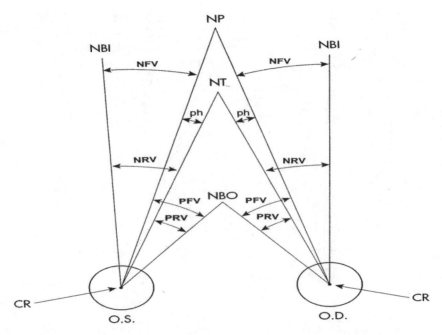

*Figure 5.2. Positions of the lines of sight of the eyes during various tests for a patient with exophoria at near. CR, center of rotation; NBI, position at near base-in blur; NT, position of near point test target; NP, near point phoria position; NBO, position at near base-out blur; ph, dissociated phoria. See text for explanations of NRV, PRV, NFV, and PFV.*

The dissociated phoria test measures the amount of fusional vergence needed to maintain single binocular vision. The dissociated phoria is the demand on fusional vergence, often simply called the demand. In the diagram in Figure 5.1, the lines of sight must be rotated from DP to DT for single binocular vision. So patients with esophoria must use part of their NFV to get to DT and have single vision. The portion of their NFV left over (the angle between DT and DBI) is known as the reserve. In esophoria, the reserve is equal to the NRV.

Figure 5.2 illustrates the position of the lines of sight during nearpoint testing in a patient with exophoria at near. NFV, PFV, NRV, and PRV are labeled in the diagram. In exophoria, part of the patient's PFV must be used to meet the demand on fusional convergence. The demand is labeled ph in the diagram for phoria, and is the angle between NT and NP. Then the reserve is the portion of the PFV left over after the lines of sight are rotated in to NT; that is, the reserve in Figure 5.2 is the angle between NT and NBO. The amount of the fusional convergence left in reserve is equal to the PRV in exophoria.

These terms can be visualized on the x,y plot of accommodation and convergence,[7-9] and we can relate these terms to the zone of clear single binocular vision (ZCSBV). The positive relative vergence (PRV) at a given level of accommodation is the horizontal distance on the graph from the demand line to the right-hand limit of the ZCSBV. The negative relative vergence (NRV) is the horizontal distance from the demand line to the left-hand limit of the

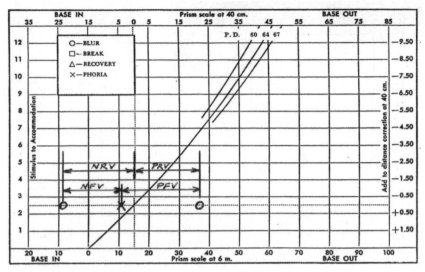

*Figure 5.3. A plot of 4Δ exo, a base-in blur of 24, and a base-out blur of 22 at 40 cm. Therefore, the NRV is 24, the NFV is 20, the PFV is 26, the PRV is 22, the demand is 4, and the reserve is 22.*

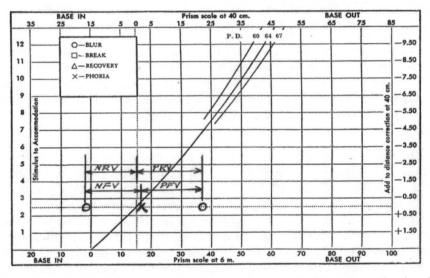

*Figure 5.4. A plot of 2Δ eso, a base-in blur of 16, and a base-out blur of 22 at 40 cm. Therefore, the NRV is 16, the NFV is 18, the PFV is 20, the PRV is 22, the demand is 2, and the reserve is 16.*

ZCSBV. The positive fusional vergence (PFV) for a given stimulus to accommodation level is the horizontal distance on the graph from the phoria line to the right-hand boundary of the ZCSBV. The negative fusional vergence (NFV) is the horizontal distance from the phoria line to the left-hand boundary of the ZCSBV.

As noted earlier, the dissociated phoria is a measure of the amount of fusional vergence required for single binocular vision at the testing distance. Thus, the demand on fusional convergence is equal to the dissociated phoria. On the

45

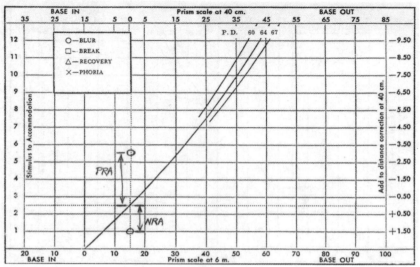

*Figure 5.5. The NRA and PRA at 40 cm for a patient with a plus to blur of +1.50 D and a minus to blur of -3.00 D.*

graph, the demand is equal to the horizontal distance from the phoria line to the demand line for testing with the patient's subjective refraction in place.

The reserve is the horizontal distance from the demand line to the right-hand limit of the ZCSBV in exophoria and to the left-hand limit in esophoria. It represents the amount of fusional vergence that can still be exerted after the demand has been met. In exophoria the reserve is equal to the base-out limit or, in other words, the PRV. In esophoria the reserve is equal to the base-in limit or NRV.

Examples of the graphical dimensions associated with these terms are presented in Figures 5.3 and 5.4. Figure 5.3 shows the graph for a patient with an exophoria of 4Δ at 40 cm. The vergence posture of the eyes during the measurement of the near phoria is dependent on tonic, proximal, and accommodative convergence. The PFV and NFV represent the fusional vergence that can be exerted in the convergent (base-out) and divergent (base-in) directions, respectively, from that point. The PRV and NRV are measurements of the patient's convergence and divergence capabilities with respect to the target; on the graph they are measured from a point on the demand line corresponding to the testing distance. Figure 5.4 illustrates an example showing near-point esophoria. The following formulas give the relationship of fusional vergence and relative vergence values:

PFV = PRV - phoria

NFV = NRV + phoria

Exophoria is a minus value in the formulas and esophoria is a plus since they represent divergent and convergent positions, respectively, in relation to the target. (This, of course, is the same sign convention as is used in the formula for calculated ACA ratio)

## NRA AND PRA

The plus to blur test is often referred to as the negative relative accommodation (NRA) test because accommodation is decreased by plus lenses. A synonym for the minus to blur test is the positive relative accommodation (PRA) test because minus lenses present a stimulus to increase accommodation. Just as we did for the fusional vergence terms, we can identify the magnitudes of the NRA and PRA on the accommodation and convergence graph. The PRA is the vertical distance upward on the graph from the demand line to the minus to blur point. The NRA is the vertical distance downward on the graph from the demand line to the plus to blur point (Figure 5.5).

## REFERENCES

1. Maddox EE. The Clinical Use of Prisms; and the Decentration of Lenses, 2nd ed. Bristol, England: John Wright & Co, 1893:83-106.
2. Schor C. Introduction to the symposium on basic and clinical aspects of vergence eye movements. Am J Optom Physiol Opt 1980;57:535-36.
3. Morgan MW. The Maddox analysis of vergence. In: Schor CM, Ciuffreda KJ, eds. Vergence Eye Movements: Basic and Clinical Aspects. Boston: Butterworth-Heinemann, 1983:15-21.
4. Stark L, Kenyon RV, Krishnan VV, Ciuffreda KJ. Disparity vergence: a proposed name for a dominant component of binocular vergence eye movements. Am J Optom Physiol Opt 1980;57:606-09.
5. Fry GA. Letter to the Editor: Disparity vergence. Am J Optom Physiol Opt 1981;58:685.
6. Stark L. Reply. Am J Optom Physiol Opt 1981; 58:686.
7. Hofstetter HW. The graphical analysis of clinical optometric findings. In: Transactions of the International Ophthalmic Optical Congress 1961. London: Lockwood, 1962:456-60.
8. Hofstetter HW. Graphical analysis. In: Schor CM, Ciuffreda KJ, eds. Vergence Eye Movements: Basic and Clinical Aspects. Boston: Butterworth-Heinemann, 1983:439-64.
9. Michaels DD. Visual Optics and Refraction-A Clinical Approach, 3rd ed. St Louis: Mosby, 1985:361-65.

## PRACTICE PROBLEMS

Determine the NRV, PRV, NFV, PFV, demand, and reserve for individuals with the following results of tests taken at 40 cm:

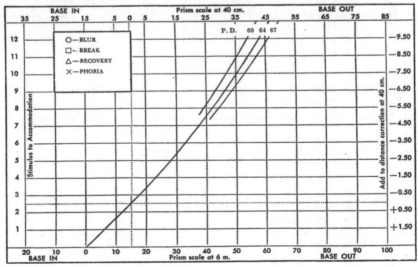

1. 8Δ exo, BI blur = 17, BO blur = 12.

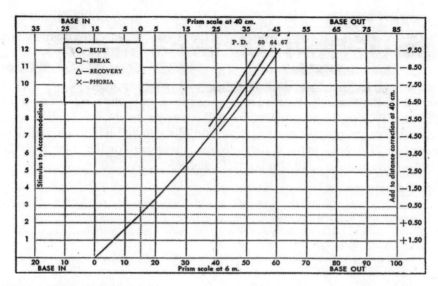

2. 3Δ eso, BI blur = 5, BO blur = 24

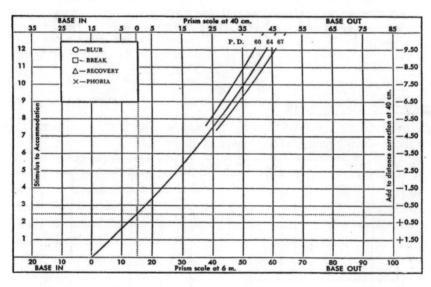

3. 2Δ exo, BI blur = 12, BO blur = 15

# Chapter 6
# Simple Guidelines for Evaluating the Stress on Fusional Vergence

The Maddox classification of vergence considers the total vergence response to be composed of tonic vergence, proximal vergence, accommodative vergence, and fusional vergence, in varying amounts depending on viewing distance, test conditions, and individual visual characteristics of the patient. Of the Maddox components, the one which can be associated with asthenopia and eyestrain when strained is fusional vergence. So various guidelines or rules of thumb have been developed to assess stress on fusional vergence. In chapter 5 we noted that the dissociated phoria is a measure of the demand on fusional vergence. We also noted that the amount of fusional vergence left in reserve is equal to the PRC in exophoria and equal to the NRC in esophoria.

Treatment regimens for vergence disorders include prisms, spherical lens adds, and vision training. Prism can be used to directly reduce the demand on fusional vergence and thus relieve symptoms. Lens adds alter the amount of accommodative convergence in the total vergence response and thereby indirectly reduce the demand on fusional vergence. Vision training or vision therapy primarily improves the reserve, thus allowing the patient to more effortlessly and efficiently handle the demand on fusional vergence.

In this chapter we will look at three simple guidelines used to assess the strain on fusional vergence.

## SHEARD'S CRITERION
Of the various guidelines for evaluating the strain on fusional vergence in lateral imbalances, the most widely used is Sheard's criterion.[1,2] The work of Hofstetter[3] suggested that application of Sheard's criterion correlates well with asthenopic symptoms and with relief of symptoms by vergence training. This was confirmed by Sheedy and Saladin,[4,5] who found that of several vergence and fixation disparity criteria, Sheard's criterion was the most effective in predicting asthenopic symptoms, and by Dalziel,[6] who reported that vision training that brought vergence findings to the point at which Sheard's criterion was met was effective in alleviating symptoms.

Sheard's postulate was that the fusional reserve should be at least twice the demand. Thus, the positive relative vergence (PRV) should be at least twice the amount of an exophoria and the negative relative vergence (NRV) should be at least twice the amount of an esophoria. In other words, according to Sheard's criterion, patients with exophoria are more likely to be symptomatic if their base-out blur (or break in the absence of a blur) is less than twice the amount of the exophoria, and patients with esophoria are more likely to be symptomatic if their base-in blur (or break in the absence of a blur) is less than twice the amount of the esophoria. A mathematical expression which describes when Sheard's criterion is met is $R \geq 2D$, where R represents the reserve and D represents the demand.

To determine how much prism correction is necessary to allow Sheard's criterion to just be met at a given distance, we can use the formula

$$P = (2/3)D - (1/3)R$$

where P represents the required prism, D is the demand, and R is the reserve. (In this formula D is always positive regardless of whether an exophoria or an esophoria is present, and R is always positive whether positive relative vergence is used, as in exophoria, or negative relative vergence is used, as in esophoria.) When P equals 0 or a negative number, Sheard's criterion is met without any prism correction. A positive number indicates that prism is necessary for the criterion to be met: base-in prism in exophoria or base-out prism in esophoria.

Sheard's criterion provides a means of estimating how much the demand would need to be decreased by prism in order to relieve symptoms. It can also theoretically provide an estimate of how much the reserve would have to be increased with vision therapy to relieve symptoms. In exophoria, vision therapy can be used to increase the base-out fusional vergence ranges, and in esophoria, vision therapy can be used to increase base-in fusional vergence ranges. Sheard's criterion predicts that in order to relieve symptoms with vision therapy, the reserve would have to be increased to the point that is at least twice the amount of the phoria (the demand).

## EXAMPLES OF THE USE OF SHEARD'S CRITERION

The rationale for prescription decisions will be developed in more detail in chapter 11. Here we will look at some examples that illustrate how Sheard's criterion can be used. In the first example, shown in Figure 6.1, exophoria is measured at both distance and near. Sheard's criterion is met at 6 m but not at 40 cm, because the base-out blur at 40 cm ($11\Delta$) is not twice the phoria ($10\Delta$ exophoria). To determine the prism correction necessary to meet Sheard's criterion at 40 cm we use the following formula:

$$P = (2/3)D - (1/3)R$$
$$= (2/3)(10) - (1/3)(11)$$
$$= 3\Delta \text{ base-in}$$

Base-in prism is used since the phoria is in the exo direction.

Another way to allow Sheard's criterion to be met is to increase the base-out blur to at least $20\Delta$ by vision training.

Figure 6.2 illustrates a case of esophoria at distance and near. Sheard's criterion is met at 6 m but not at 40 cm or 33 cm. That is, at 40 cm and at 33 cm the reserve (base-in blur) is not twice the demand (phoria). Sheard's criterion would be fulfilled at 40 cm with the following prism:

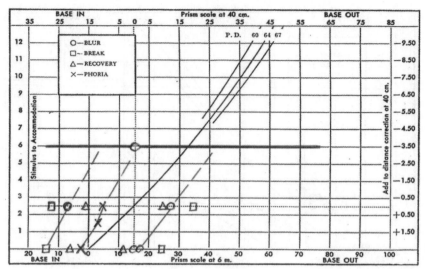

Figure 6.1. This figure illustrates the clinical findings in the table below. NRA    PRA

|  | Phoria | Base-in | Base-out | Plus to blur | Minus to blur |
|---|---|---|---|---|---|
| 6 m | 3 exo | X/14/6 | 16/24/12 |  | P |
| 40 cm | 10 exo | 22/28/16 | 12/20/10 | +2.50 | -3.50 |
| 40 cm +1.00 D add | 12 exo |  |  |  |  |

Amplitude of accommodation, 6 D.

$$P = (2/3)D - (1/3)R$$
$$= (2/3)(12) - (1/3)(12)$$
$$= 4\Delta \text{ base-out}$$

Base-out prism is required because of the esophoria.

Another form of treatment is vision training to increase the base-in limit (to at least 24 at 40 cm according to Sheard's criterion in this case). Probably the most common method of handling this type of case is to provide a plus add at near. A plus add is effective in this type of case because the ACA ratio is quite high. A high ACA ratio means that a given amount of plus add will reduce the amount of accommodative convergence considerably and thus significantly reduce the amount of the esophoria (and thus decrease the demand). The amount of plus add required to meet Sheard's criterion could theoretically be calculated by dividing the Sheard prism amount by the gradient ACA ratio, but the use of Sheard's criterion to determine add power has not been shown to be clinically effective. One of the most common ways of prescribing plus adds for nearpoint esophoria is to find the amount of plus add needed to shift the near phoria to ortho or low exo; this and other ways to determine nearpoint plus adds for esophoria at near will be discussed in more detail in chapter 11.

## EFFECTIVENESS OF SHEARD'S CRITERION
Sheard's criterion should not be viewed as an exact, mathematically derived formula, but rather as an easily applied diagnostic aid or guideline.[7] The

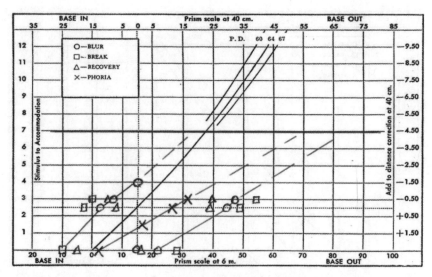

*Figure 6.2. This figure illustrates the clinical findings in the table below.*

|  | Phoria | Base-in | Base-out | Plus to blur | Minus to blur |
|---|---|---|---|---|---|
| 6 m | 2 eso | X/10/6 | 22/28/16 |  |  |
| 40 cm | 12 eso | 12/18/8 | 30/34/24 | +2.50 | -1.50 |
| 33 cm | 14 eso | 10/18/12 | 30/36/22 |  |  |
| 40 cm +1.00 D add | 12 eso |  |  |  |  |

Amplitude of accommodation, 7 D.

studies cited in the first paragraph of this chapter and clinical experience show that Sheard's criterion is a useful clinical rule of thumb. Sheedy and Saladin[4,5] found Sheard's criterion to be the best predictor of ocular symptoms overall and especially in exo deviations, but other measures were often more predictive in esophoria. Sheard's criterion often will be met in symptomatic esophoria. Saladin[8] has recommended a related guideline, the 1:1 rule, for use in esophoria.

## THE 1:1 RULE

The 1:1 rule states that the base-in recovery should be at least as great as the amount of the esophoria. The base-in recovery value can be taken from the standard prism fusional vergence ranges. Alternatively, Saladin[8] suggests that the maximum loose prism power that the patient is capable of fusing can be used as a substitute for the base-in recovery value. A formula for prism prescription with the 1:1 rule is as follows:

Base-out prism = (esophoria – base-in recovery)/2

A minus or zero value would indicate that no prism is necessary. If we apply this rule to the case depicted in Figure 6.2, we find that a base-out prism prescription of 2Δ would be recommended:

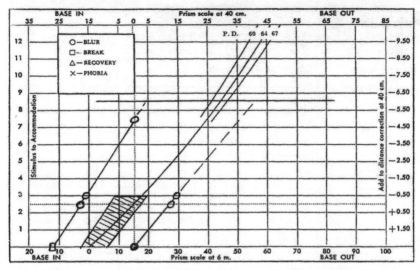

*Figure 6.3. An example of Percival's comfort zone is indicated by the cross-hatched area. Because the demand line falls within the comfort zone in this case, Percival's criterion is met with the subjective refraction lenses. The phoria line is not necessary for determining the comfort zone.*

Base-out prism = (esophoria -base-in recovery) / 2
$$= (12\Delta - 8\Delta) / 2$$
$$= 2\Delta$$

The goal of vision therapy according to the 1:1 rule would be to increase the patient's negative fusional vergence capabilities so that the base-in recovery equals or exceeds the amount of the esophoria.

## PERCIVAL'S CRITERION

Another guideline that can be used in cases of lateral imbalance is Percival's criterion.[2,9-11] Percival suggested that the positioning of the right- and left-hand boundaries of the zone of clear single binocular vision (ZCSBV) with respect to the demand line is of prime importance. Like Sheard's criterion, Percival's criterion requires separate calculations for different distances, but the criteria differ in that Percival's criterion does not take the phoria into account.

Percival defined a comfort zone, or area of comfort, that occupied the middle third of the width of the ZCSBV and extended from the zero to the 3.00D stimulus to accommodation level. The comfort zone is illustrated in Figure 6.3. Percival's criterion states that the point for a given test distance on the demand line should fall within the middle third of the ZCSBV, or, in other words, within the comfort zone. If the demand line point for a given distance between infinity and 33 cm is outside the comfort zone, Percival's criterion is not met.

The easiest way to determine whether Percival's criterion is met is to observe whether the lesser of vergence ranges (base-in or base-out) is at least half of the greater of the vergence ranges. The formula that can be used to determine the amount of prism required to meet Percivals's criterion is:
$$P = (1/3)G - (2/3)L$$

## Table 6.1.

Summary of guidelines for assessing potential strain on fusional vergence. If these conditions are not met, it is more likely that eyestrain will be present.

| Guideline Name | Guideline Application |
|---|---|
| Sheard's Criterion | In exophoria, the base-out blur (or break, if no blur reported) should be twice the amount of the exophoria.<br>In esophoria, the base-in blur (or break, if no blur reported) should be twice the amount of the esophoria. |
| 1:1 Rule | In esophoria, the base-in recovery should be at least the amount of the esophoria. |
| Percival's Criterion | When the base-in blur (or break, if no blur) is less than the base-out blur (or break, if no blur), the base-in finding should be at least half of the base-out finding.<br>When the base-out blur (or break, if no blur) is less than the base-in blur (or break, if no blur), the base-out finding should be at least half of the base-in finding. |

where P represents the prism to be prescribed, G represents the greater of the two lateral vergence range limits (base-in or base-out), and L represents the lesser of the two lateral limits (base-in or base-out). If P equals zero or a minus number, Percival's criterion is met without prism correction. To determine the minimum goal of vision training that would be required to meet Percival's criterion, the greater of the lateral limits (PRV or NRV) is divided by 2. For instance, if the base-in blur is 24 and the base-out blur is 8, then the base-out limit should be increased to at least 12 in order to allow Percival's criterion to be met.

## EXAMPLE OF THE USE OF PERCIVAL'S CRITERION

Consider the patient findings from Figure 6.2. Percival's criterion is not met at 6 m, 40 cm, or 33 cm. At 6 m, the base-in break is less than half of the base-out blur, and at both 40 cm and 33 cm, the base-in blur is less than half of the base-out blur. The amount of prism required to meet Percival's criterion at 40 cm is:

$$P = (1/3)G - (2/3)L$$
$$= (1/3)(30) - (2/3)(12)$$
$$= 2\Delta \text{ base-in}$$

For 33 cm,

$$P = (1/3)G - (2/3)L$$
$$= (1/3)(30) - (2/3)(10)$$
$$= 3.3\Delta \text{ base-in}$$

Percival's criterion could also be met at 40 cm by increasing the base-in blur to at least 15 through vision therapy and at 33 cm by increasing the base-in blur to at least 15.

## CLINICAL USAGE OF RULES OF THUMB

Sheard's criterion, the 1:1 rule, and Percival's criterion are simple guidelines or rules of thumb for evaluating strain on fusional vergence. Their main usage is a quick check of whether the stress on fusional vergence may have exceeded a threshold level likely to result in uncomfortable or inefficient vision (see Table 6.1). For example, in exophoria, we can ask: is the base-out reserve at least twice the amount of the exophoria (Sheard's criterion)? And in esophoria, we can ask: is the base-in recovery at least the amount of the esophoria (1:1 rule)?

Treatment regimens for vergence disorders include prisms, lens adds, or vision therapy. In chapters 9 and 10 we will talk about associated phoria measurements, which are generally the preferred means for deriving a prism prescription. The guidelines discussed in this chapter provide a secondary means of estimating the needed prism prescription: Sheard's criterion (particularly in exophoria) and in esophoria, the 1:1 rule.

## REFERENCES

1. Sheard C. Zones of ocular comfort. In: The Sheard Volume-Selected Writings in Visual and Ophthalmic Optics. Philadelphia: Chilton, 1957:267-285 (originally published in Am J Optom 1930;7:9-25).
2. Grosvenor T. Primary Care Optometry, 5th ed. St. Louis: Butterworth Heinemann Elsevier, 2007:259-260.
3. Hofstetter HW. The zone of clear single binocular vision. Am J Optom Arch Am Acad Optom 1945;22:361-384.
4. Sheedy JE, Saladin JJ. Phoria, vergence, and fixation disparity in oculomotor problems. Am J Optom Physiol Opt 1977;54:474-478.
5. Sheedy JE, Saladin JJ. Association of symptoms with measures of oculomotor deficiencies. Am J Optom Physiol Opt 1978;55:670-676.
6. Dalziel CC. Effect of vision training on patients who fail Sheard's criterion. Am J Optom Physiol Opt 1981;58:21-23.
7. Hofstetter HW. Objectives in optometric education. J Am Optom Assoc 1971;42:544-549.
8. Saladin JJ. Horizontal prism prescription. In: Cotter SA, ed. Clinical Uses of Prism- A Spectrum of Applications - Mosby 's Optometric Problem Solving Series. St Louis: Mosby, 1995:109-147.
9. Percival AS. The Prescribing of Spectacles, 3rd ed. Bristol, England: John Wright & Sons, 1928: 119-136.
10. Michaels DD. Visual Optics and Refraction-A Clinical Approach, 3rd ed. St Louis: Mosby, 1985:381.
11. Robertson KM. Application of Percival's criterion in correcting insignificant hyperopia in a pre-presbyope. Can J Optom 1984;46:39-40.

## OTHER SUGGESTED READING

Grisham JD. Treatment of binocular dysfunctions. In: Schor CM, Ciuffreda KJ, eds. Vergence Eye Movements: Basic and Clinical Aspects. Boston: Butterworth- Heinemann, 1983:605-646.

Sheedy JE, Saladin JJ. Validity of diagnostic criteria and case analysis in binocular vision disorders. In: Schor CM, Ciuffreda KJ, eds. Vergence Eye Movements: Basic and Clinical Aspects. Boston: Butterworth-Heinemann, 1983:517-540.

## PRACTICE PROBLEMS

For each of the following patients, answer the questions and graph your findings. Test findings were taken through the subjective refraction to best visual acuity unless otherwise noted.

1. What is the width of Percival's comfort zone at 40 cm?

2. What is the demand on fusional convergence at 40 cm?

3. What are the values for the NRV, PRV, NFV, and PFV at 40 cm?

4. What is the reserve at 40 cm?

5. Determine the calculated and gradient ACA ratio.

6. (a) Is Sheard's criterion met at distance? If not, what prism is required to meet it?
(b) Is Sheard's criterion met at 40 cm? If not, what prism is required to meet it?

7. (a) Is Percival's criterion met at distance? If not, what prism is required to meet it?
(b) Is Percival's criterion met at 40 cm? If not, what prism is required to meet it?

8. (a) Is the 1:1 rule met in the cases showing esophoria at distance? If not, what prism is required to meet? (b) Is the 1:1 rule met in the cases showing esophoria at 40 cm? If not, what prism is required to meet it?

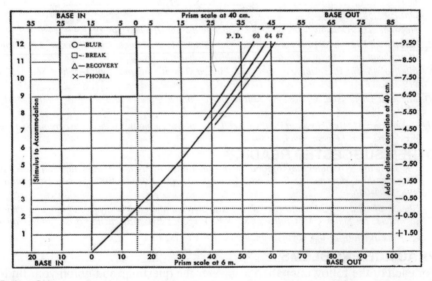

Patient GH

|  | Phoria | Base-in | Base-out | Plus to blur | Minus to blur |
|---|---|---|---|---|---|
| 6 m | 2 exo | X/10/6 | 18/22/12 |  |  |
| 40 cm | 2 exo | 14/20/12 | 24/28/20 | +2.50 | -2.00 |
| 40 cm +1.00 D add | 5 exo |  |  |  |  |

Amplitude of accommodation, 10.0 D; PD, 63 mm

Sheard's Criterion is met.

56

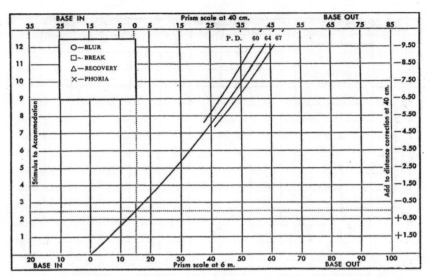

Patient JK

| | Phoria | Base-in | Base-out | Plus to blur | Minus to blur |
|---|---|---|---|---|---|
| 6 m | 4 exo | X/16/8 | 4/8/2 | | |
| 40 cm | 12 exo | 24/32/20 | 4/12/0 | +1.25 | -5.75 |
| 40 cm +1.00 D add | 14 exo | | | | |

Amplitude of accommodation, 11.0 D; PD, 64 mm.

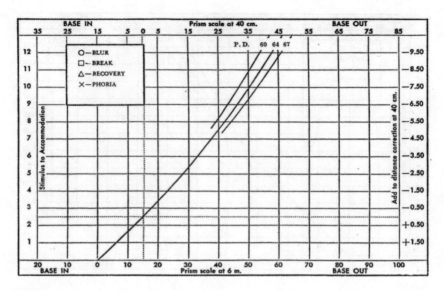

Patient RP

|  | Phoria | Base-in | Base-out | Plus to blur | Minus to blur |
|---|---|---|---|---|---|
| 6 m | Ortho | X/8/4 | 18/30/12 |  |  |
| 40 cm | 5 eso | 10/17/3 | 24/34/18 | +2.50 | -1.75 |
| 40 cm +1.00 D add | 4 exo |  |  |  |  |

Amplitude of accommodation, 9.0 D; PD, 65 mm.

58

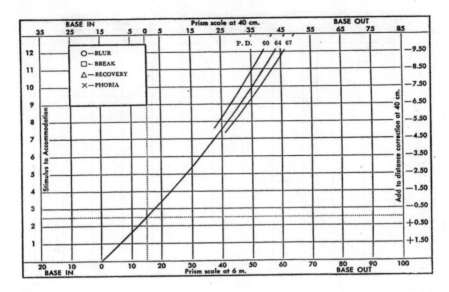

Patient LP

|  | Phoria | Base-in | Base-out | Plus to blur | Minus to blur |
|---|---|---|---|---|---|
| 6 m | 1 eso | X/8/4 | 12/21/14 |  |  |
| 40 cm | 8 exo | 20/24/8 | 8/16/-2 | +2.00 | -5.50 |
| 40 cm +1.00 D add | 10 exo |  |  |  |  |

Amplitude of accommodation, 8.0 D; PD, 62 mm.

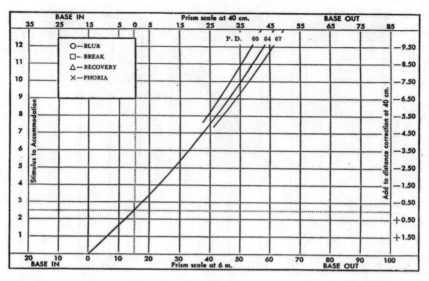

Patient MS

|  | Phoria | Base-in | Base-out | Plus to blur | Minus to blur |
|---|---|---|---|---|---|
| 6 m | 4 eso | X/8/2 | 12/22/8 | | |
| 40 cm | 6 eso | 6/14/3 | 24/32/14 | +2.25 | -1.00 |
| 40 cm +1.00 D add | 1 eso | | | | |

Amplitude of accommodation, 9.0 D; PD, 65 mm.

# Chapter 7
# Dissociated Phoria, Fusional Vergence, and Relative Accommodation Test Norms

**A**n important step in analyzing vergence and accommodation disorders is to compare individual patient findings to normal ranges. This chapter will present norms for dissociated phorias, fusional vergence ranges, and relative accommodation findings.

## MORGAN'S NORMS
The normal ranges derived by Meredith Morgan[1-5] are the most widely used values for the purpose of comparison of individual patient findings to norms. Morgan developed a set of norms from a statistical study of clinical data from a nonselected group of 800 pre-presbyopes. Although Morgan used a terminology slightly different from ours, his norms will be described with the terminology that we have developed. Morgan determined the mean and standard deviation for several findings. He arbitrarily set one-half standard deviation on either side of the mean as his normal range. The values he found are given in Table 7.1. A graph of Morgan's mean values is shown in Figure 7.1. A mental picture of this graph can be useful for comparison to the graphs of vergence disorder case types.

Besides the usefulness of Morgan's norms for assessing normalcy of test findings, we can also make a number of observations about the average test results and their variability. For example, we can find an average calculated ACA ratio

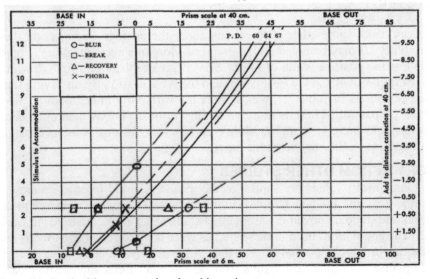

*Figure 7.1. Graph of the average values from Morgan's norms.*

using Morgan's means for distance and near phorias and assuming an average 64 mm PD:

$$\text{Calculated ACA ratio} = \frac{15 - (-1) + (-3)}{2.50} = 5.2 \ \Delta/D$$

The average calculated ACA ratio is higher than the average gradient ACA ratio of $4\Delta/D$ due to proximal convergence.

Morgan gave a normal range for the gradient ACA ratio (3 to $5\Delta/D$), but he didn't give a normal range for the calculated ACA ratio. We could compute that range using the limits of the normal ranges for phorias. The normal range for distance phorias is ortho to $2\Delta$ exo, and the normal range for near phorias is ortho to $6\Delta$ exo. So the lowest ACA ratio a patient could have and still have normal phorias would occur when the patient had a distance phoria of ortho and a near phoria of $6\Delta$ exo:

$$\text{Calculated ACA ratio} = \frac{15 - (0) + (-6)}{2.50} = 3.6 \ \Delta/D$$

And the highest calculated ACA ratio a patient could have and still have normal distance and near phorias would occur when the distance phoria is $2\Delta$ exo and the near phoria is ortho:

$$\text{Calculated ACA ratio} = \frac{15 - (-2) + (0)}{2.50} = 6.8 \ \Delta/D$$

Therefore, based on Morgan's norms, we could consider the average calculated ACA ratio to be $5.2\Delta/D$ and the normal range for calculated ACA ratios to be 3.6 to $6.8\Delta/D$.

We can make some other observations about the average findings and their variability. It may be noted on the graph of Morgan's average values (Figure 7.1) that the positive width of the ZCSBV is greater than the negative width. For example, at 40 cm the PFV is $20\Delta$ and the NFV is $10\Delta$. By observing standard deviations in Table 7.1, we can note the variability in test findings from patient to patient. There is more variability in near phorias than in distance phorias, and there is more variability on base-out fusional vergence ranges than on base-in fusional vergence ranges.

## NORMS FROM OTHER STUDIES

Morgan's mean values are similar to the means reported in other studies.[6-11] Morgan's means and standard deviations in Table 7.1 can be compared to the means and standard deviations from other studies that are summarized in Table 7.2. The populations used in these studies were from different age groups and locations in the United States. The data published by Haines[6,7] were dissociated phorias and other test results from 433 adults. Betts and Austin's data[8] were from 116 fifth grade students in Pennsylvania having a mean age of

**Table 7.1.**

Mean, standard deviation, and normal ranges for various clinical tests, as derived by Morgan.

| | Mean | Standard Deviation | Normal Range |
|---|---|---|---|
| Distance phoria | 1Δ exo | 2 | Ortho to 2 exo |
| 40 cm phoria | 3Δ exo | 5 | Ortho to 6 exo |
| Distance BI blur | X | | |
| Distance BI break | 7Δ | 3 | 5 to 9 |
| Distance BI recovery | 4Δ | 2 | 3 to 5 |
| Distance BO blur | 9Δ | 4 | 7 to 11 |
| Distance BO break | 19Δ | 8 | 15 to 23 |
| Distance BO recovery | 10Δ | 4 | 8 to 12 |
| 40 cm BI blur | 13Δ | 4 | 11 to 15, or no blur |
| 40 cm BI break | 21Δ | 4 | 19 to 23 |
| 40 cm BI recovery | 13Δ | 5 | 10 to 16 |
| 40 cm BO blur | 17Δ | 5 | 14 to 20, or no blur |
| 40 cm BO break | 21Δ | 6 | 18 to 24 |
| 40 cm BO recovery | 11Δ | 7 | 7 to 15 |
| 40 cm plus to blur  NRA | +2.00 D | 0.50 | +1.75 to +2.25 |
| 40 cm minus to blur  PRA | -2.37 D | 1.12 | -1.75 to -3.00 |
| Gradient ACA ratio | 4Δ/D | 2 | 3 to 5 |
| Amplitude of accommodation | 16.0 – (0.25)(age) | 2.00 | 16.0 - (0.25)(age) +1.00 |

11.1 years. Shepard[9] summarized test results from about 2,000 children and adults in the Chicago area. Saladin and Sheedy's data[10] were from young adult optometry students. The Jackson and Goss study[11] was done in Oklahoma with 244 school children.

The most commonly used norms are Morgan's norms. The fact that Morgan's norms are widely accepted among practitioners and that they are quite similar to the values found in other studies of various age groups suggests that they can be applied with confidence in school-age children and non-presbyopic adults.

## NORMS FOR MODIFIED THORINGTON PHORIA TEST

The values for dissociated phorias given in Table 7.2 were based on the von Graefe phoria test. The modified Thorington test is another commonly used dissociated phoria test.[12] Average values for the modified Thorington from various studies are given in Table 7.3. The means for near phoria in studies in young adults were around 2 to 3Δ exo (Table 7.1). The standard deviations are somewhat lower than the standard deviation in Morgan's norms. The means for near phorias in two studies in children were between ortho and 1Δ exo. The means for distance phorias in the two studies in children were between ortho and 1Δ eso. Average values for gradient ACA with a +1.00D

## Table 7.2.

Means (and standard deviations in parentheses) from different studies. The units for dissociated phorias and fusional vergence ranges are prism diopters and the units for the NRA and PRA are diopters.

| | Haines | Betts and Austin | Shepard | Saladin and Sheedy | Jackson and Goss |
|---|---|---|---|---|---|
| DISTANCE | | | | | |
| Phoria | 0 | 0 (2) | 1 exo (2.5) | 1 exo (3.5) | 1 exo (2) |
| BI break | 9 | 7 (3) | 9 (3) | 8 (3) | 12 (3) |
| BI recovery | 5 | 3 (2) | 4 (2) | 5 (3) | 4 (2) |
| BO blur | 9 | 7 (3) | 9 (3.5) | 15 (7) | 14 (6) |
| BO break | 22 | 21 (6) | 21 (8.5) | 28 (10) | 23 (8) |
| BO recovery | 6 | 7 (5) | 9 (4.5) | 20 (11) | 6 (5) |
| NEAR | | | | | |
| Phoria | 5 exo | 3 exo (2) | 5 exo (5) | 0.5 exo (6) | 3 exo (4) |
| BI blur | 15 | 18 (4) | 10 (3.5) | 14 (6) | 15 (6) |
| BI break | 22 | 22 (4) | 20 (5.5) | 19 (7) | 21 (4) |
| BI recovery | -- | 12 (6) | 11 (4) | 13 (6) | 9 (4) |
| BO blur | 16 | 18 (6) | 13 (5.5) | 22 (8) | 21 (8) |
| BO break | 23 | 22 (6) | 25 (11) | 30 (12) | 27 (8) |
| BO recovery | -- | 6 (7) | 13 (7.5) | 23 (11) | 10 (6) |
| NRA | -- | +2.16 (0.63) | +1.75 (0.56) | -- | +1.91 (0.54) |
| PRA | -- | -4.84 (2.34) | -2.37 (1.00) | -- | -2.14 (1.38) |

## Table 7.3.

Average values (and standard deviations in parentheses) for modified Thorington dissociated phorias from various studies.

| Study | Location | Subjects | Distance phoria mean (SD) | 40 cm phoria mean (SD) |
|---|---|---|---|---|
| Hirsch and Bing[13] | Ohio State University | 38 optometry students | -- | 3.4Δ exo (4.2) |
| Rainey et al.[14] | Indiana University | 72 optometry students | -- | 2.2Δ exo (3.1) |
| Wong et al.[15] | University of Melbourne | 72 optometry students | -- | 2.8Δ exo (3.8) |
| Lam et al.[16] | Hong Kong | 40 optometry students | -- | 2.8Δ exo |
| Jiménez et al.[17] | Spain | 1016 children, 6 to 12 yrs. old | 0.6Δ eso (1.7) | 0.4Δ exo (3.1) |
| Lyon et al.[18] | Indiana | 453 first graders and 426 fourth graders | 0Δ (2) | 1Δ exo (4) |
| Goss et al.[19] | Indiana University | 50 young adults | -- | 2.7Δ exo (4.8) |

**Table 7.4.**

Means (and standard deviations in parentheses) for prism bar vergences in various studies.

| | Wesson[22] | Scheiman et al.[23] | Scheiman et al.[23] | Jiménez et al.[17] | Lyon et al.[18] | Lyon et al.[18] |
|---|---|---|---|---|---|---|
| Location | Alabama | Philadelphia | Philadelphia | Spain | Indiana | Indiana |
| Subjects | 79 clinic patients, ages 4 to 70 yrs. | 45 children 6 yrs. old | 341 children 7 to 12 yrs. old | 1,016 children 6 to 12 yrs. old | 453 first grade children | 426 fourth grade children |
| Dist. BI break | 7 (3) | -- | -- | 6 (2) | 7 (4) | 8 (4) |
| Dist. BI recovery | 4 (2) | -- | -- | 4 (2) | 4 (3) | 5 (3) |
| Dist. BO break | 11 (7) | -- | -- | 17 (7) | 12 (7) | 12 (7) |
| Dist. BO recovery | 7 (6) | -- | -- | 11 (6) | 6 (4) | 7 (5) |
| Near BI break | 13 (6) | 12 (5) | 12 (5) | 11 (3) | 16 (7) | 13 (6) |
| Near BI recovery | 10 (5) | 6 (4) | 7 (4) | 7 (3) | 10 (5) | 9 (4) |
| Near BO break | 19 (9) | 19 (7) | 23 (8) | 18 (8) | 21 (11) | 20 (11) |
| Near BO recovery | 14 (7) | 10 (5) | 16 (6) | 13 (6) | 13 (8) | 14 (8) |

add using the modified Thorington test have ranges from 2.1 to 3.3 Δ/D in various studies.[20,21]

## NORMS FOR PRISM BAR VERGENCE RANGES

The values for vergence ranges given in Table 2 were based on phoropter rotary prism testing. Vergence ranges can also be taken using prism bars. Table 7.4 summarizes the average values for prism bar vergence ranges from various studies. A blur is recorded less often with prism bars than with rotary prisms, so blur findings are not listed in Table 7.4. If we compare the general trend of the means from these studies to Morgan's norms, we can observe that the means in Table 7.4 are fairly similar to Morgan's means for distance base-in break and recovery and for near base-out break and recovery, but less than the means from Morgan for distance base-out break and recovery and for near base-in break and recovery. The standard deviations in Table 7.4 are, for the most part, similar to the standard deviations in Tables 7.1 and 7.2, suggesting that the variability for prism bar vergence ranges is comparable to the variability in phoropter rotary prism vergence ranges.

## USE OF NORMS

Norms are used routinely to determine which test results are abnormal for a given patient. For dissociated phorias and ACA ratios we are concerned with whether they are outside the normal ranges. So any amount of esophoria at distance or near is outside Morgan's normal ranges and exophoria greater than 2Δ at distance or greater than 6Δ at near is outside Morgan's normal range. For fusional vergence ranges and relative accommodation findings, the primary concern is whether the findings are low, that is, lower than the low end of the normal range.

Part of the clinical diagnosis of vergence disorders is based on the normalcy of phorias, along with the recognition of which other test results are low. For example, a normal distance phoria and an esophoria at near suggest convergence excess. This diagnosis would be substantiated by low base-in findings at near and a low PRA. This diagnostic process will be explained in more detail in chapter 11. It is useful to have a ready familiarity with Morgan's norms for application in case analysis.

## REFERENCES

1.  Morgan MW. The clinical aspects of accommodation and convergence. Am J Optom Arch Am Acad Optom 1944;21:301-313.
2.  Morgan MW. Analysis of clinical data. Am J Optom Arch Am Acad Optom 1944;21:477-491.
3.  Morgan MW. The analysis of clinical data. Optom Weekly 1964;55(33):27-34; 55(34):23-25.
4.  Morgan MW. Accommodation and vergence. Am J Optom Arch Am Acad Optom 1968;45:417-454.
5.  Morgan MW. The Maddox analysis of vergence. In: Schor CM, Ciuffreda KJ, eds. Vergence Eye Movements: Basic and Clinical Aspects. Boston: Butterworth- Heinemann, 1983:15-21.
6.  Haines HP. Normal values of visual functions and their application in case analysis. Part IV. The analysis of findings and determination of normals. Am J Optom Arch Am Acad Optom 1941;18:58-73.
7.  Haines HP. Normal values of visual functions and their application in case analysis. Part V. Presenting a table of normal values for visual functions. Am J Optom Arch Am Acad Optom 1941;10:112-116.
8.  Betts EA, Austin AS. Seeing problems of school children. Optom Weekly 1941; 32:369-371.
9.  Shepard CF. The most probable "expecteds." Optom Weekly 1941;32:530-541.
10. Saladin JJ, Sheedy JE. Population study of fixation disparity, heterophoria, and vergence. Am J Optom Physiol Opt 1970;55:744-750.
11. Jackson TW, Goss DA. Variation and correlation of standard clinical phoropter tests of phorias, vergence ranges, and relative accommodation in a sample of school-age children. J Am Optom Assoc 1991;62:540-547.
12. Carlson NB, Kurtz D. Clinical Procedures for Ocular Examination, 3rd ed. New York: McGraw-Hill, 2004:211-213.
13. Hirsch MJ, Bing LB. The effect of testing method on values obtained for phoria at forty centimeters. Am J Optom Arch Am Acad Optom 1948;25:407-416.
14. Rainey BB, Schroeder TL, Goss DA, Grosvenor TP. Inter-examiner repeatability of heterophoria tests. Optom Vis Sci 1998;75:719-726.
15. Wong EPF, Friscke TR, Dinardo C. Interexaminer repeatability of a new, modified Prentice card compared with established phoria tests. Optom Vis Sci 2002;79:370-375.
16. Lam AKC, Lam A, Charm J, Wong K. Comparison of near heterophoria tests under varying conditions on an adult sample. Ophthal Physiol Opt 2005;25:162-167.
17. Jiménez R, Pérez MA, García JA, González MD. Statistical normal values of visual parameters that characterize binocular function in children. Ophthal Physiol Opt 2004;24:528-542.
18. Lyon DW, Goss DA, Horner DG, Downey JP, Rainey BB. Normative data for modified Thorington and step bar vergences from the Benton-IU Study. Optom 2005;76:593-599.
19. Goss DA, Reynolds JL, Todd RE. Manuscript in preparation.

20. Goss DA. *Studies on AC/A ratios determined using the modified Thorington dissociated phoria test. Indiana J Optom 2008;11:38-40.*

21. Goss DA, Moyer, BJ, Teske MC. *A comparison of dissociated phoria test findings with von Graefe phorometry and modified Thorington testing. J Behav Optom 2008;19:145-149.*

22. Wesson MD. *Normalization of prism bar vergences. Am J Optom Physiol Opt 1982;59:628-634.*

23. Scheiman M, Herzberg H, Frantz K, Margolies M. *A normative study of step vergence in elementary schoolchildren. J Am Optom Assoc 1989;60:276-280.*

## PRACTICE PROBLEMS

1. Which of the following dissociated phorias are outside the normal ranges according to Morgan's norms?
   (a) distance phoria - 1Δ exo
   (b) distance phoria - 3Δ eso
   (c) distance phoria - 4Δ exo
   (d) 40 cm phoria - 5Δ exo
   (e) 40 cm phoria - 2Δ eso
   (f) 40 cm phoria - 8Δ exo

2. Which of the following test results are low according to Morgan's norms?

|  | Patient PB | Patient RL | Patient LM | Patient LE |
|---|---|---|---|---|
| Distance base-in | X/6/3 | X/4/1 | X/7/2 | X/10/6 |
| Distance base-out | 12/20/10 | 10/22/14 | 11/17/12 | 6/12/4 |
| 40 cm base-in | 15/22/14 | 8/15/10 | 12/20/8 | 14/24/12 |
| 40 cm base-out | 6/14/2 | 20/30/17 | 15/19/10 | 12/18/2 |

3. Graph the mean values from the various studies in Table 7.2. Note how similar the form of these graphs is to the plot of Morgan's averages in Figure 7.1.

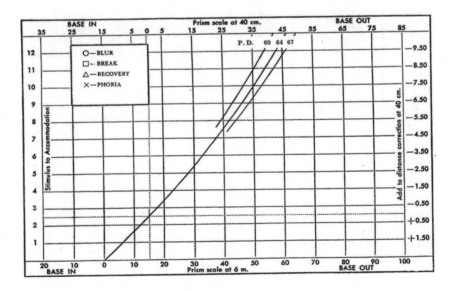

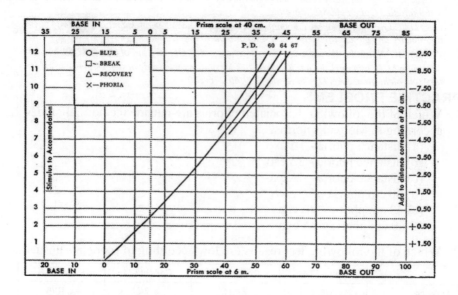

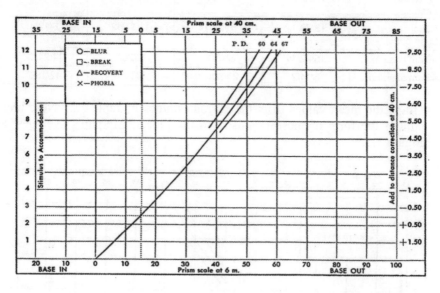

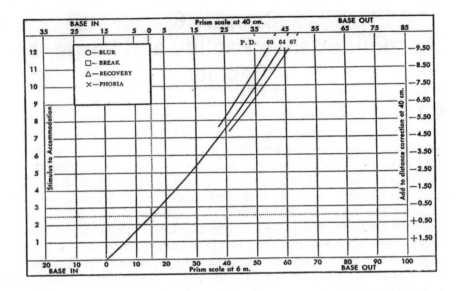

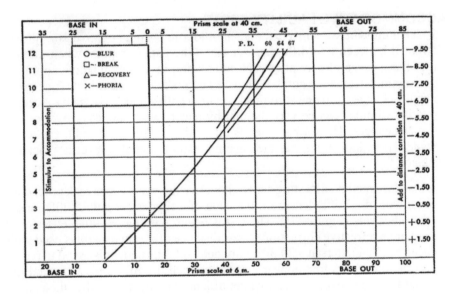

# Chapter 8
# Accommodative Facility and Vergence Facility

So far we have discussed concepts relating to the following tests: dissociated phorias, fusional vergence ranges, relative accommodation, amplitude of accommodation, and near point of convergence. Dissociated phorias provide information about vergence posture when fusion is not present. The other tests provide information about maximum accommodation and convergence levels reached under various conditions of prisms (fusional vergence ranges), lenses (relative accommodation), and changes in distance (amplitude of accommodation and near point of convergence). Note that none of these tests provide information about how quickly accommodation and convergence change. This chapter deals with accommodative facility and vergence facility tests, which provide information about the quickness of changes in accommodation and convergence.

## ACCOMMODATIVE FACILITY TESTS

For accommodative facility testing, the dioptric accommodative stimulus is alternated between two different levels.[1-4] The patient reports when a letter target first is seen clearly after each alternation in accommodative stimulus. The examiner counts the number of cycles completed in one minute (one cycle being the change from one stimulus level to the other and back again). Accommodative stimulus can be varied either by lens power changes or by viewing distance changes. The former often is referred to as *lens rock* and the latter as *distance rock*, indicating that the accommodative stimulus level is "rocked" back and forth.

The standard method of testing accommodative facility is a lens rock procedure using a pair of +2.00D lenses on one side of a flipper bar and -2.00D lenses on the other side (Figure 8.1). The test is begun with the +2.00D lenses over the patient's refractive correction. A test distance of 40 cm usually is used with reduced Snellen letters at a 20/30 acuity demand. The patient is asked to report each time the letters first appear clear after each flip of the lens bar, and the lens bar is flipped over to the other set of lenses immediately after the patient reports clarity of letters. The number of cycles per minute (cpm) is recorded. The number of cycles is the number of flips of the lens bar divided by two. In addition to determining the number of cycles, the examiner should watch the patient carefully to judge whether the patient has any greater difficulty clearing either the plus or minus side of the lens flippers.

Clinically measured lens rock accommodative facility rates correlate with objectively measured latency periods and velocities of change in accommodative response.[5,6] Children with ocular symptoms have been reported to have lower lens rock facility rates than asymptomatic children.[7]

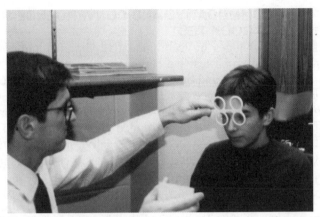

*Figure 8.1. Lens rock accommodative facility testing with a flipper bar. The patient views letters on a near point card. Each time the patient reports clarity of the letters, the lens bar is flipped to place the lenses of opposite sign in front of the patient's eyes. An accommodative facility rate in cycles per minute is recorded. One cycle is a change from plus to minus to plus. Or, in other words the number of cycles is the number of flips of the lens bar divided by two.*

Lens rock accommodative facility rates are greater if larger letters, lower power lenses, or closer test distance are used.[8] For example, on a group of 50 young adult subjects, Loerzel et al.[9] found the following mean binocular lens rock rates with different lens powers: ±1.00 D, 18.8 cpm (SD = 3.5); ±1.50 D, 15.6 cpm (SD = 3.4); ±2.00 D, 11.6 cpm (SD = 3.4). Therefore, it is important that the examiner maintain a consistent testing technique with constant letter size, lens powers, and test distance. Some clinicians have recommended using a vectographic target for binocular lens rock facility to control for suppression.[10-12]

Lens rock accommodative facility can be performed monocularly and binocularly. Binocular lens rock rates can be low without the monocular rate being low, but if the monocular rate is low, the binocular rate is usually also low. The reason for this and the diagnostic significance will be discussed later, but for the purposes of testing, the consequence is that the binocular rate is usually tested first. If the binocular rate is normal, it is not necessary to test the monocular rates because they are probably also normal. If the binocular rate is low, then the monocular rates are also tested to see if they are low as well.

On the distance rock accommodative facility test, a target with letters near the patient's best visual acuity is placed at distance and another at near. The patient is directed to alternately clear one letter on each chart as quickly as possible.[13] The examiner counts the number of alternations in viewing distance and divides by two to find the number of cycles per minute (cpm). The examiner should also watch the patient during the test to make a subjective judgment of the difficulty in changing viewing distance and of any difference in ease of shifting fixation closer or farther.

## CHANGES IN ACCOMMODATIVE AND CONVERGENCE STIMULI DURING THE LENS ROCK TEST

If we understand the changes in accommodative stimulus and convergence stimulus during the lens rock test we can see why different lens rock rates can be obtained monocularly and binocularly and why reduced binocular lens rock rates can indicate a vergence problem. For monocular testing one eye is covered. Therefore, there is no convergence stimulus. The accommodative stimulus would change as the lens bar is flipped. For example, with +2 and -2 D lenses and a 40 cm test distance the accommodative stimulus would change between 0.50 and 4.50 D. Thus the monocular lens rock is a test of accommodative facility without control of convergence.

In binocular lens rock testing we must consider convergence. We'll use testing with +2 and -2 D lenses and 40 cm target distance again as an example and we'll assume a 64 mm PD. Lenses do not affect the total convergence stimulus, so the convergence stimulus is 15Δ on both sides of the flippers. Accommodative stimulus is 0.50 D on the +2 D side of the flippers and 4.50 D on the -2 side of the flippers. Upon switch from the plus side to the minus side of the flippers, there is an increase in accommodation and a concomitant increase in accommodative convergence. To keep the total convergence constant at 15Δ, a change in fusional vergence must occur to compensate for the increase in accommodative convergence. So negative fusional vergence is used on the minus side of the flippers to keep the total amount of convergence constant.

In response to the switch to the plus side of the flippers there is a decrease in accommodation. Again due to the synkinesis of accommodation and convergence, a decrease in accommodative convergence occurs with the decrease in accommodation. To keep the total amount of convergence constant, positive fusional vergence occurs in an amount equal to the magnitude of the decrease in accommodative convergence.

Another way to look at this is that the minus side of the flippers would cause a shift in the dissociated phoria toward esophoria, so negative fusional vergence must be used to maintain fusion on the binocular lens rock. On the plus side of the flippers there would be a shift in the dissociated phoria toward exophoria, so positive fusional vergence must occur to maintain fusion. Therefore, patients with esophoria through their refractive corrections will be made more eso on the minus side of the flippers and they will be slower on the minus side of the binocular lens rock. Similarly, patients with exophoria before the start of the lens rock are likely to be slow on the plus side of the binocular lens rock.

## NORMS FOR ACCOMMODATIVE FACILITY TESTING

Mean lens rock rates reported in different studies show quite a bit of variability.[7,14-18] This can be seen in the summary of study results in Table 8.1. Cut-offs for test failure used by many clinicians using +2.00D/-2.00D flippers and a 40 cm viewing distance for patients from about 10 to 30 years of age are less than 11 or 12 cycles per minute for monocular testing and less than 8 to 10 cycles per minute for binocular testing.[1,3,7,16,19-21]

## Table 8.1.
Results of studies of lens rock accommodative facility rates with ±2.00 D flippers, 20/30 letters at 40 cm, and a one minute testing period.

| Authors | Number of subjects | Ages of subjects in years | Mean rates in cpm (standard deviation in parentheses) |
|---|---|---|---|
| Burge (1979)[11] | 30 | 6 to 30 | With polarizers, OU, 14.1 (8.5)<br>Without polarizers, OU, 18.9 (8.4) |
| Zellers et al. (1984)[15] | 100 | 18 to 30 | OD, 11.6 (5.0)<br>OS, 11.1 (5.3)<br>OU, 7.7 (5.2) |
| Hennessey et al. (1984)[7] | 50 | 8 to 14 | Symptomatic, OD, 8.6 (5.5)<br>Symptomatic, OS, 9.2 (6.5)<br>Symptomatic, OU, 4.0 (6.0)<br>Asymptomatic, OD, 11.8 (6.4)<br>Asymptomatic, OS, 12.8 (7.2)<br>Asymptomatic, OU, 7.8 (8.0) |
| Loerzel et al. (2003)[9] | 50 | 21 to 35 | OU, 11.6 (3.4) |

## Table 8.2.
Mean (and standard deviation in parentheses) ±2.00 D lens rock accommodative facility rates in cycles per minute for each of the diagnostic groups in the García et al.[22] study.

|  | Right Eye | Left Eye | Binocular |
|---|---|---|---|
| Accommodative dysfunction (n=13) | 5.7 (3.0) | 5.6 (2.9) | 7.5 (3.2) |
| Binocular dysfunction (n=11) | 12.6 (4.2) | 12.7 (3.6) | 5.2 (3.8) |
| Accommodative and binocular dysfunctions (n=12) | 8.9 (5.0) | 8.3 (4.6) | 7.1 (4.1) |
| Normal accommodation and binocularity (n=12) | 13.4 (2.2) | 13.0 (2.3) | 13.1 (2.5) |

Accommodative facility testing is associated with strong practice effects.[19,21] These practice effects can be seen on monocular lens rock rates if monocular testing is always done right eye before the left. For example, one study found a mean rate of 9.8 cpm for the right eye and 11.5 cpm for the left eye.[18] Because of this practice effect, it is possible that some patients may initially have a failing lens rock rate, but show improvement on repeated testing. Rouse et al.[21] recommended that if a failing rate is found in a one minute testing period, testing should be repeated for a second and a third minute. They suggested that test failure would be indicated if the rates remain below the cut-off for test failure in the second and third minutes of testing or if they decline over the second and third minutes of testing.

Patients with vergence disorders can have reduced binocular lens rock accommodative facility rates but normal monocular lens rock rates. This is illustrated by the results of a study by García et al.[22] They tested 48 subjects between the ages of 10 and 30 years with ±2.00 D flippers and a 40 cm testing distance. They also performed a complete accommodation and convergence diagnostic work-up to classify the patient as having an accommodative dysfunction, a

## Table 8.3.

Test distances and lens powers for the amplitude-scaled lens rock accommodative facility test recommended by Wick et al.[28] Patients who have rates less than 10 cpm with these testing parameters are likely to be symptomatic.

| Amplitude of accommodation (D) | Test distance (cm) | Lens flipper powers (D) |
|---|---|---|
| 22.25 | 10.0 | ±3.25 |
| 20.00 | 11.0 | ±3.00 |
| 18.25 | 12.0 | ±2.75 |
| 16.75 | 13.5 | ±2.50 |
| 15.50 | 14.5 | ±2.25 |
| 14.25 | 15.5 | ±2.25 |
| 13.25 | 16.5 | ±2.00 |
| 12.50 | 18.0 | ±2.00 |
| 11.75 | 19.0 | ±1.75 |
| 11.00 | 20.0 | ±1.75 |
| 10.50 | 21.0 | ±1.50 |
| 10.00 | 22.0 | ±1.50 |
| 9.50 | 23.5 | ±1.50 |
| 9.00 | 24.5 | ±1.50 |
| 8.75 | 25.5 | ±1.25 |
| 8.25 | 26.5 | ±1.25 |
| 8.00 | 28.0 | ±1.25 |
| 7.75 | 29.0 | ±1.25 |
| 7.50 | 30.0 | ±1.00 |
| 7.25 | 31.0 | ±1.00 |
| 7.00 | 32.0 | ±1.00 |
| 6.75 | 33.5 | ±1.00 |
| 6.50 | 34.0 | ±1.00 |
| 6.25 | 35.5 | ±1.00 |
| 6.00 | 37.0 | ±1.00 |
| 5.75 | 38.5 | ±1.00 |
| 5.50 | 40.5 | ±0.75 |
| 5.25 | 42.5 | ±0.75 |
| 5.00 | 44.5 | ±0.75 |
| 4.75 | 47.0 | ±0.75 |
| 4.50 | 49.5 | ±0.75 |

binocular dysfunction, both accommodative and binocular dysfunctions, or normal accommodation and binocularity. The mean lens rock facility rates for the subjects in each of these four classifications are given in Table 8.2. It may be noted that in the subjects with accommodative dysfunctions the rates are lower than the normal group both monocularly and binocularly. For the binocular dysfunction group, the binocular rate is lower than in the normal group, but the monocular rates in the binocular dysfunction group are quite close to the monocular rates in the normal group.

The García et al. study is also significant in that its data can provide a means of assessing cut-off levels for normalcy on lens rock facility. An analysis of their data found that sensitivity and specificity for a diagnosis of accommodative and/or binocular dysfunction were maximized when monocular rates were less than 11 cpm, binocular rates were less than 10 cpm, and the difference of monocular rate minus binocular rate was greater than 4 cpm.[23,24] With those cut-off levels the sensitivity and the specificity were both 91.7%. Of course, this was only one study sample of only 48 subjects; however, these monocular and binocular rate cut-offs for normalcy are close to those recommended by other sources.[1,3,7,15,19,25] So until additional study suggests otherwise, it appears reasonable to use norms of monocular 11 cpm or greater, binocular 10 or greater, monocular minus binocular 4 or less for ±2.00 D flippers with a 40 cm test distance for 10 to 30 year olds.

Some clinicians question the use of lens rock testing in children younger than about ten years of age due to the subjective nature of the test and developmental limitations in the automaticity of digit naming. Scheiman et al.[17] found an increase in lens rock rates from six years of age up to nine years of age and then fairly similar rates from 9 to 12 years. Kedzia et al.[26] suggested that the effects of time to name digits could be factored out by doing one trial with plano lenses on both sides of a flipper and then with the ±2.00 D lenses. They also developed a mechanical system for changing the lens powers in order to eliminate any effect of variability in the time it takes to handle the flipper bar.

The applicability of lens rock testing for adults over about 30 years of age may also be questioned due to the normal reduction in amplitude of accommodation with age. Siderov and DiGuglielmo[27] failed to find a significant difference in lens rock rates between symptomatic and asymptomatic 30 to 42 year old adults. To obviate difficulties relating to the amplitude of accommodation, Yothers, Wick, and colleagues[28,29] have proposed and tested an amplitude-scaled lens rock test. Preliminary testing with a group of 19 subjects suggested that the strongest association of symptoms with test results could be obtained when the test distance was such that its dioptric value was 45% of the amplitude of accommodation and the total power change on the lens flippers was 30% of the amplitude of accommodation. So for an amplitude of accommodation of 10.0 D, the test distance would be 22 cm (100/4.5 D) and the lens flipper powers would be ±1.50 D.[28] They then tested a group of 152 children, ages 6 to 16 years, and a group of 98 adults, ages 23 to 37 years, on binocular lens rock using the test distances and lens powers suggested by the amplitude-scaled values. The differences in binocular lens rock rates between symptomatic and asymptomatic children were 3.7 cpm on the amplitude-scaled test (p = 0.0004) and 2.8 cpm (p = 0.0055) on standard ±2.00 D testing at 40 cm. The differences in binocular lens rock rates between symptomatic and asymptomatic adult subjects were 4.1 cpm on the amplitude-scaled test (p = 0.0228) and 2.1 cpm (not statistically significant) on standard ±2.00 D testing at 40 cm. Table 8.3 gives the test distances and lens powers recommended for this

## Table 8.4.

Results of studies of distance rock accommodative facility rates

| Authors | Subjects | Test conditions | Mean rates in cpm (standard deviation in parentheses) |
|---------|----------|-----------------|-------------------------------------------------------|
| Haynes[13] | N = 11; 23 to 37 yrs. old | 20/25 letters, 5 minutes of arc letter separation | 26 (5) |
| Haynes [13] | N = 591 | 20/80 and 20/25 letters, 6 m and 40 cm | First graders, 14 (4) <br> Second graders, 17 (5) <br> Third graders, 19 (5) <br> Fourth graders, 22 (5) <br> Fifth graders, 24 (5) <br> Sixth graders, 26 (6) |
| Jackson and Goss[18] | N = 244; 7.9 to 15.9 yrs. old | 20/20 letters, 4 m and habitual reading distance | OD, 18.9 <br> OS, 19.9 <br> OU, 20.9 |
| Miller et al.[30] | N= 50; 21 to 36 yrs. old | 20/20 letters, 6 m and 40 cm | OD, 21.0 (4.9) <br> OS, 22.3 (4.9) <br> OU, 24.1 (4.8) |

amplitude-scaled test. Patients with rates less than 10 cpm with the indicated testing parameters are more likely to be symptomatic.[29]

Norms have not been established for the distance rock test. Studying 11 young adult subjects, Haynes[13] reported that letter size and letter separation had significant effects on distance rock rates, with higher rates found when using larger letter sizes and larger letter separations. The mean rate for 23 to 37 years old subjects was 26 cpm (SD = 5) for 20/25 letters and a letter separation of five minutes of arc. Monocular and binocular rates were combined in the computation of that mean; Haynes noted that binocular rates were slightly higher than monocular rates. Haynes[13] also discussed the results of a study of distance rock rates with 591 elementary school children. On both the distance (6 m) and near (40 cm) chart there were two horizontal rows of letters, one 20/80 row and one 20/25 row. After reading the 20/80 letters, the subjects read the 20/25 letters. Mean rates increased from 14 cpm for first graders to 26 cpm for sixth graders (Table 8.4).

Binocular distance rock rates are higher than monocular distance rock rates[18] (see Table 8.4). Distance rock rates are higher than lens rock rates. For a group of 244 school children, Jackson and Goss[18] found the mean rate on binocular ±2.00 D lens rock to be 8.9 cpm and the mean binocular distance rock rate to be 20.9 cpm. Even when the powers of the lenses used on the lens rock test are changed to give the same change in accommodative stimulus as on the distance rock test, the distance rock rates are greater than the lens rock rates.[30] The primary reason for higher rates on distance rock than on lens rock may the fact there are both proximity and blur cues for accommodation on the distance rock test, but only blur cues for accommodation on the lens rock test.[30]

Additional research will be necessary to establish normative values for distance rock accommodative facility rates. The results of four studies with published distance rock rates are summarized in Table 8.4. Rutstein and Daum[3] recommend making a qualitative judgment of whether the distance rock facility is good, fair, or poor based on clinical experience.

## VERGENCE FACILITY

Vergence facility tests are tests which evaluate the quickness of fusional vergence. Grisham[31] found that fusional vergence latencies were greater and fusional vergence velocities were less in subjects who had abnormal vergence and phoria findings based on Morgan's norms compared with subjects who had normal findings. Grisham[32] recommended an objective test in which the clinician observes the latency and velocity of a fusional vergence eye movement. A 6Δ base-out prism is introduced in front of one eye while the patient views a target at approximately 40 cm. The clinician carefully watches the eye without the prism, and subjectively evaluates the latency and velocity of the fusional vergence response. Grisham emphasized that experience with the technique is necessary to discern whether the response is slow, moderate, or fast.

Vergence facility testing is more commonly done subjectively with prism flippers.[33] The prism flippers are like the lens flippers used for accommodative facility, and like accommodative facility, vergence facility rates are recorded in cycles per minute (cpm). Buzzelli[34] tested 310 schoolchildren using 4Δ base-in/16Δ base-out flippers while they viewed an anaglyphic target at 40 cm. Test performance improved with age. For example, 5-year-olds had a mean of 7.6 cpm (SD = 1.2) and 12-year-olds had a mean of 13.0 cpm (SD = 1.2). Delgadillo and Griffin[35] tested 26 nonpresbyopic optometry students with 8Δ base-in/8Δ base-out and 5Δ base-in/15Δ base-out flippers using a vectographic target at 40 cm. Mean values were presented for both tests and for different testing sequences. The mean values were similar for the two tests, ranging from 11.3 to 14.1 cpm (SD = 4.0 to 5.7). Three unpublished studies with 8Δ BI/8Δ BO flippers found mean rates of 8.1 cpm in young adults, 6.5, 6.7, and 10.2 cpm in twelve to thirteen year olds, and 5.0 and 6.3 cpm in 9 to 12 year olds.[36]

Gall et al.[37] found that similar rates were obtained with an anaglyphic target and targets which did not have binocular suppression cues. They suggested that suppression could be monitored by lateral movement of the target. In another paper, Gall et al.[36] tested young adult subjects on sixteen combinations of prism powers ranging from 0 to 9Δ on the base-in side and 0 to 18Δ on the base-out side, and with total change in prism power ranging from 9 to 18Δ switching from one side of the flipper bar to the other for distance testing. For near testing, there were also sixteen combinations of prism powers, with the near prism powers ranging from 3 to 12Δ on the base-in side and from 3 to 27Δ on the base-out side, and with total change in prism power ranging from 15 to 30Δ switching from one side of the flipper bar to the other They found that 3Δ BI/12Δ BO best differentiated between symptomatic and asymptomatic subjects on testing at both 4 m and 40 cm. As would be expected, the rates decreased as the total power change from one side of the flippers to the other increased.

The clinical utility of vergence facility was shown in a study by Gall and Wick.[38] Eighteen of 30 young adult subjects who had asthenopic symptoms but normal dissociated phorias were found to have reduced vergence facility at distance and/or at near when tested with $3\Delta$ BI/$12\Delta$ BO prism flippers. With clinical failure criteria of 8 cpm at distance and 12 cpm at near, three subjects had failing vergence facility rates at distance only, eight had failing vergence facility rates at near only, and seven had failing rates at both distance and near. Mean near vergence facility rates were 16.1 cpm (SD = 3.5) in the asymptomatic subjects and 12.3 cpm (SD = 5.5) in the symptomatic subjects. The results of this study suggest that vergence facility should be tested when symptoms appear to be consistent with a vergence problem but dissociated phorias are normal.

In their 1998 study, Gall et al.[36] recommended a clinical failure criterion of 15 cpm for near vergence facility with $3\Delta$ BI/$12\Delta$ BO flippers, but the results of their latter study[38] suggest a failing rate of 12 cpm. Those studies were done with young adults. Somewhat lower rates would be expected for children. As with accommodative facility testing, the examiner should observe the patient during vergence facility testing to make a subjective assessment of difficulty for the patient and note whether that difficulty is more pronounced on the base-in or base-out side of the flippers.

## REFERENCES

1. Daum KM. Accommodative facility. In: Eskridge JB, Amos JF, Bartlett JD, eds. Clinical Procedures in Optometry. Philadelphia: Lippincott, 1991:687-697.

2. Goss DA. Clinical accommodation testing. Curr Opin Ophthalmol 1992;3:78-82.

3. Rutstein RP, Daum KM. Anomalies of Binocular Vision: Diagnosis & Management. St. Louis: Mosby, 1998:63-65.

4. Wick B, Yothers TL, Jiang B-C, Morse SE. Clinical testing of accommodative facility: Part I: A critical appraisal of the literature. Optom 2002;73:11-23.

5. Liu JS, Lee M, Jang J, Ciuffreda KJ, Wong JH, Grisham D, Stark L. Objective assessment of accommodation orthoptics. I. Dynamic insufficiency. Am J Optom Physiol Opt 1979;56:285-294.

6. Bobier WR, Sivak JG. Orthoptic treatment of subjects showing slow accommodative responses. Am J Optom Physiol Opt 1983;60:678-687.

7. Hennessey D, Iosue RA, Rouse MW. Relation of symptoms to accommodative infacility of school-aged children. Am J Optom Physiol Opt 1984;61:177-183.

8. Siderov J, Johnston AW. The importance of the test parameters in the clinical assessment of accommodative facility. Optom Vis Sci 1990;67:551-557.

9. Loerzel R, Tran L, Goss DA. Effect of lens power on binocular lens flipper accommodative facility rates. J Behav Optom 2003;14:7-9.

10. Pierce JR, Greenspan SB. Accommodative rock procedures in VT-a clinical guide. Part II. Optom Weekly 1971;62:776-780.

11. Burge S. Suppression during binocular accommodative rock. Optom Monthly 1979;79:867-872.

12. Scheiman M, Wick B. Clinical Management of Binocular Vision: Heterophoric, Accommodative, and Eye Movement Disorders, 2nd ed. Philadelphia: Lippincott, Williams & Wilkins, 2002:21-24.

13. Haynes HM. The distance rock test-a preliminary report. J Am Optom Assoc 1979;50:707-713.

14. Garzia P, Richman J. Accommodative facility: a study of young adults. J Am Optom Assoc 1982;53:821-825.

15. Zellers JA, Albert TL, Rouse MW. A review of the literature and a normative study of accommodative facility. J Am Optom Assoc 1984;55:31-37.

16. Levine S, Ciuffreda KJ, Selenow A, Flax N. Clinical assessment of accommodative facility in symptomatic and asymptomatic individuals. J Am Optom Assoc 1985;56:286-290.

17. Scheiman M, Herberg H, Frantz K, Margolies M. Normative study of accommodative facility in elementary schoolchildren. Am J Optom Physiol Opt 1988;65: 127-134.

18. Jackson TW, Goss DA. Variation and correlation of clinical tests of accommodative function in a sample of school-age children. J Am Optom Assoc 1991;62:857-866.

19. McKenzie KM, Kerr SR, Rouse MW, DeLand PN. Study of accommodative facility testing reliability. Am J Optom Physiol Opt 1987;64:186-194.

20. Rouse MW, DeLand PN, Chous R, Determan TF. Monocular accommodative facility testing reliability. Optom Vis Sci 1989;66:72-77.

21. Rouse MW, DeLand PN, Mozayani S, Smith JP. Binocular accommodative facility testing reliability. Optom Vis Sci 1992;69:314-319.

22. García A, Cacho P, Lara F, Megías R. The relation between accommodative facility and general binocular dysfunction. Ophthal Physiol Opt 2000;20:98-104.

23. Goss DA. The relation between accommodative facility and general binocular dysfunction. Ophthal Physiol Opt 2001;21:484-485.

24. Goss DA. Accommodative facility as an indicator of accommodative and binocular dysfunctions. Indiana J Optom 2001;4:36-39.

25. Cooper J. Accommodative dysfunction. In: Amos JF, ed. Diagnosis and Management in Vision Care. Boston: Butterworth, 1987:431-459.

26. Kędzia B, Pieczyrak D, Tondel G, Maples WC. Factors affecting the clinical testing of accommodative facility. Ophthal Physiol Opt 1999;19:12-21.

27. Siderov J, DiGuglielmo L. Binocular accommodative prepresbyopic adults and its relation to symptoms. Optom Vis Sci 1991;68:49-53.

28. Yothers T, Wick B, Morse SE. Clinical testing of accommodative facility: Part II: Development of an amplitude-scaled test. Optom 2002;73:91-102.

29. Wick B, Gall R, Yothers T. Clinical testing of accommodative facility: Part III: Masked assessment of the relation between visual symptoms and binocular test results in school children and adults. Optom 2002;73:173-181.

30. Miller KL, York RT, Goss DA. Importance of proximity cues on the distance rock accommodative facility test. J Behav Optom 1996;7:93-96.

31. Grisham JD. The dynamics of fusional vergence eye movements in binocular dysfunction. Am J Optom Physiol Opt. 1980;57:645-655.

32. Grisham JD. Treatment of binocular dysfunctions. In: Schor CM, Ciuffreda KJ, eds. Vergence Eye Movements: Basic and Clinical Aspects. Boston, MA: Butterworth- Heinemann; 1983:605-646.

33. Daum KM. Vergence facility. In: Eskridge JB, Amos JF, Bartlett JD, eds. Clinical Procedures in Optometry. Philadelphia: Lippincott, 1991:671-676.

34. Buzzelli AR. Vergence facility: developmental trends in a school age population. Am J Optom Physiol Opt 1986;63:351-355.

35. Delgadillo HM, Griffin JR. Vergence facility and associated symptoms: a comparison of two prism flipper tests. J Behav Optom 1992;3:91-94.

36. Gall R, Wick B, Bedell H. Vergence facility: establishing clinical utility. Optom Vis Sci 1998;75:731-742.

37. Gall R, Wick B, Bedell H. Vergence facility and target type. Optom Vis Sci 1998;75:727-730.

38. Gall R, Wick B. The symptomatic patient with normal phorias at distance and near: what tests detect a binocular vision problem? Optom 2003;74:309-322.

## PRACTICE PROBLEMS

1. In each of the following cases, indicate whether the +2.00 D lens rock test results suggest normal accommodative facility, an accommodative disorder, or a vergence disorder:
Patient MR: 14 cpm OD, 15 cpm OS, 12 cpm OU

Patient LG: 7 cpm OD, 7 cpm OS, 5 cpm OU
Patient TB: 12 cpm OD, 14 cpm OS, 7 cpm OU

2. Using the amplitude-scaled lens rock test, what test distances and lens powers would be used for patients with amplitudes of accommodation equal to 7.0 D?, 8.0 D ?, 9.0 D? And what would the test failure criterion rates be in each case?

# Chapter 9
## Introduction to Fixation Disparity

**F**ixation disparity is a condition in which the images of a binocularly fixated object do not stimulate exactly corresponding retinal points but still fall within Panum's fusional areas, the object thus being seen singly.[1] In other words, fixation disparity is present when the lines of sight of the two eyes do not line up exactly with the object of regard under binocular conditions, but the amount of misalignment is not large enough to result in diplopia. The existence of fixation disparity indicates that there can be a slight overconvergence (eso fixation disparity) or underconvergence (exo fixation disparity) of the lines of sight under binocular conditions. This misalignment is very small, because sensory fusion would not otherwise be possible. Fixation disparity usually is measured in minutes of arc. If it were expressed in prism diopters, it usually would be less than $0.25\Delta$ and almost always would be less than $0.75\Delta$.[2] (Ten minutes of arc, which is fairly large amount of fixation disparity, is equivalent to about $0.29\Delta$)

Fixation disparity usually is measured by subjective alignment of two small lines or bars, one seen by each eye. Other than the marks used for alignment, all features of the test target are seen binocularly. The amount of fixation disparity is the sum of the angular eccentricities of the subjectively aligned marks with respect to the convergence stimulus of the binocularly fused components of the test target (Figure 9.1). Examples of devices that can be used to measure fixation disparity are the Wesson Fixation Disparity Card,[3] the Sheedy Disparometer,[4] and the Saladin card.[5] For example, in the Disparometer and in the Saladin card, there are several pairs of marks with different preset separations; the patient is asked to pick the pair of marks which appear to be aligned. For illustration, a schematic of the Disparometer is shown in Figure 9.2.

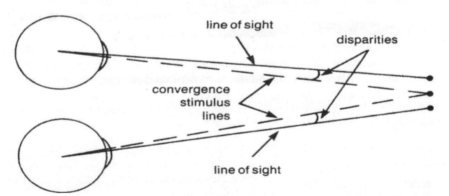

*Figure 9.1. Exo fixation disparity. The angle of disparity is the sum of the angular disparities of the two eyes. If one eye is fixating precisely, all of the disparity will be represented in the angular deviation of the other eye.*

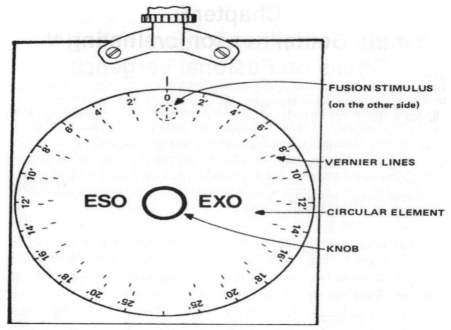

*Figure 9.2. A schematic diagram of the Sheedy Disparometer. The illustrated pairs of marks are shown to the patient one at a time in the circular window until a pair that subjectively appears aligned is chosen. The examiner can then read the actual physical separation of the lines from a window at the back of the instrument. The physical separation of the pair of lines that appears perfectly aligned is a measure of the fixation disparity. (Reprinted with permission from Sheedy JE. Fixation disparity analysis of oculomotor imbalance. Am J Optom Physiol Opt 1980;57:632-639.)*

The amount of fixation disparity measured is a function of individual characteristics of patients and testing conditions. Of the latter, the most important features are (1) the size of the area in which binocular vision is excluded, (2) the amount of fusional vergence required, and (3) if the patient is viewing through prisms, the length of time allowed for adaptation to the prisms before the fixation disparity is measured.[6-9] The larger the area without fusion clues, the greater the fixation disparity. As the amount of positive fusional vergence increases, fixation disparity shifts in the exo direction. This indicates an increasing underconvergence as the amount of convergence increases. As the amount of negative fusional vergence required for single vision increases, fixation disparity becomes more eso. Therefore, as base-in or base-out prism power is increased, fixation disparity becomes more eso or exo, respectively. As the time allowed for adaptation to the prism is increased, fixation disparity decreases.

Stress associated with the use of fusional vergence can result in asthenopia. Clinical fixation disparity measurement is a useful diagnostic tool because it is related to fusional convergence effort.[8-10] This is easily demonstrated by the observation that fixation disparity varies as a function of the prism power through which a patient views. In addition, there is a correlation of fixation disparity with dissociated phoria[11-13] (Figure 9.3).

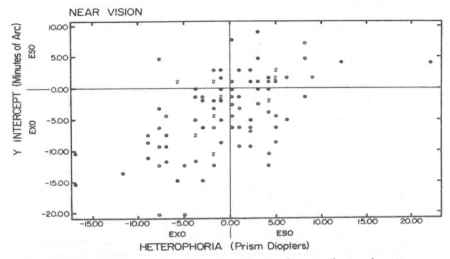

NEAR VISION

Y INTERCEPT (Minutes of Arc)

*Figure 9.3. Scatterplot showing the relationship of fixation disparity (fixation disparity curve y-intercept) with dissociated phoria. Fixation disparity in minutes of arc is plotted on the y-axis, and dissociated phoria in prism diopters is plotted on the x-axis. Each point represents findings for one individual. (Reprinted with permission from Saladin JJ, Sheedy JE. Population study of fixation disparity, heterophoria,and vergence. Am J Optom Physiol Opt 1978;55:744-750.)*

## ASSOCIATED PHORIA

Many of the clinical fixation disparity devices cannot actually measure fixation disparity; instead they detect the presence of a fixation disparity and allow the examiner to determine the prism power that reduces fixation disparity to zero. These instruments are characterized by the monocularly viewed marks being physically aligned as opposed to the varying amounts of separation in devices that allow measurement of fixation disparity. A fixation disparity exists when the patient reports that the marks or bars are not perfectly aligned perceptually. Lateral fixation disparity is zero if the patient says that the top line is directly above the bottom line. In most of these instruments, the top vertical bar is seen by the right eye and the bottom is seen by the left eye. Thus, if the patient reports the top line being to the right of the bottom line, an eso fixation disparity exists; if the top line is to the left of the bottom one, an exo fixation disparity exists. The amount of base-in prism required to reduce an exo disparity to zero or the amount of base-out prism required to reduce an eso fixation disparity to zero is referred to as the *associated phoria.*

To avoid confusion, we should distinguish between dissociated and associated phorias. Prior to this chapter, we were examining dissociated phorias. "Dissociated" refers to the fact that the eyes are dissociated; that is, binocular vision is not allowed in any part of the visual field, except, perhaps unavoidably, in the extreme peripheral portions of it. On an associated phoria measurement, binocular vision is present throughout the visual field except for a small area surrounding the two monocularly viewed testing marks. Dissociated phorias and associated phorias also differ in that dissociated phorias measure the angular misalignment of the lines of sight from the object of regard under

Most common to least: Type I > Type II > Type III, Type IV

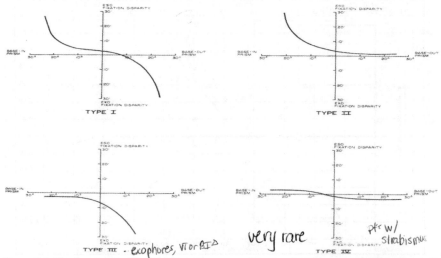

TYPE I

TYPE II

TYPE III - exophores, VI or RID          very rare          TYPE IV          pts w/ strabismus

Figure 9.4. The four types of fixation disparity curves. (Reprinted with permission from Sheedy JE. Fixation disparity analysis of coulmotor imbalance. Am J Optom Physiol Opt 1980;57:632-639.)

unfused conditions, but associated phorias do not measure binocular angular misalignment. Instead, associated phorias measure the amount of prism needed to eliminate the binocular misalignment. For these reasons, some practitioners prefer the term aligning prism over the term associated phoria.[14]

Usually, the amount of an associated phoria is less than the corresponding dissociated phoria in a given individual. Associated phorias and dissociated phorias are correlated, but some individuals yield prism values with opposite prism base orientations on the two tests. This occurrence, referred to as *paradoxical fixation disparity*, is most commonly found in patients who have received orthoptics to increase fusional vergence amplitudes. The typical paradoxical fixation disparity patient shows an exo dissociated phoria with an eso fixation disparity.[9,15]

## THE FIXATION DISPARITY CURVE AND ITS PARAMETERS

A fixation disparity curve (FDC) is a plot of the amount of fixation disparity (y-axis) obtained through various amounts of prism (x-axis). The curves for different patients vary in their configuration, slope, vertical placement, and lateral placement. Their configurations are divided into four categories, called *curve types* (Figure 9.4). The most common classification of curve types is the one described by Ogle et al.[11] Type I has a sigmoid curve shape with a steep rise in fixation disparity near both the base-in and base-out fusional limits. Approximately 60% of individuals have type I curves. Type II and type III curves have flat segments on the base-out and base-in sides, respectively. The prevalence of these types of curves is approximately 25% for Type II and 10% for type III.[16]

The configuration of FDCs is related to *prism adaptation*. Prism adaptation also is known as *vergence adaptation* or *fusional aftereffects*.[9,17-20] Prism

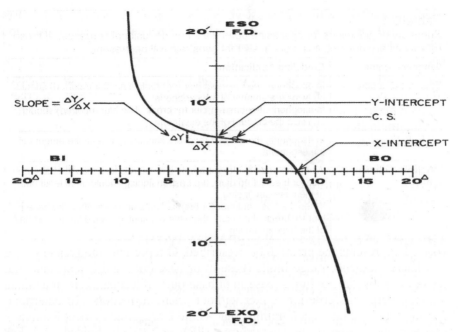

*Figure 9.5. Fixation disparity curve (FDC) parameters in a type I curve. Besides curve type, the FDC parameters are slope, y-intercept, x-intercept, and center of symmetry (CS).*

adaptation is thought to be a shift in the tonic vergence level after the use of fusional vergence. One way that it is demonstrated is to measure dissociated phorias before and after viewing through prism for some period of time. Viewing through base-out prism results in a shift of the phoria toward eso, and viewing through base-in will cause the phoria to shift in the exo direction. Prism adaptation varies from one patient to another. Schor[9,15] has found that prism adaptation and fixation disparity are inversely related and that persons with type II or III curves have asymmetric prism adaptation for convergent and divergent stimuli. Cases of greater base-out prism adaptation correspond to type II curves, and cases of greater base-in prism adaptation are found with type III curves.

The type IV curve shows changes in fixation disparity with prism in the central portion of the curve and little or no change toward the fusional limits on both sides. The prevalence of type IV curves is approximately 5%.[16] A type IV curve may indicate a deficiency of sensory and/or motor fusion.[8,9]

Other important parameters of an FDC are its slope, y-intercept, x- intercept, and center of symmetry. The *slope* is commonly derived using a best-fitting straight line through points in a range of approximately 3Δ base-in to 3Δ base-out.[13,21] The *y-intercept* is the amount of fixation disparity with zero prism. The *x-intercept* is the amount of prism that yields fixation disparity equal to zero. The *center of symmetry* is the flattest central region of the FDC. In other words, the center of symmetry is the point on the curve where the slope is closest to zero. The center of symmetry is theoretically the prism at which patients have their greatest vergence adaptation. Some optometrists suggest that the concept of the center of symmetry can be used to prescribe prism. The center of symmetry can be derived mathematically. For clinical purposes, the segment of the FDC which has the least slope can be used to derive a prism prescription. The point on the flattest segment of the curve where the prism power is the least would be used to give the amount of prism. A prism prescription based on the minimum prism value on the x-axis within the minimum slope segment of the FDC would put patients into their range of maximal vergence adaptation.

The parameters of an FDC are illustrated in Figure 9.5. The ends of the curves generally correspond to points of diplopia, and thus the x-axis values at the ends of the curves should be similar to the negative relative vergence and positive relative vergence findings.

## THE CHANGE IN FIXATION DISPARITY WITH LENSES
We can vary the relative amounts of accommodative and fusional vergence exerted under binocular conditions by placing lenses of various powers before the eyes. Because fixation disparity is related to the amount of fusional vergence being used, it will vary with lens power and sign. Plus lenses, by decreasing accommodative convergence, will increase the required positive fusional vergence for convergent stimuli and will decrease the required negative fusional vergence for divergent stimuli. Plus lenses will increase an exo fixation disparity and decrease an eso fixation disparity thus shifting the FDC down. There will also be some shift to the left because the BI and BO diplopia points (correlated with the BI and BO fusional vergence ranges) will shift to the left. By the opposite effect on accommodative convergence, minus lenses will shift the curve up and to the right. An eso fixation disparity can thus be reduced to zero with plus lenses, and an exo fixation disparity can be reduced to zero with minus lenses.

## REFERENCES
1. Cline D, Hofstetter HW, Griffin JR. Dictionary of Visual Science. 4th ed. Radnor, PA: Chilton, 1989:205.
2. Sheedy JE. Actual measurement of fixation disparity and its use in diagnosis and treatment. J Am Optom Assoc 1980;51:1079-1084.
3. Wesson MD, Koenig R. A new clinical method for direct measurement of fixation disparity. South J Optom 1983;1:48-52.
4. Sheedy JE. Fixation disparity analysis of oculomotor imbalance. Am J Optom Physiol Opt 1980;57:632-639.
5. Goss DA. A versatile new nearpoint card: the Saladin card. Indiana J Optom 2005;8:17-19.
6. Ogle KN, Mussey F, Prangen A deH. Fixation disparity and the fusional processes in binocular single vision. Am J Ophthalmol 1949;32:1069-1087.
7. Carter DB. Fixation disparity with and without foveal fusion contours. Am J Optom Arch Am Acad Optom 1964;41 :729-736.
8. Carter DB. Parameters of fixation disparity. Am J Optom Physiol Opt 1980; 57:610-617.
9. Schor CM. Fixation disparity and vergence adaptation. In: Schor CM, Ciuffreda KJ, eds. Vergence Eye Movements: Basic and Clinical Aspects. Boston: Butterworth–Heinemann, 1983:465-516.
10. Ogle KN. Researches in Binocular Vision. New York: Hafner, 1950:69-93.
11. Ogle KN, Martens TG, Dyer JA. Oculomotor Imbalance in Binocular Vision and Fixation Disparity. Philadelphia: Lea & Febiger, 1967:75-119.

12. McCullough RW. *The fixation disparity-heterophoria relationship. J Am Optom Assoc* 1978;49:369-372.

13. Saladin JJ, Sheedy JE. *Population study of fixation disparity, heterophoria, and vergence. Am J Optom Physiol Opt* 1970;55:744-750.

14. Karania R, Evans BJW. *The Mallett fixation disparity test: influence of test instructions and relationship with symptoms. Ophthal Physiol Opt* 2006;26:507-522.

15. Schor GM. *Fixation disparity: a steady state error of disparity-induced vergence. Am J Optom Physiol Opt* 1980;57:618-631.

16. Sheedy JE, Saladin JJ. *Validity of diagnostic criteria and case analysis in binocular vision disorders. In: Schor CM, Ciuffreda KJ, eds. Vergence Eye Movements: Basic and Clinical Aspects. Boston: Butterworth-Heinemann; 1983: 517-540.*

17. Carter DB. *Effects of prolonged wearing of prism. Am J Optom Arch Am Acad Optom* 1963;40:265-273.

18. Carter DB. *Fixation disparity and heterophoria following prolonged wearing of prism. Am J Optom Arch Am Acad Optom* 1965;42:141-152.

19. Alpern M. *Types of movement. In: Davson H, ed. Muscular Mechanisms. 2nd ed. Vol. 3 of The Eye. New York: Academic, 1969:65-174.*

20. Henson DB, North R. *Adaptation to prism-induced heterophoria. Am J Optom Physiol Opt* 1980;57:129-137.

21. Wick BC. *Horizontal deviations. In: Amos JF, ed. Diagnosis and Management in Vision Care. Boston: Butterworth-Heinemann, 1987:461-510.*

## OTHER SUGGESTED READING

Goss DA. *Fixation disparity. In: Eskridge JB, Amos JF, Bartlett JD, eds. Clinical Procedures in Optometry. Philadelphia: Lippincott, 1991:716-726.*

Griffin JR, Grisham JD. *Binocular Anomalies: Diagnosis and Vision Therapy, 4th ed. Amsterdam: Butterworth-Heinemann, 2002:78-92.*

## PRACTICE PROBLEMS

1. List and describe the five main parameters of FDCs.

2. What test condition factors have significant effects on the amount of fixation disparity?

3. How is vergence adaptation related to the slope of the FDC?

4. What change in fixation disparity would be expected with a plus add?

# Chapter 10
# Clinical Use of Fixation Disparity

**E**xamination of fixation disparity can be a useful adjunct to a dissociated phorias, fusional vergence, ranges, and relative accommodation findings. Because the testing conditions and the variables measured are different, analysis of fixation disparity and analysis of dissociated phorias and fusional amplitudes give somewhat different information. Schor[1] has observed that when an oculomotor imbalance has been confirmed by dissociated phorias and fusional vergence ranges in a symptomatic patient, a prism prescription can be effectively derived from fixation disparity data. Sheedy and Saladin[2,3] have shown that fixation disparity curve (FDC) data are related to the presence of ocular symptoms.

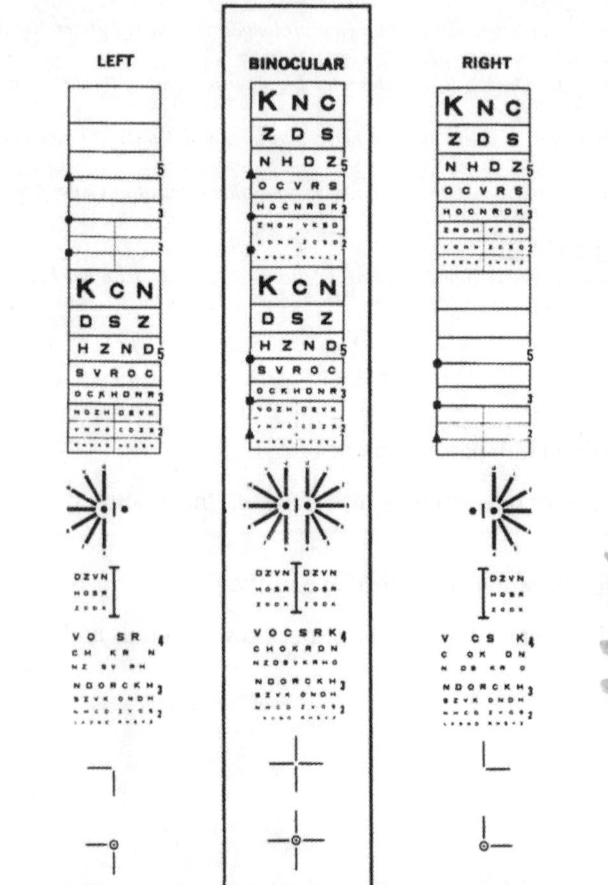

As discussed in the previous chapter, one can measure an associated phoria, the amount of prism required to eliminate fixation disparity, or one can determine an entire FDC depending on the instrumentation used. An FDC is determined by measuring the actual amount of fixation disparity when the patient views through differing amounts of prism. There are several commercially available instruments that can be used for the measurement of asso-

*Figure 10.1. The AO vectographic slide. Some portions of the chart are seen with the right eye and some with the left eye, as indicated in the diagram. On the associated phoria target the upper vertical line and the horizontal line on the right are seen with the right eye and the other two lines with the left eye when Polaroid goggles are worn.*

ciated phorias but not the amount of fixation disparity; thus they cannot be used to generate an FDC. Other instruments which provide for measurement of fixation disparity make the plotting of an FDC possible.

Fixation disparity can be used in vergence disorders in children and young adults. It can also be used to test whether the high exophoria resulting from the plus adds prescribed for presbyopia may lead to symptoms.[4,5] A very important use of fixation disparity and associated phoria data is the prescription of prism. Many practitioners view the associated phoria as the preferred method for deriving the power of a prism prescription. There

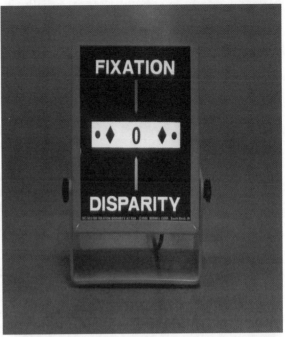

Figure 10.2. The Bernell lantern farpoint associated target. The upper line is seen with the right eye when the appropriate polaroid goggles are worn.

are also guidelines for the determination of prism prescription power from the fixation disparity curve (FDC). This chapter discusses the instrumentation and methods for measurement and interpretation of associated phorias and fixation disparity.

## MEASUREMENT OF ASSOCIATED PHORIAS

Instrumentation for the measurement of distance-associated phorias include targets in projector systems, such as American Optical (AO) vectographic slide, or free-standing instruments, such as the Bernell lantern far-point target and the Mallett far-point testing unit (Figures 10.1, 10.2, and 10.3, respectively).[6-9] The AO vectographic slide is designed for use in the AO projector. The Bernell test lantern

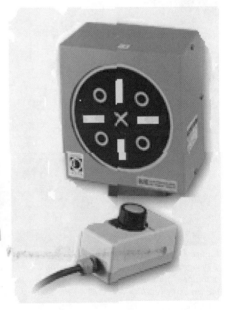

Figure 10.3. Mallett unit for distance associated phoria measurement. The patient is questioned about alignment of the vertical and horizontal lines when polaroid goggles are worn.

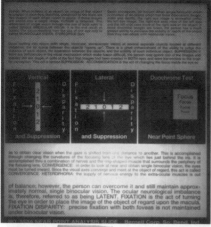

Figure 10.4. *Nearpoint slide for the Bernell lantern. The associated phoria targets are in the middle (lateral associated phoria) and in the left center (vertical associated phoria) of the slide.*

usually is placed on a table, and the Mallett unit for far-point testing can be placed on a table or mounted on a wall.

Instruments that can be used to measure near associated phorias include the Bernell lantern nearpoint target, the Mallett nearpoint units, and the Borish card[6-10] (Figures 10.4, 10.5, and 10.6). The Bernell test lantern has a nearpoint slide that can be alternated with the farpoint associated phoria slide. As noted above, it usually is used on a table, but can be hand-held for nearpoint testing. The Mallett nearpoint unit is hand-held or placed on a table. The Borish card can be hand-held or placed on a phoropter reading rod.

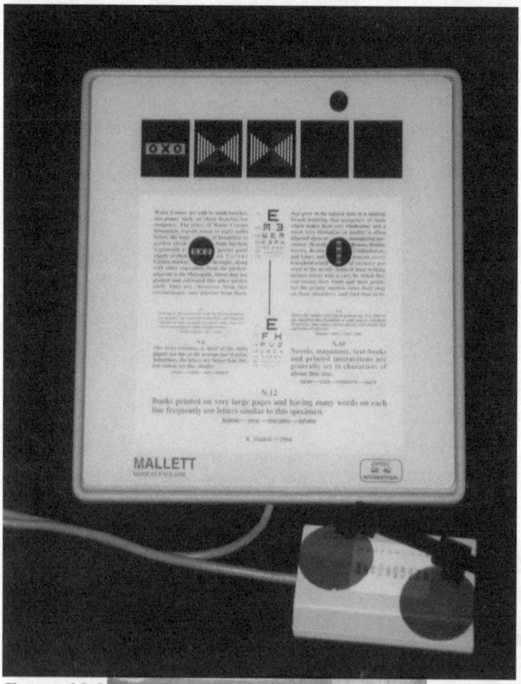

For use of each of these devices the patient must view through polaroid filter test goggles or the polaroid filter setting in the phoropter. The vertical lines are used for the measurement of the horizontal-associated phoria. On most instruments, the upper line is seen by the right eye, and the lower line is seen by the left eye. Most of the other features in the targets are seen by both eyes, and thus serve as "fusion locks." Targets with centrally placed fusion locks are preferable to those with fusion locks only in the periphery of the device.

The examiner asks the patient whether the top line is directly above or to the right or left of the lower line. If it is directly above the lower line the associated phoria is zero. If the top line is to the left of the bottom line, an exo fixation disparity exists and the minimum amount of base-in prism that aligns the two vertical lines is the associated phoria. If the top line is to the right, the associated phoria is

Figure 10.5. *A Mallett unit for nearpoint testing. This unit is designed to be handheld or placed on a table. There are associated phoria targets in the circular windows within the areas of reading text and on the upper left portion of the unit.*

90

the amount of base-out prism that neutralizes the eso fixation disparity. If either of the lines moves so that there is only temporary alignment, that should be considered misalignment, and the aligning prism recorded for the associated phoria should

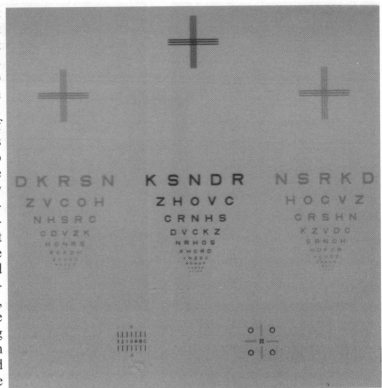

*Figure 10.6. One side of the Borish nearpoint chart. The vertical and horizontal lines for lateral and vertical associated phoria measurements, respectively, are on the lower right part of the card.*

be the amount of prism needed for the patient to maintain the lines in alignment.[11]

Distance associated phoria measurements taken with the AO vectographic slide agree well with those measured with the distance Mallett unit.[8] Associated phorias at near using the Borish card are similar to those obtained with the near-point Bernell unit[8] and with the near-point Mallett unit.[12]

## PRESCRIPTION FROM ASSOCIATED PHORIAS

Associated phorias are expected to be zero. A non-zero value can be a sign of a vergence disorder. Mallett[6,7] introduced the idea that the existence of fixation disparity indicates that fusional convergence has not adequately compensated for a heterophoria. An individual with an uncompensated phoria is one who has dissociated and associated phorias with the same prism base orientations. The following definitions come from that concept:

- Compensated exophoria – exo dissociated phoria with zero fixation disparity and thus zero associated phoria
- Uncompensated exophoria – exo dissociated phoria with exo fixation disparity and thus a base-in associated phoria

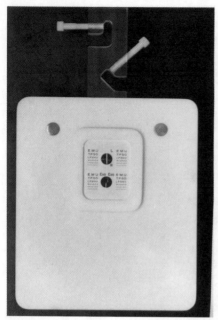

Figure 10.7. Patient's side of the Sheedy Disparometer. Pairs of lines are rotated through the round windows until the patient reports that they are aligned. Pairs of vertical lines for lateral fixation disparity are visible in the lower window. The upper window contains targets for vertical fixation disparity.

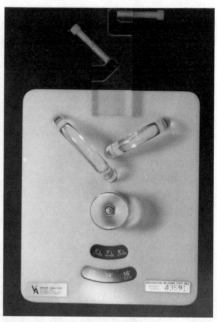

Figure 10.8. Examiner's side of the Sheedy Disparometer. The separations of the target lines are changed using the knob in the center until the patient reports alignment. The amount of fixation disparity is then read from the center of the display at the bottom of the instrument.

| DISTANCE: | 40 CM (16 INCHES) | | 25 CM (10 INCHES) |
|---|---|---|---|
| | ↑ | F.D. (MIN. ARC) | F.D. (MIN. ARC) |
| RED | 0 | 0 | 0 |
| | ½ | 4.3' | 6.9' |
| GREEN | 1 | 8.6' | 13.7' |
| | 1½ | 12.9' | 20.6' |
| ORANGE | 2 | 17.2' | 27.5' |
| BLACK | 3 | 25.8' | 41.2' |
| BLACK | 4 | 34.4' | 55' |

ESO F.D.: ARROW TO LEFT
EXO F.D.: ARROW TO RIGHT

See look can
one baby run
is help play
dark was what

Smash empty safe stone
grove desire ocean
begin bench damp
against gentle

WESSON FIXATION DISPARITY CARD ©

Figure 10.9. Wesson fixation disparity card. The arrow at the bottom of the polarized area in the center of the card is seen by the left eye when the patient wears polaroid goggles. The lines above the arrow are seen by the right eye. The patient reports the line to which the arrow appears to be pointing. Each of the marks represents a particular amount of fixation disparity calibrated for test distances of 25 cm and 40 cm as shown in the upper right corner of the card.

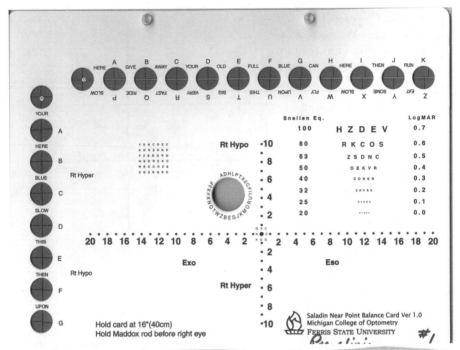

*Figure 10.10. Saladin card. The series of circles across the top of the card are used for measurement of lateral fixation disparity. The patient reports the circle within which the lines appear to be aligned. The examiner then looks at the chart on the back of the card to find the amount of fixation disparity corresponding to that circle. The circles along the left hand side of the card can be used to measure vertical fixation disparity.*

- Compensated esophoria – eso dissociated phoria with zero fixation disparity and thus zero associated phoria
- Uncompensated esophoria – eso dissociated phoria with eso fixation disparity and thus a base-out associated phoria

Using the concept of compensated and uncompensated phorias, Mallett recommended some prescription guidelines. For uncompensated exophoria, Mallett recommended base-in prism equal in amount to the associated phoria or vision training to improve positive fusional convergence. In a patient with uncompensated esophoria at distance, the treatment of choice is the base-out prism of the associated phoria. For patients with uncompensated esophoria at near, the plus add that eliminates the fixation disparity or a combination of a plus add and base-out prism can be used.

## DETERMINATION OF FIXATION DISPARITY CURVES

Devices for the measurement of associated phorias indicate whether the lines of sight of the two eyes are aligned, but they do not indicate the amount of misalignment of the lines of sight; the prism added to achieve alignment is then the associated phoria. In contrast, when we measure fixation disparity we are measuring the amount of misalignment of the lines of sight with respect to the convergence stimulus presented by the target distance. Instruments that allow a measurement of fixation disparity at near-point include the Sheedy Disparometer (Figures 10.7 and 10.8), the Wesson fixation disparity card (Figure 10.9), and the Saladin card (Figure 10.10).[8,9,13-15]

Polaroid testing goggles or the polaroid filter setting in the phoropter is necessary for the use of the Sheedy Disparometer, the Wesson fixation disparity card, or the fixation disparity measurements on the Saladin card. When using the Sheedy Disparometer, the examiner rotates pairs of vertical lines (see Figure 9.2) through the window visible to the patient (see Figure 10.7). The patient reports when the top line is directly above the bottom line. The amount of misalignment indicated on the back of the Disparometer (see Figure 10.8) provides a measure of the amount of fixation disparity in minutes of arc. Testing with the Wesson fixation disparity card involves asking the patient to which of the upper lines the arrow is pointing (see Figure 10.9). The exam-

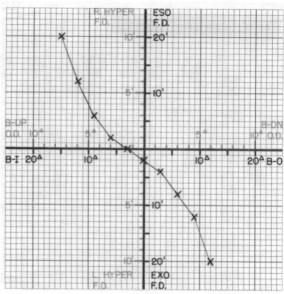

Figure 10.11. An FDC plotted from the following data:

| Prism Setting (in prism diopters) | Fixation Disparity (in minutes of arc) |
|---|---|
| 0 | 2 exo |
| 3 BI | 0 |
| 3 BO | 4 exo |
| 6 BI | 2 eso |
| 6 BO | 8 exo |
| 9 BI | 6 eso |
| 9 BO | 12 exo |
| 12 BI | 12 eso |
| 12 BO | 20 exo |
| 15 BI | 20 eso |
| 15 BO | diplopia |
| 18 BI | diplopia |

iner can then refer to the table in the upper right corner of the card to note the amount of the fixation disparity. On the Saladin card, the patient reports the circle in which the two lines appear to be exactly aligned. All three devices can either be hand-held or mounted on the phoropter reading rod.

To plot an FDC, fixation disparity is measured at several different prism settings. Prism power can be set by the phoropter rotary prism or by placing loose prisms in a trial frame.[16] Sheedy[14] has recommended measuring fixation disparity with zero prism, then with base-in prism, increasing the power in 3 prism diopter increments to diplopia, and then with base-out prism in 3Δ increments to diplopia. Wick[17] prefers to alternate base-in and base-out prism in

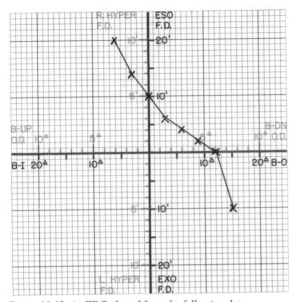

*Figure 10.12. An FDC plotted from the following data:*

| Prism Setting (in prism diopters) | Fixation Disparity ( in minutes of arc) |
|---|---|
| 0 | 10 eso |
| 3 BI | 14 eso |
| 3 BO | 6 eso |
| 6 BI | 20 eso |
| 6 BO | 4 eso |
| 9 BI | diplopia |
| 9 BO | 2 eso |
| 12 BI | diplopia |
| 12 BO | 0 |
| 15 BI | diplopia |
| 15 BO | 10 exo |
| 18 BI | diplopia |
| 18 BO | diplopia |

the following order: 0, 3Δ base-in, 3Δ base-out, 6Δ base-in, 6Δ base-out, 9Δ base-in, 9Δ base-out, etc., to diplopia with both base-in and base-out. Using the latter order, if diplopia occurs much earlier on one prism base direction than on the other, alternation can be continued with the use of a prism power that can just be fused on the side with the lower fusional range; this may serve to limit an effect of increasing prism adaptation on the shape of the curve.[18]

The x-axis on an FDC is the amount of prism in prism diopters. Base-in is to the left on the x-axis. Base-out increases to the right on the FDC graph. The FDC graph is designed this way because greater base-out represents a greater convergence stimulus. The amount of the fixation disparity in minutes of arc is plotted on the y-axis. Eso fixation disparity (the eyes slightly convergent with respect to the convergence stimulus) is above the x-axis. Exo fixation disparity (slight divergence of the lines of sight with respect to the target) is below the x-axis.

The parameters of the FDC (curve type, slope, y-intercept, x-intercept, and center of symmetry) were defined in Chapter 9. Because the x-intercept is the point where fixation disparity is equal to zero, the x-value (prism setting) might be thought to be equal to the associated phoria. However, FDC x-intercepts usually are greater in magnitude than the associated phorias measured with the near-point Bernell target, the Borish card, or the Mallett near-point unit.[8,19]

The position of the center of symmetry is mathematically derived. In a clinical setting, Sheedy's criterion, which will be described below, is easier to determine and can be used instead of the center of symmetry.

## PRESCRIPTION FROM FIXATION DISPARITY CURVES

The following guidelines for prescribing from FDCs are summarized from Sheedy,[13,14] Sheedy and Saladin,[20] Schor,[21] and Wick.[17] Curve type may be the best diagnostic parameter of the FDC. Persons with type I curves usually are asymptomatic, while those with types II, III, and IV curves are more likely to be symptomatic. The type I FDC patient who does have asthenopia usually has an FDC with a high slope and is managed well with vision training. A successful vision training program is correlated with a flattening of the FDC slope and a widening of the FDC.

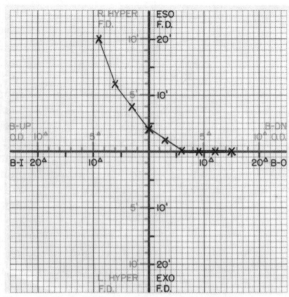

Figure 10.13. An FDC plotted from the following data:

| Prism Setting (in prism diopters) | Fixation Disparity ( in minutes of arc) |
|---|---|
| 0 | 4 eso |
| 3 BI | 8 eso |
| 3 BO | 2 eso |
| 6 BI | 12 eso |
| 6 BO | 0 |
| 9 BI | 20 eso |
| 9 BO | 0 |
| 12 BI | diplopia |
| 12 BO | 0 |
| 15 BI | diplopia |
| 15 BO | 0 |
| 18 BI | diplopia |
| 18 BO | diplopia |

Most type II FDCs occur in patients with esophoria.[22] Patients with type II curves respond better to prism prescription and plus lens adds than to vision therapy. Type III curves usually are associated with exophoria.[22] Patients with type III curves can be managed with prism prescription or vision therapy, although vision therapy is less likely to be successful than in type I curve patients.

**Table 10.1**
Clinical fixation disparity curve parameters.
Curve type
Slope
x-intercept
y-intercept
Sheedy's criterion

96

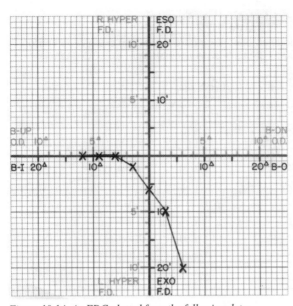

*Figure 10.14. An FDC plotted from the following data:*

| Prism Setting (in prism diopters) | Fixation Disparity (in minutes of arc) |
|---|---|
| 0 | 6 exo |
| 3 BI | 2 exo |
| 3 BO | 10 exo |
| 6 BI | 0 |
| 6 BO | 20 exo |
| 9 BI | 0 |
| 9 BO | diplopia |
| 12 BI | 0 |
| 12 BO | diplopia |
| 15 BI | diplopia |

Prism prescriptions from fixation disparity curves can be based on the amount of prism that allows the patient to operate at a flat portion of the curve. If the center of symmetry was derived, it could be used to prescribe prism power. However, a simpler approach is to identify the flattest segment of the curve and then find the point on that segment closest to the y-axis, in other words, the lowest x (prism) value on that flat segment. In Sheedy's words, one can "prescribe prism to a flat portion of the curve."[14] Griffin and Grisham[23] have suggested that this minimum amount of prism on the flat segment of the curve can be called "Sheedy's criterion." For clinical purposes we can substitute Sheedy's criterion for the center of symmetry as one of the five FDC parameters.

There is no general agreement among clinicians whether prism or vision therapy is preferable for patients with type IV curves based on the FDC alone. A type IV curve may indicate poor sensory or motor fusion, or both.

Patients with steeper FDC slopes are more likely to be symptomatic. Flatter slopes are correlated with higher levels of prism adaptation.[24] A high value for the y-intercept also can be a sign of an oculomotor problem. Slope and y-intercept can be useful for diagnostic evaluation, but they do not directly yield a numerical value for lens or prism prescription.

Some patients complain of instability of the nonius lines during fixation disparity testing. This can result in an irregularly shaped FDC. An irregular FDC can be an indication of an accommodation problem. If so, vision training to improve accommodation can result in a smoothing of the FDC.

## Table 10.2

Mean FDC x-intercepts in various studies. Standard deviations are given in parentheses. Units are prism diopters. BI prism is negative in sign, and BO prism is positive.

| Study | Sheedy Disparometer | Wesson Card | Saladin card |
|---|---|---|---|
| Saladin and Sheedy[25] (n=103) | -3.3 (11.0) | -- | -- |
| Wesson and Koenig[15] (n=10) | -0.9 (1.8) | -0.9 (1.4) | -- |
| Wildsoet and Cameron[19] (n=10) | -0.9 (3.6) | -- | -- |
| Van Haeringen et al.[26] (n=18) | +3.5 (6.4) | -3.1 (4.1) | -- |
| Brownlee and Goss[8] (n=89) | +0.4 (10.2) | -- | -- |
| Brownlee and Goss[8] (n=14) | 0 (7.3) | -2.3 (3.9) | -- |
| Dittemore et al.[27] (n=30) | -0.2 | -2.5 | -- |
| Goss and Patel[28] – OK data (n=96) | +2.3 (7.1) | -1.5 (4.4) | -- |
| Goss and Patel[28] – IN data (n=37) | +1.1 (6.5) | -4.0 (5.1) | -- |
| Ngan et al.[29] (n=42) | -- | -2.9 (5.8) | +0.4 (5.8) |

## Table 10.3

Mean FDC y-intercepts in various studies. Standard deviations are given in parentheses. Units are minutes of arc. Exo fixation disparity is negative in sign, and eso fixation disparity is positive.

| Study | Sheedy Disparometer | Wesson Card | Saladin card |
|---|---|---|---|
| Saladin and Sheedy[25] (n=103) | -3.5 (5.9) | -- | -- |
| Wesson and Koenig[15] (n=10) | 0 (2.3) | -1.7 (2.9) | -- |
| Wildsoet and Cameron[19] (n=10) | -4.5 (4.4) | -- | -- |
| Van Haeringen et al.[26] (n=28) | +1.7 (3.4) | -1.5 (5.5) | -- |
| Brownlee and Goss[8] (n=89) | -1.4 (5.9) | -- | -- |
| Brownlee and Goss[8] (n=14) | +1.4 (3.8) | -1.8 (3.5) | -- |
| Dittemore et al.[27] (n=30) | -1.1 (4.1) | -3.3 (3.7) | -- |
| Goss and Patel[28] – OK data (n=96) | +0.5 (5.4) | -2.6 (7.3) | -- |
| Goss and Patel[28] – IN data (n=38) | -0.7 (6.6) | -5.7 (13.7) | -- |
| Ngan et al.[29] (n=50) | -- | -10.2 (13.4) | -0.2 (2.8) |
| Corbett and Maples[30] (n=28) | -- | -- | -1.9 (2.7) |

## CLINICAL FIXATION DISPARITY CURVE PARAMETERS

Sheedy's criterion can be more readily recognized on a clinically plotted fixation disparity curve than the center of symmetry. Therefore, we will modify our earlier list of fixation disparity curve parameters for clinical purposes to replace center of symmetry with Sheedy's criterion. Clinical FDC parameters are listed in Table 10.1.

## EXAMPLES

Figures 10.11 through 10.14 show examples of fixation disparity curves. The FDC in Figure 10.11 is a type I curve. The slope using points from from $3\Delta$ base-in to $3\Delta$ base-out is:

## Table 10.4

Mean FDC slopes in various studies. Standard deviations are given in parentheses. Units are minutes of arc per prism diopter.

| Study | Sheedy Disparometer | Wesson Card | Saladin Card |
|---|---|---|---|
| Saladin and Sheedy[25] (n=103) | -0.7 (0.7) | -- | -- |
| Wesson and Koenig[15] (n=10) | -0.8 (0.4) | -0.8 (0.5) | -- |
| Wildsoet and Cameron[19] (n=10) | -1.0 (0.3) | -- | -- |
| Van Haeringen et al.[26] (n=28) | -0.4 (0.3) | -0.9 (0.6) | -- |
| Brownlee and Goss[8] (n=89) | -0.5 (0.5) | -- | -- |
| Brownlee and Goss[8] (n=14) | -0.6 (0.8) | -1.1 (1.1) | -- |
| Dittemore et al.[27] (n=30) | -0.7 (0.7) | -1.0 | -- |
| Goss and Patel[28] – OK data (n=96) | -0.6 (0.7) | -0.9 (1.1) | -- |
| Goss and Patel[28] – IN data (n=38) | -0.7 (0.6) | -1.4 (1.7) | -- |
| Ngan et al.[29] (n=49) | -- | -1.3 (1.5) | -0.2 (0.4) |

Slope = (4 exo – 0) / 6Δ = (-4-0) / 6Δ = -0.67 minutes of arc per prism diopter

The y-intercept in Figure 10.11 is 2 minutes of arc exo, and the x-intercept is 3Δ base-in. There is no portion of the curve that is completely flat. It is flattest from 6Δ base-in to 3Δ base-out. Because that segment includes zero, Sheedy's criterion would be zero. The fairly low magnitude slope, low exo y-intercept, and Sheedy's criterion equal to zero suggest good vergence function.

In the FDC in Figure 10.12, the curve type is I. The fixation disparity is 6 minutes of arc eso at 3Δ BO and 14 minutes of arc eso at 3Δ BI, so the slope is -8 minutes of arc divided by 6Δ, or -1.3 minutes of arc per prism diopter. The x-intercept is 12Δ BO, and the y-intercept is 10 minutes of arc eso fixation disparity. The flattest segment of the curve extends from 3Δ BO to 12Δ BO, so Sheedy's criterion is 3Δ BO. The type I curve suggests that vision therapy may be a good treatment approach. It is likely that the fairly high magnitude slope would be decreased with vision therapy. Another potentially useful treatment approach would be a plus add to reduce or eliminate the eso fixation disparity.

In the curve in Figure 10.13, the curve type is II. Fixation disparity measures 2 minutes of arc eso at 3Δ BO and 8 minutes of arc eso at 3Δ BI, so the slope is -6 minutes of arc divided by 6Δ, which is equal to -1 minute of arc per prism diopter. The x-intercept is 6Δ BO, and the y-intercept is 4 minutes of arc eso. The curve is flat from 6Δ BO to 15Δ BO, so Sheedy's criterion is 6Δ BO. Treatment options could include a plus add and/or base-out prism.

In the curve in Figure 10.14, the curve type is III. Fixation disparity measures 10 minutes of arc exo at 3Δ BO and 2 minutes of arc exo at 3Δ BI, so the slope is -8 minutes of arc divided by 6Δ, which is equal to -1.3 minute of arc per prism diopter. The x-intercept is 6ΔBI, and the y-intercept is 6 minutes of arc exo fixation disparity. The curve is flat from 6Δ BI to 12Δ BI, so Sheedy's criterion is 6Δ BI. Treatment options include vision therapy or base-in prism.

## COMPARISON OF FINDINGS WITH DIFFERENT FIXATION DISPARITY INSTRUMENTS

Comparison studies have shown that the clinical FDC parameters found with the Disparometer differ from those found with the Wesson card, as can be seen from the results of studies summarized in Tables 10.2, 10.3, and 10.4. Compared to the Disparometer, the Wesson card shows a more base-in x-intercept, a more exo y-intercept, and steeper slope. These differences exist when all subjects are considered together and when exophoric and esophoric subjects are considered separately.[28] Results on the Wesson card also differ from the results on the Saladin card.[29] There are currently no widely agreed upon norms for FDC parameters, perhaps in part due to the variability of results from study to study. Another reason may be that it is important to consider all of the FDC parameters and the curve shape together rather than looking at single FDC parameters in isolation. However, the means and standard deviations given in Tables 10.2, 10.3, and 10.4 may be helpful in recognizing normal and abnormal findings. The Saladin card is newer than the Disparometer and Wesson card, so there are less published data for it. Patients with esophoria may tend to be symptomatic at a lower magnitude slope threshold than patients with exophoria.[2]

## REFERENCES

1. Schor CM. Fixation disparity: a steady state error. Am J Optom Physiol Opt 1980;57:618-631.
2. Sheedy JE, Saladin JJ. Phoria, vergence, and fixation disparity in oculomotor problems. Am J Optom Physiol Opt 1977;54:474-478.
3. Sheedy JE, Saladin JJ. Association of symptoms with measures of oculomotor deficiencies. Am J Optom Physiol Opt 1978;55:670-676.
4. Sheedy JE, Saladin JJ. Exophoria at near in presbyopia. Am J Optom Physiol Opt 1975;52:474-481.
5. Sheedy JE. Analysis of oculomotor balance. Rev Optom 1979;116:44-45.
6. Mallett RFJ. Fixation disparity in clinical practice. Aust J Optom 1969;52: 97-109.
7. Mallett RFJ. Fixation disparity-its genesis in relation to asthenopia. Ophthalmic Optician 1974; 14:1159-1168.
8. Brownlee GA, Goss DA. Comparisons of commercially available devices for the measurement of fixation disparity and associated phorias. J Am Optom Assoc 1988;59:451-460.
9. Goss DA. Fixation disparity. In: Eskridge JB, Amos JF, Bartlett JD, eds. Clinical Procedures in Optometry. Philadelphia, PA: Lippincott, 1991:716-726.
10. Borish IM. The Borish nearpoint chart. J Am Optom Assoc 1978;49:41-44.
11. Karania R, Evans BJW. The Mallett fixation disparity test: influence of test instructions and relationship with symptoms. Ophthal Physiol Opt 2006;26:507-522.
12. Yee L. Comparison of nearpoint techniques. J Am Optom Assoc 1981;52: 5.79-582.
13. Sheedy JE. Fixation disparity analysis of oculomotor imbalance. Am J Optom Physiol Opt 1980;57:632-639.
14. Sheedy JE. Actual measurement of fixation disparity and its use in diagnosis and treatment. J Am Optom Assoc 1980; 51: 1079-1084.
15. Wesson MD, Koenig R. A new clinical method for direct measurement of fixation disparity. South J Optom 1983;1:48-52.
16. Frantz KA, Scharre JE. Comparison of Disparometer fixation disparity curves as measured with and without the phoropter. Optom Vis Sci 1990;67: 117-122.
17. Wick BC. Horizontal deviations. In: Amos JF, ed. Diagnosis and Management in Vision Care. Boston: Butterworth-Heinemann, 1987:461-510.

Assoc. Phoria - do not have eso or exo. It is an amount of prism.

18. Scheiman M, Wick B. *Clinical Management of Binocular Vision-Heterophoric, Accommodative, and Eye Movement Disorders*, 2nd ed. Philadelphia: Lippincott, 2002: 433-434.

19. Wildsoet CF, Cameron KD. The effect of illumination and foveal fusion lock on clinical fixation disparity measurements with the Sheedy Disparometer. *Ophthal Physiol Opt* 1985;5:171-178.

20. Sheedy JE, Saladin JJ. Validity of diagnostic criteria and case analysis in binocular vision disorders. In: Schor CM, Ciuffreda KJ, eds. *Vergence Eye Movements: Basic and Clinical Aspects*. Boston: Butterworth-Heinemann, 1983: 517-540.

21. Schor CM. Fixation disparity and vergence adaptation. In: Schor CM, Ciuffreda KJ, eds. *Vergence Eye Movements: Basic and Clinical Aspects*. Boston: Butterworth-Heinemann, 1983:465-516.

22. Saladin JJ. Phorometry and stereopsis. In: Benjamin WJ, ed. *Borish's Clinical Refraction*, 2nd ed. St. Louis: Butterworth Heinemann Elsevier, 2006:899-960.

23. Griffin JR, Grisham JD. *Binocular Anomalies: Diagnosis and Vision Therapy*, 4th ed. Amsterdam: Butterworth-Heinemann, 2002:85-92.

24. Schor CM. The influence of rapid prism adaptation upon fixation disparity. *Vision Res* 1979; 19:757-765.

25. Saladin JJ, Sheedy JE. Population study of fixation disparity, heterophoria, and vergence. *Am J Optom Physiol Opt* 1978;55:744-750.

26. van Haeringen R, McClurg P, Cameron KD. Comparison of Wesson and modified Sheedy fixation disparity tests. Do fixation disparity measures relate to normal binocular visionstatus? *Ophthal Physiol Opt* 1986;6:397-400.

27. Dittemore D, Crum J, Kirschen D. Comparison of fixation disparity measurements obtained with the Wesson Fixation Disparity Card and the Sheedy Disparometer. *Optom Vis Sci* 1993;70:414-420.

28. Goss DA, Patel J. Comparison of fixation disparity curve variables measured with the Sheedy Disparometer and the Wesson Fixation Disparity Card. *Optom Vis Sci* 1995;72:580-588.

29. Ngan J, Goss DA, DeSpirito J. Comparison of fixation disparity curve parameters with the Wesson and Saladin fixation disparity cards. *Optom Vis Sci* 2005;82:69-74.

30. Corbett A, Maples WC. Test-retest reliability of the Saladin card. *Optom* 2004;75:629-639.

## PRACTICE PROBLEMS

1. Give the Mallett classification for each of the following sets of test findings. (In addition to the Mallett categories, you can also use paradoxical fixation disparity in your answers)

| Dissociated phoria | Associated phoria | Mallett Classification |
|---|---|---|
| 8Δ exo | 0 | compensated exophoria |
| 3Δ eso | 0 | " esophoria |
| 9Δ exo | 3Δ BI | uncompensated exophoria |
| 6Δ eso | 2Δ BO | " esophoria |
| 6Δ exo | 2Δ BO | paradoxical fixation disparity |

2. List some instruments that can be used to measure associated phorias and some instruments that can be used to measure fixation disparity.

3. How does the design of instruments that can be used to measure fixation disparity differ from the design of instruments that are used to measure associated phorias?

4. List the clinical FDC parameters.

5. Plot FDCs using the following data. What are the curve type, slope, y-intercept, x-intercept, and Sheedy's criterion for each curve?

$$\text{Slope} = \frac{\text{fd } 3\text{BO} - \text{fd } 3\text{BI}}{6^\triangle}$$

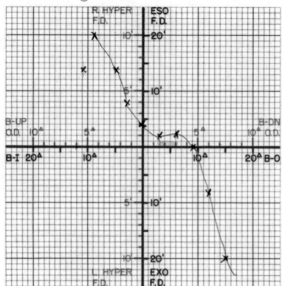

Patient PM

| Prism Setting (in prism diopters) | Fixation Disparity ( in minutes of arc) |
|---|---|
| 0 | 4 eso |
| 3 BI | 8 eso |
| 3·BO | 2 eso |
| 6 BI | 14 eso |
| 6 BO | 2 eso |
| 9 BI | 20 eso |
| 9 BO | 0 |
| 12 BI | diplopia |
| 12 BO | 8 exo |
| 15 BI | diplopia |
| 15 BO | 20 exo |
| 18 BI | diplopia |
| 18 BO | diplopia |

Curve Type I

$$\text{Slope} = \frac{3\text{BO} - \cancel{\text{fd}} 3\text{BI}}{6^\triangle}$$

$$= \frac{2' - 8'}{6^\triangle}$$

$$= \frac{-6'}{6^\triangle} = -1\,'/\!\!\triangle$$

y int = 4' eso fd.

x int = 9△ BO

— Sheady's Criterion
  best prism adaptation.
  3△ BO = (point on the
  flattest seg of the
  curve, closest to the
  y-axis

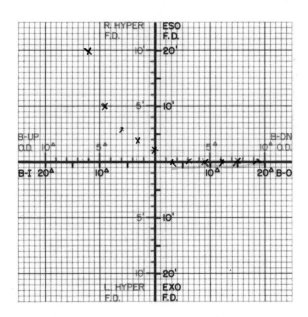

Patient CR

| Prism Setting (in prism diopters) | Fixation Disparity ( in minutes of arc) |
|---|---|
| 0 | 2 eso |
| 3 BI | 4 eso |
| 3 BO | 0 |
| 6 BI | 6 eso |
| 6 BO | 0 |
| 9 BI | 10 eso |
| 9 BO | 0 |
| 12 BI | 20 eso |
| 12 BO | 0 |
| 15 BI | diplopia |
| 15 BO | 0 |
| 18 BI | diplopia |
| 18 BO | 0 |
| 21 BI | diplopia |
| 21 BO | diplopia |

$$Slope = \frac{0-4'}{6^\triangle} = \frac{-4'}{6^\triangle}$$

$$= -0.7\,'/\triangle$$

y-int. = 2' eso fd

x-int = $3^\triangle$ BO

— Sheady's Criterion
$3^\triangle$ BO (point of flat part of the curve which is closest to the y-int.)

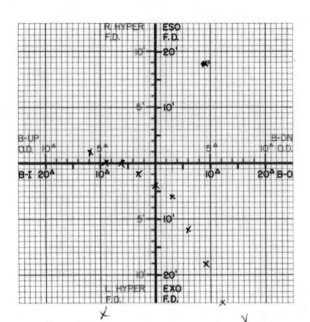

Patient JB

| Prism Setting (in prism diopters) | Fixation Disparity ( in minutes of arc) |
|---|---|
| 0 | 4 exo |
| 3 BI | 2 exo |
| 3 BO | 6 exo |
| 6 BI | 0 |
| 6 BO | 12 exo |
| 9 BI | 0 |
| 9 BO | 18 exo |
| 12 BI | 2 eso |
| 12 BO | 25 exo |
| 15 BI | 2 eso |
| 15 BO | diplopia |
| 18 BI | 2 eso |
| 18 BO | diplopia |
| 21 BI | diplopia |
| 21 BO | diplopia |

Type II

$$\text{slope} = \frac{-6-(-2)}{6^\Delta}$$

$$= \frac{-4'}{6^\Delta} = -0.7\,'/_\Delta$$

y-int = 4' exo fd
x-int = 6$^\Delta$ BI
Sheedy's Criterion
6 BI

104

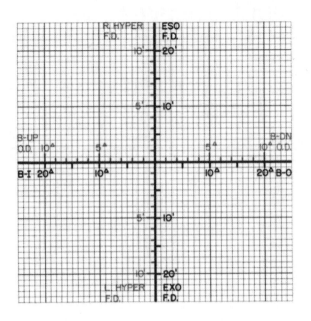

Patient RM

| Prism Setting (in prism diopters) | Fixation Disparity ( in minutes of arc) |
|---|---|
| 0 | 0 |
| 3 BI | 0 |
| 3 BO | 0 |
| 6 BI | 4 eso |
| 6 BO | 2 exo |
| 9 BI | 8 eso |
| 9 BO | 4 exo |
| 12 BI | 12 eso |
| 12 BO | 6 exo |
| 15 BI | 25 eso |
| 15 BO | 12 exo |
| 18 BI | diplopia |
| 18 BO | 20 exo |
| 21 BI | diplopia |
| 21 BO | diplopia |

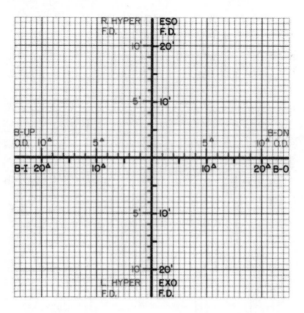

Patient BP

| Prism Setting (in prism diopters) | Fixation Disparity ( in minutes of arc) |
|---|---|
| 0 | 4 exo |
| 3 BI | 2 exo |
| 3 BO | 10 exo |
| 6 BI | 2 exo |
| 6 BO | 20 exo |
| 9 BI | 0 |
| 9 BO | diplopia |
| 12 BI | 4 eso |
| 12 BO | diplopia |
| 15 BI | 8 eso |
| 15 BO | diplopia |
| 18 BI | 12 eso |
| 18 BO | diplopia |
| 21 BI | 20 eso |
| 21 BO | diplopia |

# Chapter 11
# Diagnosis and Prescription Guidelines in Vergence Disorders

**H**aving covered concepts of ACA ratios, Maddox classification of convergence, vergence testing procedures and norms, the zone of clear single binocular vision, guidelines for assessing strain on fusional vergence, accommodative facility, vergence facility, and fixation disparity, we are now ready to apply those concepts to the recognition of vergence disorder case types. Vergence disorders can be classified into one of eight case types. This classification is based on distance and near phorias, ACA ratios, and characteristic patterns of findings on fusional vergence ranges, relative accommodation, facility tests, near point of convergence, and other tests. Identification of the vergence disorder case type is helpful in designing treatments for patients with vergence problems, because the applicability and efficacy of the different treatments for vergence disorders varies with the ACA ratio and direction of the phoria.[1-5]

Treatments for vergence disorders include lens adds, prism, and vision therapy. Lens adds can be useful in reducing strain on fusional vergence by changing accommodation and as a result changing accommodative convergence also. The change in accommodative convergence changes the amount of fusional vergence needed to have the total amount of convergence required for fusion. Lens adds are most effective when the ACA ratio is high because a small amount of add power will cause a relatively larger shift in phoria. Prism prescriptions reduce the strain on fusional vergence by changing the vergence stimulus. Prisms can be useful in several of the vergence disorders. A moderate ACA ratio makes a prism prescription more convenient because the recommended prism amounts for distance and near may be similar, making it possible to provide prism in one pair of glasses for full-time wear. Vision therapy is useful for vergence disorders because patients can increase their fusional vergence capabilities. Vision therapy can be used in any of the vergence disorders. However, some practitioners emphasize vision therapy more for exophoria than for esophoria, because positive fusional vergence is easier to increase with vergence training than is negative fusional vergence.[6]

The vergence disorder case types described below are (1) convergence insufficiency, (2) convergence excess, (3) divergence insufficiency, (4) divergence excess, (5) basic exo, (6) basic eso, (7) fusional vergence dysfunction, and (8) pseudoconvergence insufficiency. The ACA ratio is high in convergence excess and divergence excess, and low in convergence insufficiency and divergence insufficiency. Normal ACA ratios are found in basic exo, basic eso, and reduced fusional vergence case types. In pseudoconvergence insufficiency, there is an accommodative insufficiency, and the patient exhibits dissociated phorias and some other findings similar to those in convergence insufficiency.

## ANALYSIS OF VERGENCE DISORDERS

We can use the knowledge gained from the preceding chapters as part of a comprehensive approach to the analysis of vergence disorders. The steps in this system are as follows:

1. Use the normal ranges from Morgan's norms to determine whether the distance and near dissociated phorias are normal (ortho to $2\Delta$ exo at distance and ortho to $6\Delta$ exo at near). Tentatively identify the case type based on the normalcy of the phorias.

2. Confirm or revise the tentative case type diagnosis by determining which of the fusional vergence, relative accommodation, facility, near point of convergence (NPC), etc., findings are low. Morgan's norms and the other norms presented previously are useful for this purpose. In addition, the graph of the zone of clear single binocular vision (ZCSBV) can be used to assess the pattern and consistency of findings. The findings typical of each of the vergence disorders are summarized in Table 11.1.

3. Use the case type as a guide for the preferred method of treatment (lens add, prism, and/or vision therapy) or alternative treatments. If a lens add or prism is chosen as the treatment, the power of the add or prism can be suggested from the appropriate guideline or test.

### Convergence Insufficiency

Convergence insufficiency is a common condition, with prevalences reported in the literature ranging from about 2 to 8% in children and young adults.[7-9] Convergence insufficiency is characterized by a normal distance phoria and a high exophoria at near. Other test results that help to identify cases of convergence insufficiency are low base-out vergence ranges at near and a receded NPC. The literature does not agree on a particular cut-off for the NPC to indicate convergence insufficiency,[10] but the general guidelines suggested by the authors of the NPC studies summarized in Table 3.1 are that a break greater than 5 or 6 cm can be considered abnormal. However, a survey of optometrists involved in the management of binocular vision disorders found that a break value of 10 cm on the NPC was the most frequent cut-off used in the diagnosis of convergence insufficiency, and the average cut-off was a break of 9.3 cm.[11] Some convergence insufficiency patients can achieve a normal NPC with extra effort, so some clinicians note not only the numerical value of the NPC, but also the apparent effort exerted by the patient on the NPC test. The ACA ratio is low in convergence insufficiency. Accommodation findings are normal. Common symptoms of convergence insufficiency include ocular discomfort during reading and other near-point tasks, headaches, diplopia, blurred vision, and fatigue.[12,13] Some patients do not have asthenopia because they avoid near-point tasks.

The treatment of choice for convergence insufficiency is vision therapy to improve positive fusional vergence function. Vision therapy has a very high rate of success in relieving the symptoms of convergence insufficiency.[14-20] Grisham[18] summarized the results of several studies and reported that 72%

**Table 11.1**

Summary of diagnostic findings and treatments for each of the vergence disorder case types. The process of making a diagnosis and deciding on a treatment proceeds from left to right in the columns of the table. A tentative diagnosis is made based on the phorias and ACA ratio. Then this diagnosis may or may not be confirmed by other test findings and the pattern of the ZCSBV.

| Case type | Distance phoria | Near phoria | ACA Ratio | Other test findings | Pattern of ZCSBV | Treatment options |
|---|---|---|---|---|---|---|
| Convergence insufficiency | normal | high exo | low | low BO ranges at near, receded NPC, normal lag of accommodation | less tilted to the right than normal | 1) vision therapy 2) BI for near based on associated phoria or Sheard's criterion |
| Convergence excess | normal | eso | high | low BI ranges at near, low PRA, slow on minus side of binocular lens rock | more tilted to the right than normal | 1) plus add which makes near dissociated phoria normal or which reduces near eso fixation disparity to zero 2) vision therapy |
| Divergence insufficiency | eso | normal | low | low BI ranges at distance | lateral position shifted to the right compared to normal, less tilted than normal | 1) BO prism based on distance associated phoria or 1:1 rule 2) vision therapy |
| Divergence excess | high exo | normal | high | low BO ranges at distance | lateral position shifted to the left compared to normal, more tilted than normal | 1) vision therapy 2) BI prism for distance based on distance associated phoria or Sheard's criterion 3) minus add for distance, sometimes with plus add for near |
| Basic exophoria | high exo | high exo | normal | low BO ranges at distance and near, low NRA, slow on plus side of binocular lens rock | entire zone shifted to the right compared to normal, tilt normal | 1) vision therapy 2) BI prism based on associated phorias or Sheard's criterion |
| Basic esophoria | eso | eso | normal | low BI ranges at distance and near, low PRA, slow on minus side of binocular lens rock | entire zone shifted to the right compared to normal, tilt normal | 1) BO prism based on associated phorias or 1:1 rule 2) vision therapy |
| Fusional vergence dysfunction | normal | normal | normal | all vergence ranges low, reduced vergence facility, low NRA and PRA | Positive and negative widths both less than normal, tilt normal | vision therapy |
| Pseudo convergence insufficiency | normal | high exo | appears low due to poor accommodative response | receded NPC, NPC improves with plus add, low BO ranges at near, high lag of accommodation, amplitude of accommodation often low | tilt of left and right sides normal, phoria line less tilted than normal | plus add for near and/or vision therapy |

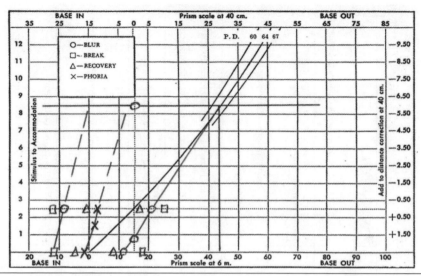

Figure 11.1. An example of a ZCSBV in convergence insufficiency. The graph of the ZCSBV is plotted from the data in the following table.

|  | Phoria | Base-in | Base-out | Plus to blur | Minus to blur |
|---|---|---|---|---|---|
| Distance | 1 exo | X/12/4 | 12/18/8 |  |  |
| 40 cm | 12 exo | 24/28/16 | 6/10/2 | +1.75 | -6.00 |
| 40 cm +1.00 | 13 exo |  |  |  |  |

Amplitude of accommodation = 8.50 D; PD = 64 mm; NPC = 12 cm; near associated phoria = 4Δ base-in.

of patients were "cured" and 91% of patients were either cured or improved with vision therapy. Vergence training for convergence insufficiency results in reduced symptoms, increases in base-out vergence ranges, and improvements in the NPC.[17]

An alternative treatment for convergence insufficiency is a prism prescription for near use. If the patient is unwilling or unable to do vision training, a base-in prism prescription for wear during near work may be helpful. One study found statistically significant improvements in reading performance in convergence insufficiency patients with base-in prism,[21] although another study did not find a significant reduction in symptoms with base-in prism compared to control subjects.[22] The prism prescribed for reading and nearpoint activities can be based on the near associated phoria. If associated phoria findings are not available, other procedures for finding potential prism power include Sheard's criterion for near or Sheedy's criterion from the near fixation disparity curve.

An example of convergence insufficiency is given in Figure 11.1. We can use the steps outlined above to analyze this case. The distance phoria is within Morgan's norms. The near phoria is more exo than Morgan's norms. The ACA ratios are low: calculated ACA = 1.6 Δ/D; gradient ACA = 1Δ/D. We can thus tentatively identify the case type as convergence insufficiency. The base-out blur, break, and recovery at near are all abnormally low based on Morgan's norms. The NPC is somewhat receded. When we examine the graph of the

ZCSBV (see Figure 11.1), we can see that the findings are consistent with each other in that the expected double parallelogram pattern of the ZCSBV is observed. Because the ACA is low, the ZCSBV does not tilt very much to the right. The low base-out findings at near, the receded NPC, and the ZCSBV tilting to the right less than normal confirm the tentative diagnosis of convergence insufficiency.

We can use Sheard's criterion to assess the strain on fusional vergence in exophoria. For Sheard's criterion to be met, the magnitude of the PRV should be twice the amount of the exophoria. In this case it is not, which suggests significant strain on positive fusional vergence. In the case in Figure 11.1, the prism recommended by Sheard's criterion for near would be:

$$P = (2/3)(12) - (1/3)(6) = 6\Delta \text{ base-in}$$

Because of the diagnosis of convergence insufficiency in the case in Figure 11.1, vision therapy to improve fusional vergence function can be recommended. If the patient did not wish to do vision therapy, a second alternative would be a prism prescription for near use. The near associated phoria suggests that the prism prescription should be $4\Delta$ base-in.

## Convergence Excess

Convergence insufficiency and convergence excess are the most common vergence disorders. The prevalence of convergence excess in clinic populations has been reported from about 6 to 8%.[7,9,23,24]

Convergence excess is characterized by a normal distance phoria, esophoria at near, and a high calculated ACA ratio. Low base-in vergence ranges at near (NRV) are typical of convergence excess. Positive relative accommodation (PRA) is low because of its relation to negative fusional vergence. Convergence excess patients are slow on the minus side of lens rock binocular accommodative facility and slow on the base-in side of vergence facility. Common symptoms of convergence excess include ocular discomfort and headaches following short periods of reading and occasional blurred vision or diplopia associated with near-point tasks.

The most common treatment for convergence excess is prescription of a plus add for near.[25,26] The near plus add can be provided in single vision reading glasses, bifocal lenses, or progressive addition lenses. A plus add is particularly effective because the ACA ratio is high. Another possible treatment is vision therapy to improve negative fusional vergence function. Although this is somewhat more difficult than improving positive fusional vergence, vision therapy is effective in increasing negative fusional vergence ranges.[6,27-30] Vision therapy for convergence excess has been reported to result in relief of symptoms in 66 to 84% of cases.[28,29]

An effective amount of plus lens addition to prescribe is the amount of plus that shifts the near phoria to ortho or a small amount of exo (shifts it into the normal range). The add that would shift the near phoria to ortho could be derived by dividing the amount of esophoria by the gradient ACA ratio,

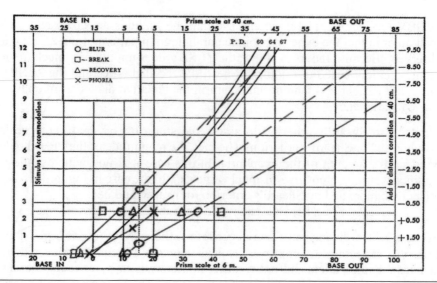

Figure 11.2. An example of convergence excess. The graph of the ZCSBV is plotted from the data in the following table.

|  | Phoria | Base-in | Base-out | Plus to blur | Minus to blur |
|---|---|---|---|---|---|
| Distance | 1 exo | X/6/4 | 11/20/10 |  |  |
| 40 cm | 5 eso | 6/12/2 | 20/27/14 | +2.00 | -1.25 |
| 40 cm +1.00 | 2 exo |  |  |  |  |

Amplitude of accommodation = 11.00 D; PD = 64 mm; NPC = 1cm.

assuming accurate measurements of the near phoria and gradient ACA ratio. So a near add could be found using the following formula and then rounding up to the nearest 0.25D, if necessary:

plus add = amount of esophoria/gradient ACA ratio

For example, if the near phoria is 7 eso and the gradient ACA ratio is 8Δ/D, the add would be +1.00D. Because the near phoria and the ACA ratio covary, the power of the plus adds thus derived do not show much variation. Most adds for convergence excess are in the neighborhood of +1.00 or +1.25D.

Another way of deriving the power of the plus add is to use fixation disparity. The power of the add should be the minimum plus that reduces the eso fixation disparity to zero. This can be done with an associated phoria target. Plus can be added until the patient reports the vertical lines to be aligned.

An example of convergence excess is shown in Figure 11.2.

The distance phoria is normal and the near phoria is eso. The ACA ratios are high: calculated ACA = 7.1 Δ/D; gradient ACA = 7 Δ/D. The phorias and the high ACA ratio suggest convergence excess. The fact that the base-in vergence ranges at near are low and the PRA is low confirms convergence excess. The ZCSBV conforms fairly closely to the double parallelogram configuration, suggesting that the test findings are internally consistent. The tilting of the ZCSBV to the right is characteristic of convergence excess. The

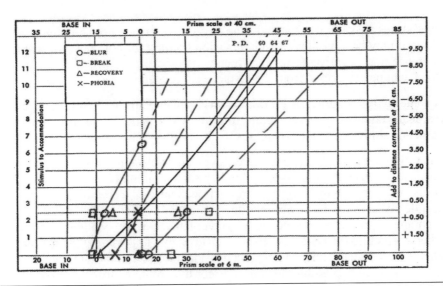

Figure 11.3. An example of divergence insufficiency. The graph of the ZCSBV is plotted from the data in the following table.

|  | Phoria | Base-in | Base-out | Plus to blur | Minus to blur |
|---|---|---|---|---|---|
| Distance | 6 eso | X/2/-1 | 17/24/14 |  |  |
| 40 cm | 1 exo | 12/17/10 | 15/22/12 | +2.50 | -4.00 |
| 40 cm +1.00 | 3 exo |  |  |  |  |

Amplitude of accommodation = 11.00 D; PD = 62 mm; distance associated phoria = 3Δ base-out.

most common treatment in convergence excess is a plus add. The near phoria through the subjective refraction to best visual acuity is 5 eso and the gradient ACA ratio is 7Δ/D, so the add that would be predicted as producing ortho-phoria at near would be +0.71 D:

$$\text{plus add} = (5\Delta) / (7\Delta/D) = 0.71 \text{ D}$$

Using that formula, an add of +0.75 D would be recommended as it would be expected to yield a near phoria within the normal range.

## Divergence Insufficiency

Divergence insufficiency is characterized by esophoria at distance and a normal near phoria. The ACA ratio is low. Distance base-in vergence ranges are low. Symptoms of divergence insufficiency may include occasional diplopia at distance, headaches, ocular discomfort, and ocular fatigue associated with distance vision. The distance diplopia in divergence insufficiency is occa-sional and long standing. In contrast, a sudden onset distance diplopia with esotropia at distance can be a sign of a serious condition such as sixth nerve palsy or divergence paralysis.[31] Divergence insufficiency is the least common of the vergence disorders.

A common treatment for divergence insufficiency is base-out prism.[25,32] The base-out prism can be used only for distance or can be prescribed for full-time wear. Full-time wear is not a problem if the patient's positive fusional vergence capabilities are sufficient to handle the increased convergence stimulus at near; if not, it may be advisable to include vision training for both positive fusional vergence and negative fusional vergence along with the prism prescription. Prism can be prescribed from the distance associated phoria.

An alternative to prism prescription is vision therapy to improve negative fusional vergence. Vision therapy improves the patient's negative fusional vergence abilities and thus increases the base-in vergence ranges.

Alteration of the spherical lens power is not a feasible approach in esophoria at distance because accommodation should be at a minimum level while viewing at distance through the subjective refraction. Thus, an increase in plus power or a decrease in minus power over the subjective refraction will not decrease accommodation or accommodative convergence for far viewing. However, when correcting the refractive error, it is advisable to prescribe the maximum plus to best visual acuity to keep accommodation at a minimum level. Thus it is important, if possible, to fully correct hyperopia or to be careful not to overminus myopia.

Figure 11.3 shows a case of divergence insufficiency. The distance phoria is a high eso and the near phoria is normal. The calculated ACA ratio is 3Δ/D and the gradient ACA ratio is 2Δ/D. The distance base-in vergence ranges are low. The negative number on the distance base-in recovery means that the recovery occurred with base-out prism. The double parallelogram appearance of the ZCSBV suggests that the test findings are internally consistent. The tilt of the ZCSBV is consistent with a low ACA ratio; that along with the shift in the lateral position of the zone to the right is consistent with divergence insufficiency. In divergence insufficiency a common treatment is base-out prism. The distance associated phoria indicates a prism prescription of 3Δ base-out. The 1:1 rule would recommend a prism prescription of 3.5Δ base-out:

$$\text{Prism} = [(6)-(-1)] / 2 = 3.5\Delta$$

The prism could be worn for distance only. But if the 3Δ base-out prism is worn full-time, it probably will not induce near problems. This prediction is based on the following reasoning. The near phoria through the subjective refraction is 1Δ exo. This represents a stimulus to positive fusional vergence of 1Δ. With the addition of a 3Δ base-out prism the stimulus to positive fusional convergence is 4Δ. At near the reserve convergence is 15 (the base-out blur at 40 cm through the subjective refraction). The 3Δ base-out prism will reduce the reserve by 3Δ to 12Δ. Considering that Sheard's criterion (a demand of 4Δ and a reserve of 12Δ) would be met, we could predict that no difficulty at near would be induced by the prism.

## Divergence Excess

Divergence excess is characterized by a high exophoria at distance and a normal near phoria. Distance base-out vergence ranges are low. The stimulus ACA ratio is high. Symptoms can include occasional diplopia at distance and asthenopia, but patients with divergence excess are also often asymptomatic.[33]

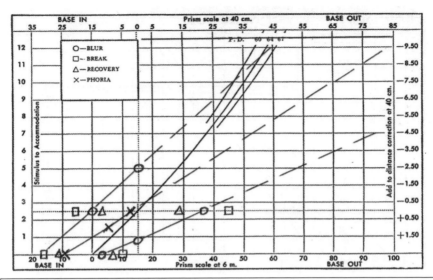

*Figure 11.4. An example of divergence excess. The graph of the ZCSBV is plotted from the data in the following table.*

|  | Phoria | Base-in | Base-out | Plus to blur | Minus to blur |
|---|---|---|---|---|---|
| Distance | 9 exo | X/17/11 | 3/10/6 |  |  |
| 40 cm | 2 exo | 15/21/12 | 22/30/14 | +1.75 | -2.50 |
| 40 cm +1.00 | 9 exo |  |  |  |  |

Amplitude of accommodation = 12.50 D; PD = 62 mm; distance associated phoria = 4Δ base-in.

Vision training for divergence excess is quite successful and can be considered the treatment of choice.[15,34-36] Base-in prism for distance prescribed using the distance associated phoria is another potential treatment.

Because the ACA ratio is high in divergence excess, a decrease in plus power or an increase in minus power can be effective in reducing the distance exophoria. It should be kept in mind that the minus lens addition requires additional accommodation and will make the near phoria as well the distance phoria more convergent. If the minus add strains accommodation or induces an esophoria at near it may be advisable to prescribe a plus add at near in bifocal form. Hyperopia is often undercorrected in divergence excess. Myopia is generally not overcorrected in divergence excess, except occasionally when the divergence excess results in intermittent exotropia at distance and even then sometimes only to maintain more consistent fusion until vision therapy can be instituted. Although strabismus is beyond the scope of this manual, it can be pointed out that all practitioners do not agree on the value of lens adds in divergence excess intermittent exotropia. Some writers who see divergence excess intermittent exotropia as an adaptation to esophoria at near recommend nearpoint plus adds along with vision therapy,[37] and others recommend minus adds for distance and/or base-in prism for distance when patients are uncooperative or unsuccessful in vision therapy.[38]

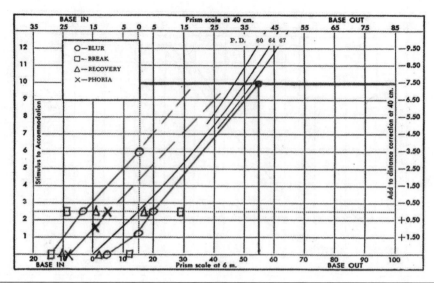

Figure 11.5. An example of basic exophoria. The graph of the ZCSBV is plotted from the data in the following table.

| | Phoria | Base-in | Base-out | Plus to blur | Minus to blur |
|---|---|---|---|---|---|
| Distance | 8 exo | X/14/10 | 4/12/2 | | |
| 40 cm | 10 exo | 18/24/14 | 5/14/2 | +1.25 | -3.50 |
| 40 cm +1.00 | 14 exo | | | | |

Amplitude of accommodation = 10.0 D; PD = 64 mm; NPC = 9 cm; distance associated phoria = 4Δ base-in; 40 cm associated phoria =3Δ base-in; monocular lens rock normal, but can't clear plus side on binocular lens rock with +2.00 D flippers.

Figure 11.4 illustrates a case of divergence excess. The distance phoria is high exo. The near phoria is within the normal range. Distance base-out vergence ranges are low. The phoria line and the ZCSBV are tilted quite a bit to the right, indicating a high ACA ratio. The lateral position of the ZCSBV is shifted to the left, indicating exo at distance. The calculated ACA ratio is 8.6 Δ/D. The gradient ACA ratio is 7 Δ/D.

Sheard's criterion is met at 40 cm. Sheard's criterion is not met at 6 m, suggesting strain on fusional vergence at distance. The distance associated phoria is 4Δ base-in, indicating uncompensated exophoria at distance. In the case that vision therapy would not be undertaken, the distance associated phoria gives a value for prism prescription of 4Δ BI. Sheard's criterion at 6 m would suggest a prism prescription of approximately 5Δ BI at distance:

$$P = (2/3)(9) - (1/3)(3) = 5\Delta\ BI$$

## Basic Exophoria

Basic exophoria is characterized by greater than normal exophoria at both distance and near. The stimulus ACA ratio is at approximately normal levels. Base-out fusional vergence ranges are lower than normal. The plus-to-blur finding is usually low. The near point of convergence is receded. Patients with basic exophoria are slow on the plus side of binocular lens rock accommodative facility and slow on the base-out side of vergence facility. Symptoms

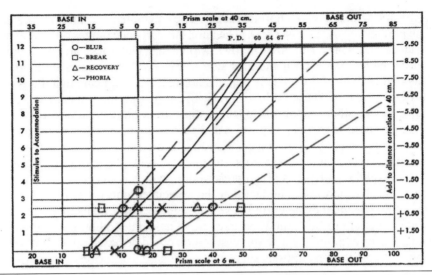

*Figure 11.6. An example of basic esophoria. The graph of the ZCSBV is plotted from the data in the following table.*

|  | Phoria | Base-in | Base-out | Plus to blur | Minus to blur |
|---|---|---|---|---|---|
| Distance | 8 eso | X/2/-1 | 18/24/17 |  |  |
| 40 cm | 8 eso | 5/12/0 | 25/34/20 | +2.50 | -1.00 |
| 40 cm +1.00 | 4 eso |  |  |  |  |

Amplitude of accommodation = 12.0 D; PD = 64 mm; NPC = 2 cm; distance associated phoria = 4Δ base-out; 40 cm associated phoria =3Δ base-out; monocular lens rock normal, but can't fuse minus side on binocular lens rock with +2.00 D flippers.

of basic exophoria may include eye strain or headaches associated with near work or the use of distance vision. The patient also may complain of occasional blurred vision or diplopia associated with either distance or near vision tasks.

Basic exophoria is fairly frequently seen, but is not as common as convergence insufficiency. One study of a clinical population of children found a prevalence of only 0.3%.[24] A small study of university students reported a prevalence of 3.1%.[7] In a report of exo patients that included both strabismic and non-strabismic cases, 62% were classified as having convergence insufficiency, 28% were in the basic exo category, and 10% were classified as having divergence excess.[39]

Vision training for basic exophoria has a high rate of success,[15,40] and many practitioners consider it to be the treatment of choice for basic exophoria. If the associated phorias are similar in magnitude at distance and near, a base-in prism prescription for full-time wear from the associated phoria findings is a convenient alternative. The minus add from undercorrecting a hyperopia may be helpful if there is no accompanying accommodative problem.

A case of basic exophoria is shown in Figure 11.5. The distance and near dissociated phorias show a greater than normal amount of exophoria when compared with Morgan's normal ranges. The calculated ACA ratio is 5.2 Δ/D. The gradient ACA ratio is 4 Δ/D. The base-out vergence ranges are low at both distance and near. The NRA is low. Monocular lens rock rates are normal, but the patient can't clear the plus side of the +2.00 D flippers on binocular lens rock. The tilt of the ZCSBV looks normal, but it appears that the zone is shifted to the left. These findings indicate basic exophoria. Sheard's criterion is not met at either 6 m or 40 cm, suggesting strain on fusional vergence. The finding of base-in associated phorias at distance and near indicates uncompensated exophoria at both distance and near. Vision training to increase positive fusional vergence would be a good treatment option. An additional treatment option would be a base-in prism prescription, which could be given based on the associated phorias. The fact that the associated phorias are very close to the same amount at distance and at 40 cm suggests that a convenient treatment would be prism in full-time wear glasses. If associated phoria measurements had not been available, the prism prescription could be based on Sheard's criterion. The prism prescriptions suggested by Sheard's criterion in this case are:

$$6 \text{ m: } P = (2/3)(8) - (1/3)(4) = 4\Delta \text{ base-in}$$
$$40 \text{ cm: } P = (2/3)(10) - (1/3)(5) = 5\Delta \text{ base-in}$$

## Basic Esophoria

In basic esophoria, esophoria is found at distance and near, and the ACA ratio is approximately normal. Base-in fusional vergence ranges are lower than normal. The minus-to-blur finding is usually low. Basic eso patients are slower on the minus side on binocular lens rock accommodative facility and slow on the base-in side on vergence facility. Nearpoint asthenopia is a common complaint in basic esophoria. Symptoms also may include occasional blurred vision or diplopia during distance or near viewing. Prevalences of about 1% have been reported.[7,24]

The most common treatment for basic esophoria is base-out prism. The prism can be prescribed using the associated phorias measured at distance and near. If the distance and near associated phorias are not equal, the lower amount of the two is usually prescribed or an amount can be decided upon by trial-framing. Another treatment option is vision training to improve negative fusional vergence. Hyperopic refractive error should be completely corrected.

If a patient has esophoria which is significantly greater at near than at a distance, a plus add for near can be incorporated along with base-out prism or base-in vision training. This situation incorporates aspects of treatment of both basic esophoria and convergence excess. Sometimes basic eso patients will manifest symptoms only at near even though significant esophorias are found at both distance and near. In such cases, the use of plus add for near may be sufficient treatment by itself. When plus adds are used for basic esophoria, the powers can be derived in the same ways as in convergence excess.

Figure 11.6 illustrates an example of basic esophoria. The dissociated phorias at distance and near show equal amounts of esophoria. The base-in vergence findings and the PRA are lower than normal. The calculated ACA ratio is 6

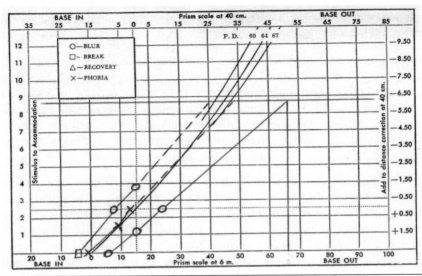

*Figure 11.7. An example of fusional vergence dysfunction. The graph of the ZCSBV is plotted from the data in the following table.*

|  | Phoria | Base-in | Base-out | Plus to blur | Minus to blur |
|---|---|---|---|---|---|
| Distance | 1 exo | X/4/2 | 6/12/4 |  |  |
| 40 cm | 2 exo | 7/12/4 | 8/14/3 | +1.25 | -1.25 |
| 40 cm +1.00 | 6 exo |  |  |  |  |

Amplitude of accommodation = 8.75 D; PD = 64 mm; NPC = 7 cm.

$\Delta$/D. The gradient ACA ratio is 4 $\Delta$/D. The patient shows normal lens rock accommodative facility rates monocularly, but cannot fuse the -2.00 D side of the lens rock binocularly. Neither Sheard's criterion nor the 1:1 rule are met at either distance or near. The associated phorias are base-out at distance and near, indicating uncompensated esophoria. The tilt of the ZCSBV is approximately the same as the tilt of the demand line, but it appears shifted to the right compared with normal. These findings indicate basic esophoria. One way of managing basic esophoria is base-out prism. Prism could be prescribed based on the associated phorias. Alternately, the prism prescription could be based on the 1:1 rule. The prism recommended by the 1:1 rule would be:

$$6 \text{ m: } P = [8 - (-1)]/2 = 4.5\Delta \text{ BO}$$
$$40 \text{ cm: } P = (8 - 0)/2 = 4\Delta \text{ BO}$$

## Fusional Vergence Dysfunction

In the fusional vergence dysfunction case type, distance and near dissociated phorias are normal and the ACA ratio is normal, but both base-in and base-out fusional vergence ranges are below normal.[41,42] NRA and PRA are usually low. Amplitude of accommodation and lag of accommodation are normal. Vergence facility rates are low. Other terms have been used for fusional vergence dysfunction. It has been called reduced fusional vergence. Schapero[43] referred to it as restricted zone cases, and Griffin and Grisham[44] called it basic orthophoria with restricted zone. Asthenopic symptoms often are associated with reading or near work.

Fusional vergence dysfunction may be a primary condition, or it may be secondary to impediments to sensory fusion, such as uncorrected refractive error, aniseikonia, or suppression, or it may be secondary to uncorrected vertical deviations.[43,45] Treatment should include correction of any accompanying refractive problems or vertical deviations. Once such conditions are ruled out or ameliorated, treatment for fusional vergence dysfunction is vision therapy to improve positive and negative fusional vergence.

The test findings in a case of fusional vergence dysfunction are shown in Figure 11.7. The dissociated phorias at both distance and near are normal. The calculated ACA ratio is 5.6 $\Delta$/D. The gradient ACA ratio is 4 $\Delta$/D. The base-in vergence ranges, base-out vergence ranges, NRA, and PRA are all low. The tilt of the ZCSBV appears normal, but the zone is very narrow. The findings and the pattern of the ZCSBV indicate the fusional vergence dysfunction case type.

## Pseudoconvergence Insufficiency

In pseudoconvergence insufficiency, phoria findings are like those in convergence insufficiency: normal at distance and high exophoria at near. Base-out ranges at near are usually low. Amplitude of accommodation is often low. The lag of accommodation is abnormally high.

Examination of the ZCSBV shows that the left and right sides of the zone show a normal amount of tilt to the right. The phoria line is less tilted than the sides of the zone.[26] As discussed in Chapter 4, this occurs because accommodative response is reduced, and thus accommodative vergence is reduced, during measurement of the near phoria. The ACA ratio appears low because the lag of accommodation is abnormally high when the near phoria is taken. The NPC is receded. An interesting phenomenon that occurs in pseudoconvergence insufficiency is that the NPC improves with a plus add.[46] This paradoxical result is thought to be due to increased accommodative accuracy with the plus add, allowing accommodation and accommodative convergence to increase as the target is moved closer to the patient.

Pseudoconvergence insufficiency actually is an accommodative insufficiency rather than a 'true' convergence insufficiency. Therefore, treatment is aimed largely at managing the accommodative problem. Treatment often also includes vision therapy to improve positive fusional vergence. A high lag of accommodation usually is treated with a plus add for near-point. A common way to assess the lag of accommodation is monocular estimation method (MEM) dynamic retinoscopy. Normal lags of accommodation with MEM retinoscopy are usually between zero and 0.75 D. In pseudo convergence insufficiency, the lag will be greater than 0.75 D, whereas in a 'true' convergence insufficiency, the lag of accommodation will be normal.

### Table 11.2.

Ratings of Griffin and Grisham[51] of their confidence in different clinical methods of prescribing prism based on their clinical experience. The number 3 indicates best, 2 indicates good, and 1 indicates fair. They did not include the 1:1 rule in their ratings.

| Test | Exophoria | Esophoria |
|------|-----------|-----------|
| Sheard's criterion | 3 | X2 |
| Percival's criterion | 1 | 2 |
| Associated phoria | 3 | 3 |
| Sheedy's criterion | 2 | 2 |
| Prism confirmation procedure | 3 | 3 |
| Prism adaptation test | 1 | 1 |

Another treatment option in addition to a plus add is vision therapy to improve accommodative function. If accommodative function is improved with vision therapy, the phoria will tilt further to the right than before therapy so that it roughly parallels the left and right sides of the ZCSBV. Incorporation of vision therapy to improve positive fusional vergence will also result in the right hand of the ZCSBV shifting to the right and the zone becoming wider. An example of pseudoconvergence insufficiency was shown previously in Figure 4.1.

## COMMENTS

The identification of appropriate treatments for each of the case types is related to ACA ratio in that phorias are most easily shifted to normal levels by lens adds when the ACA ratio is high. Vision therapy can be used in any of the vergence disorders. However, some practitioners are more likely to recommend vision therapy for exophoria than for esophoria because vision training usually is more effective in improving positive fusional vergence than negative fusional vergence. The test findings, ZCSBV pattern, and recommended treatments for each of the vergence disorder case types are summarized in Table 11.1.

The efficacy of prism correction in relieving oculomotor symptoms has received only limited controlled study. In a study by Worrell et al,[47] subjects wore either glasses without prism or identical-appearing glasses with prism, as indicated by Sheard's criterion. The subjects participated in the study for two weeks, wearing one type of glasses the first week and the other type the following week. At the end of this time the subjects indicated which glasses they preferred. Although the sample size was small, the results suggested that prism corrections are best tolerated in esophoria at distance. The results also suggested that presbyopes with exo deviations at near tolerate prisms, but younger persons do not. Payne et al.[48] described a study in which ten symptomatic patients preferred spectacles prescribed from near Mallet unit associated phorias over spectacles with no prism. Each pair of spectacles was worn for one week. Nine of the ten subjects had exo fixation disparity at near. Stavis et al.[21] found base-in prism to be an effective treatment for convergence insufficiency. O'Leary and Evans[49] found that subjects with a near associated phoria on the Mallett unit of 2.5Δ BI or more had improved reading test scores when they wore the prism measured with the Mallett unit.

Carter[50] noted that when prism is given to a person who exhibits prism adaptation, that individual indicates a need for a larger prism at the next examination. He suggested that this should not be a problem if the practitioner does not prescribe prism for an asymptomatic person or for an individual without a significant distance heterophoria. Prism adaptation also can be tested for by remeasuring the phorias after the patient reads for a few minutes while using the proposed prism prescription. A significant change in the phorias indicates prism adaptation, in which case the prism prescription may be contraindicated. Griffin and Grisham[51] refer to this as the prism adaptation test. It has been noted that the use of fixation disparity and associated phorias for prescribing prism is effective because fixation disparity is affected by prism adaptation.[52]

The standard method for measuring phorias taught at many schools is the von Graefe prism dissociation technique. If there is some question about the validity of a phoria measurement using the von Graefe technique with the refractor, then the measurement can be repeated and/or other subjective and objective testing methods (such as modified Thorington test, stereoscope, and cover test prism neutralization) can be used. It also should be verified that in high refractive errors inaccuracy in the phoria measurement did not result from a tilt of the refractor or the use of an improper inter-pupillary distance.

In cases where the ACA ratio is high, spherical lens power alterations will be effective in changing convergence posture. Since this is not true for patients with low ACA ratios, prism correction or vision training is preferable to lens power changes when the ACA ratio is low. Prism correction may be more conveniently incorporated in spectacles for full-time wear if the ACA ratio is moderate and thus the phorias are similar at different distances. Spherical lens power alterations that would compromise clear vision or a comfortable range of accommodation should not be used.

When using a device that measures only associated phorias (as opposed to the entire fixation disparity curve), a prism prescription can be based on the associated phoria. If an entire fixation disparity curve is derived, the prism prescription can be based on Sheedy's criterion. In the absence of associated phoria data, prism prescriptions can also be based on Sheard's criterion in exophoria and the 1:1 rule in esophoria. It is also useful to observe the patient's subjective response to the prism being considered. Griffin and Grisham[51] call this a prism confirmation procedure. The patient views through a loose prism with the power and base direction being considered for prescription and the patient is asked whether print or letters appear clearer and whether vision seems more comfortable. Positive responses confirm the potential usefulness of the prism. To rule out a placebo effect, the base direction is then reversed without the patient's knowledge and the same questions are asked. It is expected that reversal of the base direction should reduce clarity and/or comfort. Table 11.2 shows the ratings of confidence in various methods of prescribing prism given by Griffin and Grisham.[51] Many practitioners would rate associated phorias higher than Sheard's criterion, particularly in esophoria. Griffin and Grisham

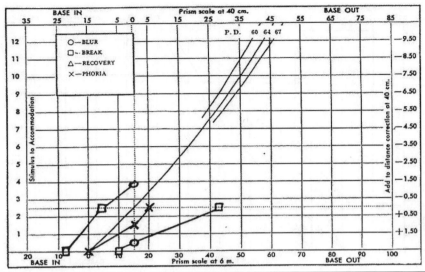

Figure 11.8. Test findings and ZCSBV for patient AG.

|  | Phoria | Base-in | Base-out | Plus to blur | Minus to blur |
|---|---|---|---|---|---|
| Distance | Ortho | X/8/4 | X/10/0 |  |  |
| 40 cm | 5 eso | X/10/2 | X/28/20 | +2.00 | -1.25 |
| 40 cm +1.00 | Ortho |  |  |  |  |

PD = 59 mm; eso fixation disparity with plano sphere OU, zero fixation disparity with +1.00 D sphere OU.

did not rate the 1:1 rule, but it has been suggested to be useful because Sheard's criterion is sometimes met in symptomatic esophoria.

When prism is prescribed for non-strabismic disorders, it is generally split between the two eyes. Prism is prescribed primarily when the patient is experiencing asthenopia or withdraws from visual tasks. Obviously, a careful case history[53-57] is indispensable in evaluating the patient's visual needs and complaints.

There have been many different schemes proposed by various authors for establishing the phoria levels that define each of the vergence disorder case types. The classification scheme described above is perhaps the easiest to remember because it is based on the well-known Morgan normal ranges for phorias. There will be occasional cases which do not exactly fit the exact specifications described here, but the principles developed here can still be applied. For instance, a case with 5Δ exo at distance and 15Δ exo at near would not exactly fit either convergence insufficiency or basic exo, but could be considered as a combination of the two and treatment plans derived accordingly; vision therapy would be a good treatment alternative. Similarly, a case with 5Δ eso at distance and 12Δ eso at near could be analyzed as a combination of basic eso and convergence excess; treatment options could include a plus add for near combined with BO prism or vision therapy.

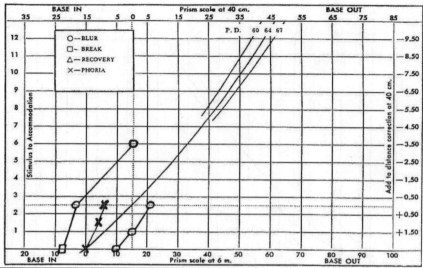

Figure 11.9. Test findings and ZCSBV for patient FN.

|  | Phoria | Base-in | Base-out | Plus to blur | Minus to blur |
|---|---|---|---|---|---|
| Distance | Ortho | X/8/4 | 10/18/6 |  |  |
| 40 cm | 9 exo | 18/22/12 | 6/18/0 | +1.50 | -3.50 |
| 40 cm +1.00 | 11 exo |  |  |  |  |

PD = 62 mm; amplitude of accommodation = 10.0 D; NPC = 9 cm.

The guidelines above are for patients without strabismus or sensory anomalies such as amblyopia. Many of the same basic principles apply to patients with strabismus, but treatment also must include treatment for sensory anomalies, such as amblyopia, suppression, etc. Strabismus and amblyopia are beyond the scope of this manual, and comprehensive sources on those conditions should be consulted for further information.[58-62]

## CASE REPORTS

AG, an 11-year-old boy, complained of blurred near vision. He stated that letters ran together. He did not wear spectacles. Unaided visual acuities were 6/6-2/6 OD, 6/6 OS, 6/6-2/6 OU at distance, and 20/20-2/8 OD, 20/20-3/8 OS at near. The cover test showed orthophoria at distance and a small esophoria at near. Near point of convergence was to the bridge of the nose. The subjective refraction was plano D sphere OU. Salient examination findings are shown in Figure 11.8. The phoria findings and the high ACA ratio suggest convergence excess. This is confirmed by noting the low base-in findings at near, the low PRA, an eso fixation disparity at near, and the fact that the ZCSBV tilts to the right, as shown in Figure 11.8. It may be noted that the 1:1 rule is not met at 40 cm. A +1.00 D add was sufficient to shift the esophoria at near to orthophoria. An eso fixation disparity was noted with no lenses in place. Fixation disparity was reduced to zero with +1.00 D spheres. The patient was asked to look at magazine print with +1.00 D lenses held in front of his eyes, and he stated that he could read finer print with the lenses. It also was demonstrated that these lenses made distance vision blurry. The options of single vision reading lenses, bifocals, and progressive addition lenses were explained to AG and his family, and they decided on single vision reading lenses. Lenses with powers of +1.00 D sphere were prescribed. AG subsequently reported that he could read much more easily with his spectacles.

Patient FN, a 28-year-old female graduate student, complained of afternoon headaches, a vague tiredness around the eyes, and a pulling sensation around the eyes. She had one-year-old glasses for distance vision which she wore on a full-time basis. The powers of the lenses in the glasses were -2.25-0.50 X 175 OD, -2.25-0.25 X 10 OS. Distance visual acuities with these lenses were 6/4.5-2/6 OD, 6/4.5-3/6 OS, 6/4.5-1/6 OU. Aided near acuities were 20/20 OD and OS. The cover test with the habitual correction revealed ortho at distance and a moderately large exophoria at near. The NPC was 9 cm. The subjective refraction was -2.50-0.25 X 170 OD (6/4.5-1/6), -2.25-0.25 X 15 OS (6/4.5-1/6). This patient's ZCSBV is shown in Figure 11.9. The phorias, the receded NPC, the low PRV, the low NRA, and the pattern of the ZCSBV indicate convergence insufficiency. It may be noted that Sheard's criterion was not met at 40 cm. The patient was started on a vision therapy program that included daily at-home work on a Brock string and Tranaglyphs and once a week office visits for additional training. After a few weeks of training, the patient reported that her headaches and eyestrain were much less frequent. The base-out fusional vergence range at 40 cm had improved to 20/27/8, the NRA had improved to +2.00D, and the NPC was found to be 4.5 cm.

## REFERENCES

1. Saladin JJ. Horizontal prism prescription. In: Cotter SA, ed. Clinical Uses of Prism-A Spectrum of Applications-Mosby's Optometric Problem Solving Series. St Louis: Mosby-Year Book, 1995:109-147.

2. Rutstein RP, Daum KM. Anomalies of Binocular Vision: Diagnosis and Management. St. Louis: Mosby, 1998:154-183.

3. Newman JM. Analysis, interpretation, and prescription for the ametropias and heterophorias. In: Benjamin WJ, ed. Borish's Clinical Refraction, 2nd ed. St. Louis: Butterworth Heinemann Elsevier, 2006:963-1025.

4. Griffin JR, Grisham JD. Binocular Anomalies: Diagnosis and Vision Therapy, 4th ed. Amsterdam: Butterworth-Heinemann, 2002:92-97.

5. Scheiman M, Wick B. Clinical Management of Binocular Vision-Heterophoric, Accommodative, and Eye Movement Disorders, 2nd ed. Philadelphia: Lippincott Williams & Wilkins, 2002: 71-79.

6. Daum KM. The course and effect of visual training on the vergence system. Am J Optom Physiol Opt 1982;59:223-227.

7. Porcar E, Martinez-Palomera A. Prevalence of general binocular dysfunction in a population of university students. Optom Vis Sci 1997;74:111-113.

8. Rouse MW, Borsting E, Hyman L, et al. Frequency of convergence insufficiency among fifth and sixth graders. Optom Vis Sci 1999;76:643-649.

9. Montés-Mico R. Prevalence of general dysfunctions in binocular vision. Ann Ophthalmol 2001;33:205-208.

10. Daum KM. Characteristics of convergence insufficiency. Am J Optom Physiol Opt 1988;65:426-438.

11. Rouse MW, Hyman L, Hussein M, et al. How do you make the diagnosis of convergence insufficiency?: Survey results. J Optom Vis Dev 1997;28:91-97.

12. Cooper J, Duckman R. Convergence insufficiency: incidence, diagnosis, and treatment. J Am Optom Assoc 1978;49:673-680.

13. Daum KM. Convergence insufficiency. Am J Optom Physiol Opt 1984;61:16-22.

14. Cooper J, Selenow A, Ciuffreda KJ, et al. Reduction of asthenopia in patients with convergence insufficiency after fusional vergence training. Am J Optom Physiol Opt 1983;60:982-989.

15. Daum KM. Characteristics of exodeviations. II. Changes with treatment with orthoptics. Am J Optom Physiol Opt 1986;63:244-251.

16. Suchoff IB, Petito GT. The efficacy of visual therapy: accommodative disorders and non-strabismic anomalies of binocular vision. J Am Optom Assoc 1986;57:119-125.

17. Griffin JR. Efficacy of vision therapy for nonstrabismic vergence anomalies. Am J Optom Physiol Opt 1987;64:411-414.

18. Grisham JD. Visual therapy results for convergence insufficiency: a literature review. Am J Optom Physiol Opt 1988;65:448-454.

19. Scheiman M, Mitchell GL, Cotter S, et al. A randomized clinical trial of treatments for convergence insufficiency in children. Arch Ophthalmol 2005;123:14-24.

20. Scheiman M, Mitchell GL, Cotter S, et al. A randomized clinical trial of vision therapy/orthoptics versus pencil push-ups for the treatment of convergence insufficiency. Optom Vis Sci 2005;82:583-593.

21. Stavis M, Murray M, Jenkins P, et al. Objective improvement from base-in prisms for reading discomfort associated with mini-convergence insufficiency type exophoria in school children. Bin Vis Strab Quart 2002;17:135-142.

22. Scheiman M, Cotter S, Mitchell GL, et al. Randomised clinical trial of the effectiveness of base-in prism reading glasses versus placebo reading glasses for symptomatic convergence insufficiency in children. Br J Ophthalmol 2005;89:1318-1323.

23. Hokoda SC. General binocular dysfunctions in an urban optometry clinic. J Am Optom Assoc 1985;56:560-562.

24. Scheiman M, Gallaway M, Coulter R, et al. Prevalence of vision and ocular disease conditions in a clinical pediatric population. J Am Optom Assoc 1996;67:193-202.

25. Wick BC. Horizontal deviations. In: Amos JF, ed. Diagnosis and Management in Vision Care. Boston: Butterworth-Heinemann, 1987:461-510.

26. Grosvenor T. Primary Care Optometry, 5th ed. St. Louis: Butterworth Heinemann Elsevier, 2007:260-264.

27. Daum KM. Negative vergence training in humans. Am J Optom Physiol Opt 1986;63:487-496.

28. Shorter AD, Hatch SW. Vision therapy for convergence excess. N Engl J Optom 1993;45:51-53.

29. Gallaway M, Scheiman M. The efficacy of vision therapy for convergence excess. J Am Optom Assoc 1997;68:81-86.

30. Ficarra AP, Berman J, Rosenfield M, Portello JK. Vision training: Predictive factors for success in visual therapy for patients with convergence excess. J Optom Vis Dev 1996;27:213-219.

31. Scheiman M, Wick B. Clinical Management of Binocular Vision-Heterophoric, Accommodative, and Eye Movement Disorders, 2nd ed. Philadelphia: Lippincott Williams & Wilkins, 2002:249-253.

32. Scheiman M, Gallaway M, Ciner E. Divergence insufficiency: characteristics, diagnosis, and treatment. Am J Optom Physiol Opt 1986;63:425-431.

33. Rutstein RP, Daum KM. Anomalies of Binocular Vision: Diagnosis & Management. St. Louis: Mosby, 1998:162-163.

34. Pickwell LD. Prevalence and management of divergence excess. Am J Optom Physiol Opt 1979;56:78-81.

35. Daum KM. Divergence excess: characteristics and results of treatment with orthoptics. Ophthal Physiol Opt 1984;4: 15-24.

36. Scheiman M, Wick B. Clinical Management of Binocular Vision-Heterophoric, Accommodative, and Eye Movement Disorders, 2nd ed. Philadelphia: Lippincott Williams & Wilkins, 2002:289-290.

37. Flax N. Management of divergence excess intermittent exotropia. J Behav Optom 1996;7:66,72-73.

38. Cooper J. A viewpoint: intermittent exotropia of the divergence excess type. J Behav Optom 1996;7:67-72.

39. Daum KM. Characteristics of exodeviations: I. A comparison of three classes. Am J Optom Physiol Opt 1986;63:237-243.

40. Daum KM. Equal exodeviations: characteristics and results of treatment with orthoptics. Aust J Optom 1984;67:53-59.

41. Grisham JD. The dynamics of fusional vergence eye movements in binocular dysfunction. Am J Optom Physiol Opt 1980;57:645-655.

42. Grisham JD. Treatment of binocular dysfunctions. In: Schor CM, Ciuffreda KJ, eds. Vergence Eye Movements: Basic and Clinical Aspects. Boston: Butterworth-Heinemann, 1983:605-646.

43. Schapero M. The characteristics of ten basic visual training problems. Am J Optom Arch Am Acad Optom 1955;32:333-342.

44. Griffin JR, Grisham JD. Binocular Anomalies: Diagnosis and Vision Therapy, 4th ed. Amsterdam: Butterworth-Heinemann, 2002:96.

45. Scheiman M, Wick B. Clinical Management of Binocular Vision-Heterophoric, Accommodative, and Eye Movement Disorders, 2nd ed. Philadelphia: Lippincott Williams & Wilkins, 2002:306-15.

46. Richman JE, Cron MT. Guide to Vision Therapy. South Bend, IN: Bernell Corporation, 1987:17-18.

47. Worrell BE Jr, Hirsch MJ, Morgan MW. An evaluation of prism prescribed by Sheard's criterion. Am J Optom Arch Am Acad Optom 1971;48:373-376.

48. Payne CR, Grisham JD, Thomas KL. A clinical evaluation of fixation disparity. Am J Optom Physiol Opt 1974;51:88-90.

49. O'Leary CI, Evans BJW. Double-masked randomized placebo-controlled trial of the effect of prismatic corrections on rate of reading and the relationship with symptoms. Ophthal Physiol Opt 2006;26:555-565.

50. Carter DB. Effects of prolonged wearing of prism. Am J Optom Arch Am Acad Optom 1963;40:265-273.

51. Griffin JR, Grisham JD. Binocular Anomalies-Diagnosis and Vision Therapy, 4th ed. Amsterdam: Butterworth-Heinemann, 2002:90-92.

52. Schor CM. Fixation disparity and vergence adaptation. In: Schor CM, Ciuffreda KJ, eds. Vergence Eye Movements: Basic and Clinical Aspects. Boston: Butterworth-Heinemann, 1983:465-516.

53. Borish IM. Clinical Refraction, 3rd ed. Chicago: Professional Press, 1970:307-344.

54. Grosvenor T. Primary Care Optometry, 5th ed. St. Louis: Butterworth Heinemann Elsevier, 2007:99-111.

55. Birnbaum MH. Optometric Management of Nearpoint Vision Disorders. Boston: Butterworth-Heinemann, 1993:89-96.

56. Amos JF. Patient history. In: Eskridge JB, Amos JF, Bartlett JD, eds. Clinical Procedures in Optometry. Philadelphia: Lippincott, 1991:3-16.

57. Haine CL. The ophthalmic case historian. In: Benjamin WJ, ed. Borish's Clinical Refraction, 2nd ed. St. Louis: Butterworth Heinemann Elsevier, 2006:195-216.

58. Getz DJ. Strabismus and Amblyopia, revised ed. Santa Ana, CA: Optometric Extension Program, 1990.

59. Caloroso EE, Rouse MW. Clinical Management of Strabismus. Boston: Butterworth-Heinemann, 1993.

60. Rutstein RP, Daum KM. Anomalies of Binocular Vision: Diagnosis & Management. St. Louis: Mosby, 1998.

61. Griffin JR, Grisham JD. Binocular Anomalies-Diagnosis and Vision Therapy, 4th ed. Amsterdam: Butterworth-Heinemann, 2002.

62. von Noorden GK, Campos EC. Binocular Vision and Ocular Motility-Theory and Management of Strabismus, 6th ed. St Louis: Mosby, 2002.

## PRACTICE PROBLEMS

For each of the following cases:

    a. Plot the findings.

b. What is the calculated ACA ratio?

c. What is the gradient ACA ratio?

d. Is Sheard's criterion met at distance and at 40 cm? If not, what prism would be necessary to meet it?

e. Is Percival's criterion met at distance and at 40 cm? If not, what prism would be necessary to meet it?

f. Is the 1:1 rule met at distance and at 40 cm in esophoria cases? If not, what prism would be necessary to meet it?

g. Which of the vergence disorder case types do the findings indicate?

h. What is the Mallett classification at distance and at 40 cm?

i. What treatments are used for this case type?

j. If prism or a lens add is indicated, what power would be appropriate?

All test findings were taken through the distance subjective refraction except for near phorias taken through an add as noted.

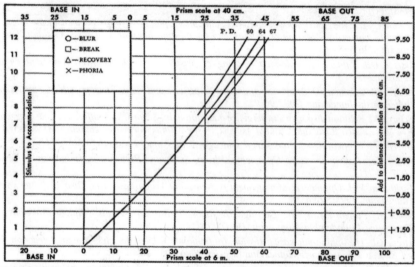

| Patient RP | | | | | | |
|---|---|---|---|---|---|---|
| | Phoria | Base-in | Base-out | Plus to blur | Minus to blur |
| Distance | ortho | X/8/4 | 12/18/8 | | |
| 40 cm | 10 exo | 17/24/8 | 8/14/2 | +2.25 | -7.50 |
| 40 cm +1.00 D add | 11 exo | | | | |

PD, 64 mm; Amplitude of accommodation, 10.0 D; NPC, 12 cm; Distance associated phoria, 0; 40 cm associated phoria, 3Δ BI; MEM, 0.25 D lag.

$$\text{Calc. ACA} = \frac{15 - 0 + (-10)}{25} = \frac{5^{\Delta}}{2.5} = 2.0^{\Delta}/D$$

$$\text{Gradient ACA} = \frac{(-10) - (-11)}{-1} = \frac{+1^{\Delta}}{+1D} = 1^{\Delta}/D$$

128

Conv. Excess L

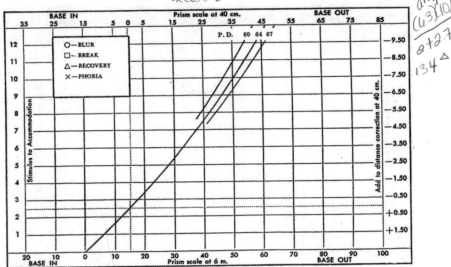

| Patient DE | | | | | |
|---|---|---|---|---|---|
| | Phoria | Base-in | Base-out | Plus to blur | Minus to blur |
| Distance | ortho | X/8/6 | 10/20/8 | | |
| 40 cm | 7 eso | 8/18/4 | 25/36/18 | +2.25 | -1.50 |
| 40 cm +1.00 D add | 1 exo | | | | |

PD, 63 mm; Amplitude of accommodation, 12.5 D; NPC, 2 cm; Distance associated phoria, 0; 40 cm associated phoria, 2△ BO; slow on minus side of binocular lens rock.

$$Calc\ ACA = \frac{14.75 - 0 + 7}{2.5} = \frac{21.75^△}{2.5D} = 8.7^△/D$$ (63mm @ 40)

O — for low findings

$$Gradient\ ACA = \frac{7-(-1)}{+1} = \frac{8^△}{1} = 8^△/D$$

* Better opt for conv.
excess = plus add for
near 2° = VT

R must be twice the demand

Sheard Crit. (not met @ near) = 2/3(7) - 1/3(8) = 14/3 - 8/3 = 2△ BO

1-1 rule (BC it's eso)
P = (7-4)/2 = 3/2 = 1 1/2 BO

Perc = met @ near
= not met @ distance

P = 1/3 G - 2/3 L = 1/3(25) - 2/3(8) = 25/3 - 16/3 = 9/3 = 3△ BO

RT

Ex: RP

Conv. Ampl.
$$\frac{(64)(10)}{12 + 2.7} = \frac{640}{14.7} = 43.5 D$$

Mallett would recomm
3△ BI

Sheard's Cri

P = 2/3D - 1/3R =
2/3(10) - 1/3(8) = 20/3 - 8/3
= 4△ BI

**129** Perc = 1/3 G - 2/3 L = 1/3(17) - 2/3(8)
= 17/3 - 16/3 = 1/3△ BI

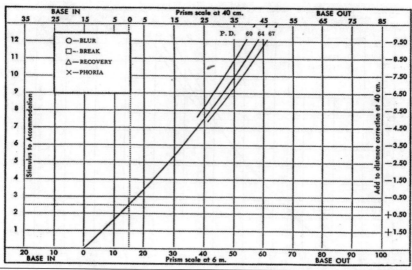

| Patient AT | | | | | |
|---|---|---|---|---|---|
| | Phoria | Base-in | Base-out | Plus to blur | Minus to blur |
| Distance | (6 eso) | (X/4/0) | 22/32/14 | | |
| 40 cm | ortho | 12/19/10 | 18/22/12 | +2.50 | -4.50 |
| 40 cm +1.00 D add | 3 exo | | | | ~ |

PD, 62 mm; Amplitude of accommodation, 11.0 D; NPC, 6 cm; Distance associated phoria, 3Δ BO; 40 cm associated phoria, 0.

$$\text{Calc ACA} = \frac{14.5 - 64 + 0}{25} = \frac{8.5}{2.5D} = 3.4^\triangle/D \text{ (a little low)}$$

$$\text{Grad ACA} = \frac{0 - (-3)}{+1} = 3^\triangle/D \text{ (lower end of nom)}$$

Tent. Diag. Divergence Insuff.

Sheard's Criterion $P = \frac{2}{3}(6) - \frac{1}{3}(4) = \frac{12}{3} - \frac{4}{3} = \frac{8}{3}$

Percival Crit $= \frac{1}{3}G - \frac{2}{3}L = \frac{1}{3}(22) - \frac{2}{3}(4) = \frac{22}{3} - \frac{8}{3} = \frac{14}{3}$

$$P = \frac{6 - 0}{2} = \frac{6}{2} = 3$$

↑ACA tells you how much to change phoria.

(+) add is a great tx option.

Eso means you don't want to undercorrect a hyperope.

130

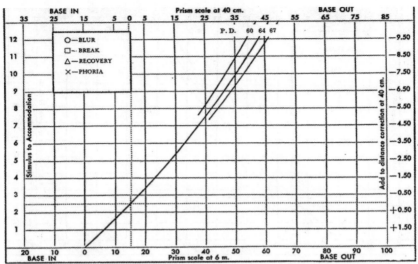

| Patient BC | | | | | |
|---|---|---|---|---|---|
| | Phoria | Base-in | Base-out | Plus to blur | Minus to blur |
| Distance | 8 exo | X/10/6 | 5/12/7 | | |
| 40 cm | 1 exo | 14/22/10 | 18/24/12 | +1.75 | -2.75 |
| 40 cm +1.00 D add | 8 exo | | | | |

PD, 60 mm; Amplitude of accommodation, 14.3 D; NPC, 3 cm; Distance associated phoria, 3Δ BI ; 40 cm associated phoria, 0.

$$Gradient\ ACA = 7\ (abnormal)$$

$$Calc\ ACA = \frac{14.1 - (-8) + (-1)}{2.5} = 8.4\,°/_D \quad Tent. Diag.\ Div. Excess$$
(Low BO @ distance)

(-) adds risks strain on acc. bc (-) adds increase accomm.

Tx: ① VT
② undercorrect a hyperope

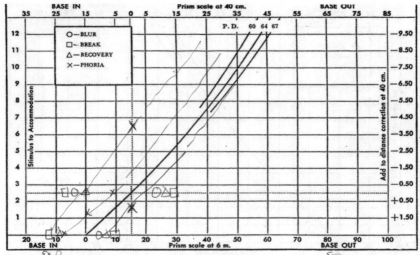

**Patient DW**

|  | Phoria | Base-in | Base-out | Plus to blur | Minus to blur |
|---|---|---|---|---|---|
| Distance | 7 exo | X/12/8 | 5/10/6 |  |  |
| 40 cm | 11 exo | 18/22/15 | 8/14/7 | +1.25 | -4.25 |
| 40 cm +1.00 D add | 14 exo |  |  |  |  |

PD, 60 mm; Amplitude of accommodation, 12.0 D; NPC, 8 cm; Distance associated phoria, 3Δ BI ; 40 cm associated phoria, 4Δ BI; slow on plus side of binocular lens rock.

High Exo Distance + near ( Div Excess)

(60mm PD)

Calc ACA = $\dfrac{14.1 - (-7) + (-11)}{2.5}$ = 4.0 $^{\Delta}$/D

Grad ACA = 3

Tent Dx: Basic Esophoria

P = 2/3(7) - 1/3(5) = 14/3 - 5/3 = 3$^{\Delta}$BI

P = 2/3(11) - 1/3(8) = 22/3 - 8/3 = 14/3 = 4 2/3 $^{\Delta}$BI

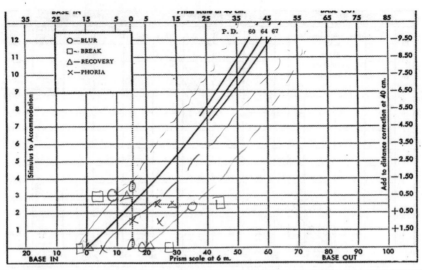

| Patient HH | | | | | |
|---|---|---|---|---|---|
| | Phoria | Base-in | Base-out | Plus to blur | Minus to blur |
| Distance | 7 eso | X/3/0 | 18/28/20 | | |
| 40 cm | 8 eso | 6/12/2 | 24/30/14 | +2.50 | -1.25 |
| 40 cm +1.00 D add | 3 eso | | | | |

PD, 64 mm; Amplitude of accommodation, 14.3 D; NPC, 1 cm; Distance associated phoria, 3Δ BO; 40 cm associated phoria, 3Δ BO; slow on minus side of binocular lens rock.

$$\text{Calc ACA} = \frac{15-7+8}{2.50} = \frac{16^\Delta}{2.5D} = 6.4^\Delta/D$$

Tent Dx:

Basic ESO

$$\text{Grad ACA} = \frac{(+8)-(+3)}{+1} = 5^\Delta/1D = 5^\Delta/D$$

$$P = 2/3 (7) - 1/3 (3) = 14/3 - 8/3 = 11/3 = 3.3^\Delta BO$$

$$P = 2/3 (8) - 1/3 (6) = 16/3 - 6/3 = 10/3 = 3.3^\Delta BO$$

$$P = 1/3 (18) - 2/3 (3) = 18/3 - 6/3 = 12/3 = 4^\Delta BO$$

$$P = 1/3 (24) - 2/3 (6) = 24/3 - 12/3 = 4^\Delta BO$$

$$P = (7-0)/2 = 3.5^\Delta BO$$

$$P = (8-2)/2 = 3^\Delta BO$$

$$8 \text{ eso} / 5^\Delta/D = 1.6D \rightarrow 1.75D \text{ (As long as there is no distance complaint, this is an option.)}$$

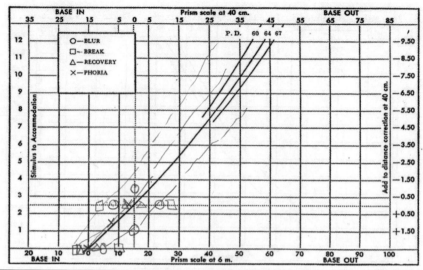

| Patient SM | | | | | | |
|---|---|---|---|---|---|---|
| | Phoria | Base-in | Base-out | Plus to blur | Minus to blur |
| Distance | ortho | X/3/1 | 5/10/4 | | |
| 40 cm | 2 exo | 6/11/3 | 8/12/2 | +1.50 | -1.25 |
| 40 cm +1.00 D add | 6 exo | | | | |

PD, 64 mm; Amplitude of accommodation, 11.0 D; NPC, 10 cm; Distance associated phoria, 0; 40 cm associated phoria, 0; poor vergence facility.

$$Calc\ ACA = \frac{15 - 0 + (-2)}{2.5} = \frac{13^{\triangle}}{2.5D} = 5.2^{\triangle}/D \quad All\ vergences\ are\ low.$$

$$Grad\ ACA = \frac{-2 - (-6)}{+1} = 4^{\triangle}/1D = 4^{\triangle}/D$$

134

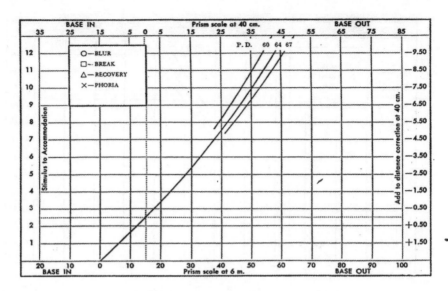

| Patient JH | | | | | |
|---|---|---|---|---|---|
| | Phoria | Base-in | Base-out | Plus to blur | Minus to blur |
| Distance | ortho | X/8/3 | 10/20/12 | | |
| 40 cm | 10 eso | 6/10/2 | 24/30/18 | +2.25 | -1.25 |
| 40 cm +1.00 D add | 2 eso | | | | |

PD, 62 mm; Amplitude of accommodation, 15.0 D; NPC, 1 cm; Distance associated phoria, 0; 40 cm associated phoria, 4Δ BO; +1.25 D reduces eso fixation disparity to zero.

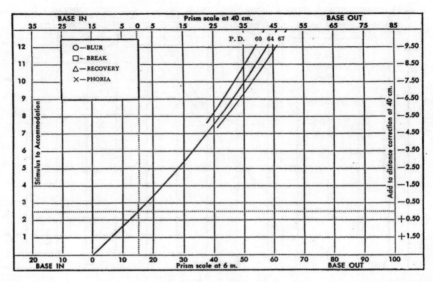

| Patient JP | | | | | |
|---|---|---|---|---|---|
| | Phoria | Base-in | Base-out | Plus to blur | Minus to blur |
| Distance | ortho | X/7/4 | 10/14/8 | | |
| 40 cm | 9 exo | 15/22/14 | 6/12/4 | +2.00 | -7.50 |
| 40 cm +1.00 D add | 10 exo | | | | |

PD, 63 mm; Amplitude of accommodation, 14.0 D; NPC, 11 cm; Distance associated phoria, 0; 40 cm associated phoria, 3Δ BI; MEM, 0.50 D lag.

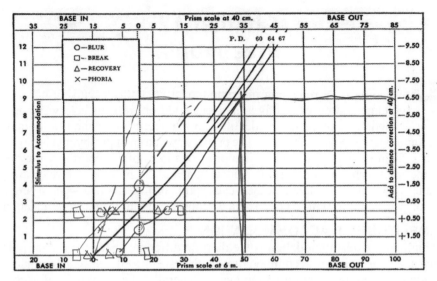

| Patient NE | | | | | |
|---|---|---|---|---|---|
| | Phoria | Base-in | Base-out | Plus to blur | Minus to blur |
| Distance | ortho | X/7/4 | 9/18/6 | | |
| 40 cm | 10 exo *High* | 12/20/10 | (10/14/6) | +1.75 | (1.50) |
| 40 cm +1.00 D add | 11 exo | | | | |

PD, 62 mm; Amplitude of accommodation, 9.2 D; NPC, 10 cm; Distance associated phoria, 0; 40 cm associated phoria, 2Δ BI; MEM, 1.50 D lag.

$$CALC\ ACA = \frac{14.5 - 0 + (-10)}{2.5} = 4.5^\Delta / 2.5D = 1.8^\Delta / D$$

$$Grad\ ACA = \frac{-10 - (-11)}{+1} = 1^\Delta / 1D = 1^\Delta / D$$

Tent. Dx: Pseudo conv. Insuff.

# Chapter 12
# Presbyopia

**P**resbyopia is "a reduction in accommodative ability occurring normally with age and necessitating a plus lens addition for satisfactory seeing at near, sometimes quantitatively identified by the recession of the near-point of accommodation beyond 20 cm."[1] The primary symptom of presbyopia is blurred near vision or difficulty reading fine print. Patients often report that they get some improvement in clarity of reading material by holding it further away. Patients occasionally state that their eyes "pull" or feel strained when trying to read. The defining sign of presbyopia is reduced amplitude of accommodation.

## AMPLITUDE OF ACCOMMODATION

Amplitude of accommodation is the dioptric difference between the far point and the near point of accommodation with respect to the spectacle plane or some other reference point of the eye.[2] Generally, the amplitude of accommodation is measured by noting the distance from the punctum proximum or near-point of accommodation to the spectacle plane while the patient wears the correction for ametropia. The near-point of accommodation usually is determined by a pushup test performed monocularly with each eye and binocularly, and it is the closest of the three measurements thus derived.[3,4] The distance measured can then be converted into diopters. If the patient is not wearing lenses equal to the subjective refraction during the test, then adjustment must be made to the dioptric value obtained: an increase for any amount of uncorrected hyperopia, or a decrease for any amount of uncorrected myopia. A formula for amplitude of accommodation in diopters is as follows:

Amplitude of accommodation = [100 / NPA in cm] + [RE - L]

where NPA represents the near-point of accommodation (usually measured in cm), RE represents the patient's refractive error in diopters, and L represents the power in diopters of the lens worn while the measurement of the near-point of accommodation was taken.

There is a predictable normal gradual decline in amplitude throughout one's life. Various tables of amplitude norms for given ages are available. Formulas for the expected changes in amplitude of accommodation with age also can be used. Hofstetter[5,6] derived the following formulas (also shown in Figure 12.1) for expected amplitudes from the data of Donders, Duane, and Kaufman:

Maximum amplitude = 25 − (0.4) (age)

Probable amplitude = 18.5 − (0.3) (age)

Minimum amplitude = 15 − (0.25) (age)

These formulas are applicable up to about 60 years of age. At approximately 60 years of age, absolute presbyopia, in which accommodative ability is completely absent,[1] has been reached. Patients with absolute presbyopia often will have amplitude of accommodation measurements up to about 1.00

D because of the depth of focus of the eye.

If we look again at the definition of presbyopia that opened this chapter, we can see the last part of the definition states that presbyopia is "sometimes quantitatively identified by the recession of the near point of accommodation beyond 20 cm." In other words, the amplitude of accommodation has declined to less than 5 D. If we put 5 D into the probable amplitude formula above, we find an age of 45 years. Typical ages when presbyopia is first seen clinically in regions with temperate climates are 40 to 45 years.[7] The onset of presbyopia is earlier in areas closer to the equator.[7] The earliest known quantification of the advance of presbyopia with age has been attributed to Daza de Valdes in 1623.[8]

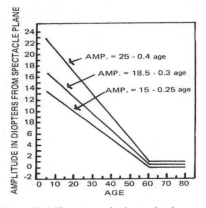

Figure 12.1 The expected relationship between amplitude of accommodation in diopters and age in years, according to Hofstetter's formulas. (Reprinted with permission from Hofstetter HW. A useful age-amplitude formula. Pennsylvania Optom 1947;7:5-8)

## RULES AND TESTS FOR PRESCRIBING PRESBYOPIC ADDS

Various rules of thumb can be applied, along with a consideration of the patient's needs and preferences and the previous prescription, to determine the power of the add to be prescribed.[9-13] One such rule is to keep half the amplitude in reserve. In other words, for most visual tasks the patient should not be required to use more than half the amplitude of accommodation. The use of this rule necessitates the accurate determination of the patient's habitual preferred working distances. A formula for the rule can be written as follows:

Add = Stimulus to accommodation at working distance – (amplitude of accommodation / 2)

For instance, if an individual's usual working distance is 40 cm and the amplitude of accommodation is 1.50 D, the add proposed by this rule is calculated as

Add = (100 / 40cm) – (1.50 D / 2)

Add = 2.50 D – 0.75 D

Add = 1.75 D

A second rule used to determine an add involves balancing the plus-lens-to-blur (negative relative accommodation) and the minus-lens-to-blur (positive relative accommodation) findings. It states that the proper add allows the absolute value of the negative relative accommodation (NRA) finding to be equal to the absolute value of the positive relative accommodation (PRA) finding; if this value cannot be achieved by an add that is a multiple of 0.25 D, then the NRA should be 0.25 D larger than the PRA. The latter qualifier is used because adds are available only in 0.25 D steps. It is implied that this criterion refers to the patient's usual working distance. It may be noted as long as the PRA and NRA points on the graph fall at the top (amplitude of accommodation line) and bottom of the zone of clear single binocular vision (ZCSBV), respectively, rather than at the left and right sides of the ZCSBV, respectively, the add proposed by this rule will be the same as the add proposed by keeping half the amplitude in reserve. An example of the use of the rule is

Working distance = 40 cm

NRA at 40 cm through +2.00 add = +0.50 D

PRA at 40 cm through +2.00 add = -1.00 D

Add suggested = +1.75 D

If a + 1.75 D add is used, the result will be an interval of 0.75 D to both the NRA endpoint and the PRA endpoint.

The near binocular cross cylinder (BCC) test yields the lens power with which the retina is conjugate to the test target. Some practitioners use the BCC test to derive a tentative presbyopic add, which then can be refined by additional testing, such as the NRA, PRA, and accommodative ranges. By itself, the BCC often will give an add power that is too high for a beginning presbyope, but is quite close to the final prescription for the advanced presbyope.

Another useful test is the plus build-up test. The test is started with the distance subjective refraction lenses. The patient is instructed to look at the 20/20 letters or letters at the patient's best acuity level on a reduced Snellen card at 40 cm or the patient's usual working distance. Plus is added in 0.25 D steps. The patient is instructed to report when the letters are first readable. The clinician notes this add amount. Then more plus is added in 0.25 D steps, and the patient reports when the letters are seen most clearly. This lens power can be refined by additional add testing, such as the NRA, PRA, and accommodative ranges. The final prescription is usually about 0.50 D more plus than the "first readable" lens add level on the plus build-up test, and the final prescription usually is also equal to the patient's preferred add level on the test.

## ACCOMMODATIVE RANGES

An additional test that some practitioners use is the measurement of accommodative ranges through the near correction.[14] This test involves the determination of a near-point and far-point of accommodation through the proposed near correction. Because a range of accommodation (linear distance from near-point to far-point) is not directly converted into amplitude of accommodation in diopters, the data obtained from the ranges cannot be directly interpreted to yield a value for an add. The actual purpose of the test, as used by most practitioners, is to demonstrate to patients the distances over which they can expect to have clear vision and to give the examiner confidence that previous testing has resulted in an acceptable nearpoint add. Most commonly, the tentative near-point prescription is placed in a trial frame, and subjective comments as well as the near-point and far-point are elicited by moving the test card nearer

**Table 12.1 Methods for deriving presbyopic add power**

(1) Balance the NRA and PRA
Find the plus add from which $|NRA| = |PRA|$
Or $|NRA| = |PRA| + 0.25 D$
(2) Keep half the amplitude in reserve
Add = Accommmodative stimulus for working distance – (Amplitude of accommodation / 2)
(3) Binocular cross cylinder test
(4) Plus build-up test
(a) +0.50 D over the minimum plus to 20/20 at near
(b) increase plus to maximum clarity of nearpoint letters
(5) Age

to the patient and then moving it farther away. The add can be increased or decreased to alter the range and/or to improve the subjective reports of the patient.

## RELATIONSHIP OF PRESCRIBED ADD TO AGE

Because the amplitude of accommodation declines with age, the power of the presbyopic reading addition will increase with age. Several texts contain tables with expected add as a function of age.[9,10,13] It is helpful to consider age as a factor to check the proposed add, but the clinician should not rely on age over carefully performed testing in prescribing adds for presbyopia. A list of methods of deriving presbyopic add power is summarized in Table 12.1.

## OTHER CONSIDERATIONS IN PRESCRIBING FOR PRESBYOPIA

There are many factors to consider in prescribing for presbyopia. As a result, it is difficult to identify a single rule of thumb as being used consistently by most optometrists.[15] Such subjective factors as the patient's previous prescription, visual symptoms, and habitual working distance must be taken into account.[10,13] Patients' complaints that they must hold near work farther away than they would like indicate that an increase in plus power is advisable, whereas lens power changes when patients are satisfied with a previous prescription may cause patient dissatisfaction, regardless of the fact that the change may be indicated by a rule of thumb. Power changes should be large enough to alleviate the patient's complaints, but should not be so large that adaptation difficulties would result.[16] Even factors such as the physical build of the patient may be of importance. For example, a smaller individual with shorter arms may have presbyopic symptoms earlier than a taller person of comparable age and amplitude because the person with shorter arms holds reading material closer.[7] Refractive error can also affect the onset of presbyopia with potentially earlier onset in hyperopia because the accommodative demand at the principal plane of the eye is greater for spectacle corrected hyperopes than for spectacle corrected myopes for the same distance from the spectacle plane.[17,18] The patient's pupil size can also be a factor in that persons with smaller pupils have greater depths of focus and may have later onset of presbyopic symptoms.

Some general guidelines for the management of presbyopia which can be briefly summarized are as follows:

1. Don't delay prescription of the first bifocal or progressive addition lens for too long. Adaptation to the lenses can become more difficult when the add power is greater.

2. Think in terms of total nearpoint power rather than just the power of the add. In some cases a change in distance correction while maintaining the same add power may be the best way to solve a nearpoint problem.

3. The case history is very important in deciding whether a change in total nearpoint power is needed.

4. If emmetropic patients with presbyopia want single vision reading glasses, be sure to warn them that distance vision will be blurry with the lenses.

5. In general, prescribe the least amount of total nearpoint power that provides maximum visual acuity and optimum visual performance.

6. "Trial framing" the proposed total nearpoint power is a very useful way of demonstrating ranges of clear vision to the patient and of subjectively confirming the nearpoint prescription.

7. Proper location of the reading portion of the lens and proper frame adjustment are essential for acceptable use of bifocals or progressive addition lenses.

8. Consider the nature and working distances of the patient's occupational tasks and recreational activities.

There are several texts and resources that give detailed discussions of these and other factors to be considered in prescribing for presbyopia.[10,19-23] A text on the treatment of computer-related vision problems includes a chapter on computer use by the patient with presbyopia.[24]

## NEARPOINT PHORIA AND VERGENCE RANGE TESTING IN PRESBYOPIA

Dissociated phorias and vergence ranges can be tested at near using the same procedures in presbyopic patients as in non-presbyopic patients with one exception. Testing must be done through a plus add. This is sometimes referred to as the tentative add. It can be derived, for example, by using the binocular cross cylinder test or by using the keep half the amplitude in reserve calculation. In other words, the near phoria and near vergence ranges can be taken through the binocular cross cylinder test endpoint or through the add that would keep half the amplitude in reserve. The tentative add is often the starting point for NRA and PRA testing in presbyopes.

## EXOPHORIA IN PRESBYOPIA

Because plus adds are necessary for clear vision in presbyopia, patients will often show a high exophoria on dissociated phoria testing at near. The high nearpoint exophoria often associated with presbyopic adds may or may not be associated with diplopia or asthenopic symptoms. Presbyopes with high nearpoint exophoria are less often symptomatic than are nonpresbyopes with comparable amounts of exophoria. This situation can be explained by the

**Table 12.2. Summary of the characteristics of high exophoria at near in presbyopia**

- A natural consequence of the nearpoint plus add for presbyopia
- Usually does not cause symptoms
- Morgan's norms and Sheard's criterion not used in presbyopia
- Zero associated phoria at near is usually correlated with lack of symptoms. A non- zero associated phoria at near can be used as a guide for prescribing base-in prism for near.
- Potential treatments if the nearpoint exophoria is a problem:
  Decenter reading segments in for a base-in prism effect
  Single vision reading glasses with base-in prism
  Base-in prism in the reading segments
  Vision therapy to improve positive fusional vergence

theory that presbyopes can use accommodative convergence at near to help maintain fusion.[25] Presbyopia occurs due to changes in the accommodative apparatus within the eye, not the innervation going to the eye. Therefore, stimulation of the near triad may result in limited accommodation, but accommodative convergence will still occur. Thus the individual with presbyopia can use accommodative convergence to supplement positive fusional vergence.

When the exophoria does result in asthenopia, alternatives available for correction are: (1) segments decentered to get a base-in effect (it may be necessary to use a wider segment when it is decentered so that the patient is not looking through the edge of the segment); (2) a separate prescription for near work, with base-in prism or decentering to obtain a base-in effect; (3) vision therapy; or (4) base-in prism in the reading segments.[26] Vision therapy to increase positive fusional vergence has a high success rate in presbyopia.[27-31]

Sheedy[32] emphasized that it should be determined whether the patient has an exo fixation disparity when a large nearpoint exophoria is present. No correction may be necessary when an exo fixation disparity is not uncovered. Thus whenever a high exophoria is found, testing with an associated phoria device may be warranted. If a non-zero associated phoria is found, vision therapy may be indicated or the amount of base-in prism from the associated phoria can be prescribed. The characteristics of nearpoint exophoria in presbyopia are summarized in Table 12.2.

## ZONE OF CLEAR SINGLE BINOCULAR VISION IN PRESBYOPIA

The presbyopic ZCSBV may show only a decrease in height without any other apparent change in the five fundamental variables of the zone.[33] Associated either directly or indirectly with the decrease in amplitude of accommodation are several apparent variations in the results of conventional clinic tests and in the appearance of the ZCSBV:

1. An increase in exophoria or a decrease in esophoria in the near-point tests attributable to a lower amount of accommodative convergence, because a plus add substitutes for accommodation.

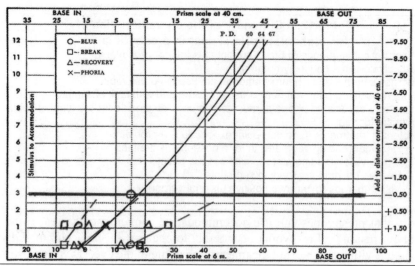

Figure 12.2 An example of findings in presbyopia.

|  | Phoria | Base-in | Base-out | NRA | Minus to blur |
|---|---|---|---|---|---|
| Distance | 1 exo | X/8/4 | X/18/12 |  |  |
| 40 cm +1.25 D add | 8 exo | 17/22/14 | X/12/6 | +1.25 | -1.75 |

Amplitude of accommodation = 3.00 D; working distance = approximately 40 cm; BCC = +1.25 D add; 40 cm associated phoria with +1.00 D add = 0.

2. An increase in the nearpoint base-in blur, break, and recovery and a decrease in the base-out blur, break, and recovery also resulting from the reduction in accommodative convergence associated with the plus add.

3. The base-out limit possibly showing a break without a blur because the presbyope may not be able to accommodate sufficiently to obtain a blur on this test.

4. A lower minus-lens-to-blur directly attributable to the reduction in the amplitude of accommodation.

5. The possible addition of a rightward extension to the upper right corner of the zone. This tail, or spike, occurs only in some individuals, and only when a base-out limit is taken at a stimulus to accommodation level at or near the patient's amplitude of accommodation. One possible explanation for this extension is that a greater accommodative convergence occurs because an increased innervation to accommodation is necessary for an accommodative response at or near the amplitude.[34,35]

6. Because the height of the ZCSBV is reduced in presbyopia due to the low amplitude of accommodation, relatively short line segments determine the base-in, phoria, and base-out lines. As a result, a small error can cause a relatively large distortion of the slope of the zone in presbyopia.[36] These distortions can be particularly pronounced if near tests are performed through adds that require presbyopes to use almost all their amplitudes of accommodation. Because of these distortions, the ZCSBV is not as useful for advanced presbyopes as it is for non-presbyopes.

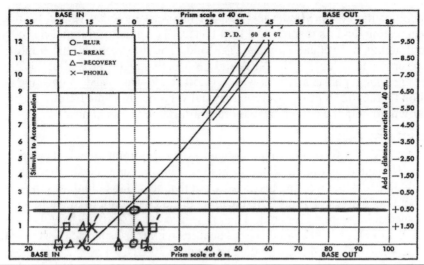

Figure 12.3 Another example of findings in presbyopia.

| | Phoria | Base-in | Base-out | NRA | Minus to blur |
|---|---|---|---|---|---|
| Distance | 2 exo | X/10/6 | X/19/10 | | |
| 40 cm +1.50 D add | 14 exo | X/22/17 | X/6/2 | +1.00 | -1.00 |

Amplitude of accommodation = 2.00 D; working distance = approximately 40 cm; BCC = +1.50 D add; 40 cm associated phoria with +1.50 D add = 3Δ BI.

## EXAMPLES

The individual whose findings are depicted in Figure 12.2 has a working distance of 40 cm and an amplitude of accommodation of 3.00 D. If half the amplitude is kept in reserve, the suggested add is

Add = 2.50 D – (3.00 D / 2)

Add = 2.50 D - 1.50 D

Add = +1.00 D

The binocular cross cylinder test yielded an add of +1.25 D, and that add was used for nearpoint phoria and vergence range testing. The NRA and PRA starting from a +1.25 D add were +1.25 D and -1.75 D, respectively. Those results indicate that the NRA and PRA would be balanced with an add of +1.00 D. The rule keep half the amplitude in reserve and balancing the NRA and PRA both suggest an add of +1.00 D. The associated phoria at 40 cm with a +1.00 D add is zero, indicating that the patient is unlikely to have symptoms associated with the higher exophoria at near with the plus add.

Test findings for a second example appear in Figure 12.3. With a working distance of 40 cm and an amplitude of accommodation of 2.00 D, keeping half the amplitude in reserve indicates an add of +1.50 D:

Add = 2.50 D – (2.00 D /2)

Add = 2.50 D – 1.00 D

Add = +1.50 D

The binocular cross cylinder test was used to derive a tentative add for near-point testing, and its result was +1.50 D add. The plus-to-blur and minus-to-blur findings were equal with that +1.50 add. The rule keep half the amplitude in reserve and balancing the NRA and PRA both suggest an add of +1.50 D. The associated phoria at 40 cm with a +1.50 D add was 3Δ BI, suggesting that vision therapy to improve positive fusional vergence or some base-in prism at near would help the patient have more comfortable vision at near.

## CASE REPORTS

Patient GV, a 48-year-old male college professor, complained of nearpoint blur. He stated that he now had to hold reading material out farther than he would like to when wearing his glasses, but that he had to hold things too close without his glasses. His preferred reading distance was approximately 40 cm. His spectacles were 4 years old. Their powers were -2.25-0.50 X 5 OD, -3.00-0.25 X 175 OS, +1.00 D add. Visual acuities with these spectacles were 6/4.5 OD, 6/4.5-1/6 OS, 6/4.5 OU at distance and 20/30 OD, 20/30 + 2/8 OS, 20/30 + 2/8 OU at near. The cover test with the current correction revealed ortho at distance and a slight exophoria at near. The subjective refraction findings were -2.50-0.25 X 165 OD (6/4.5), -3.00-0.50 X 160 OS (6/4.5). The distance disso-ciated phoria with these lenses was 1Δ eso. The distance fusional vergence ranges were base-in X/8/2, base-out 8/24/12. The near BCC test yielded a +1.50 D add. The NRA and PRA starting from this add were +0.75 D and -0.75 D, respectively. Through the +1.50 D add the dissociated phoria at 40 cm was zero. This patient had no distance vision complaint. This is consistent with the minimal change from the distance portion of the habitual prescription to the subjective refraction (the change in spherical equivalent was -0.12D for both OD and OS). The case history and the test findings suggest an increase in the plus add. Balancing the NRA and PRA suggests a +1.50 D add over the subjective refraction. This is a change of +0.37 D OD and OS in the spherical equivalent total near-point power from the habitual prescription. The patient reported that the subjective refraction lenses in a trial frame gave good distance vision and that the +1.50 D add over that provided clear comfortable near vision. Progressive addition lenses with those powers were ordered.

Patient JK, a 43-year-old female nurse, complained of some difficulty seeing fine print. She had spectacles that were several years old and that she wore them only to drive. These spectacles had powers of -0.50 D sphere OD, -1.00 D sphere OS. Unaided visual acuities were 6/6 OD, 6/7.5 + 3/6 OS, 6/6 OU at distance, and 20/40 - 2/6 OD, 20/30 - 2/8 OS, 20/30 OU. The cover test without correction showed ortho at distance and near. The subjective refrac-tion findings were plano sphere OD (6/6 + 2/6), -0.50 D sphere OS (6/6 + 3/6). The distance dissociated phoria with these lenses was 1Δ eso. The distance fusional vergence ranges were base-in X/12/4, base-out 18/24/4. The plus build-up indicated a minimum plus of +0.75 D add over the distance refractive correction to read 20/20 at 40 cm. The BCC result was a +1.50 D add. The dissociated phoria and fusional vergence ranges at 40 cm through the + 1.50 D add from the BCC test were 4Δ exo; base-in 16/20/14, base-out 10/16/4. The

NRA and PRA findings were +1.00 D and -1.25 D, respectively, over the BCC finding. Balancing the NRA and PRA suggests a plus add of +1.25 D. This is a total near-point power of +1.25 D OD, +0.75 D OS. When JK looked at magazine print through these lenses in a trial frame, she reported that the print was easy to read. She wanted to get glasses that would help her at near and for occasional distance use. Progressive addition lenses with powers of plano sphere OD, -0.50 D sphere OS, +1.25 D add were ordered.

## ETIOLOGY OF PRESBYOPIA

Literature reviews[37,38] that have evaluated the reasons for the age-related decline in amplitude of accommodation have concluded that it is most likely that the important factors are:

(a) increase in crystalline lens size and volume,

(b) decrease in flexibility of the crystalline lens, and

(c) decrease in elasticity of the lens capsule.

Possible additional contributors to presbyopia are:

(a) decreased leverage in the zonules due to change in the geometry of their attachments as a result of the change in crystalline lens size and shape,

(b) changes in ciliary muscle geometry (decreased length and perhaps increased width),

(c) decreased number, density, and integrity of equatorial zonules, and

(d) decreased elasticity of the choroid.

These reviews concluded that the following are not factors in presbyopia:

(a) ciliary muscle contractile force,

(b) zonule elasticity, and

(c) neural control of accommodation.

## REFERENCES

1. Hofstetter HW, Griffin JR, Berman MS, Everson RW. Dictionary of Visual Science and Related Clinical Terms, 5th ed. Boston: Butterworth-Heinemann, 2000:407.

2. Hofstetter HW, Griffin JR, Berman MS, Everson RW. Dictionary of Visual Science and Related Clinical Terms, 5th ed. Boston: Butterworth-Heinemann, 2000:19.

3. Carlson NB, Kurtz D, Heath DA, Hines C. Clinical Procedures for Ocular Examination. Norwalk, CT: Appleton & Lange, 1990:11-12.

4. London R. Amplitude of accommodation. In: Eskridge JB, Amos JF, Bartlett JD, eds. Clinical Procedures in Optometry. Philadelphia: Lippincott, 1991:69-71.

5. Hofstetter HW. A comparison of Duane's and Donders' tables of the amplitude of accommodation. Am J Optom Arch Am Acad Optom 1944;21:345-363.

6. Hofstetter HW. A useful age-amplitude formula. Pennsylvania Optom 1947;7:5-8.

7. Ciuffreda KJ. Accommodation, the pupil, and presbyopia. In: Benjamin WJ, ed. Borish's Clinical Refraction. Philadelphia: Saunders, 1998:77-120.

8. Pointer JS. The presbyopic add. I. Magnitude and distribution in a historical context. Ophthal Physiol Opt 1995;15:235-240.

9. Borish IM. Clinical Refraction, 3rd ed. Chicago: Professional Press, 1970:178-184.

10. Patorgis CJ. Presbyopia. In: Amos JF, ed. Diagnosis and Management in Vision Care. Boston: Butterworth-Heinemann, 1987:203-238.

11. Hanlon SD, Nakabayashi J, Shigezawa G. A critical view of presbyopic add determination. J Am Optom Assoc 1987;58:468-472.

12. Grosvenor TP. Primary Care Optometry, 5th ed. St. Louis: Butterworth Heinemann Elsevier, 2007:254-256.

13. Fannin TE. *Presbyopic addition. In: Eskridge JB, Amos JF, Bartlett JD, eds. Clinical Procedures in Optometry. Philadelphia: Lippincott, 1991:198-205.*

14. Hofstetter HW. *The accommodative range through the near correction. Am J Optom Arch Am Acad Optom 1948;25:275-285.*

15. Hofstetter HW. *A survey of practices in prescribing presbyopic adds. Am J Optom Arch Am Acad Optom 1949;26:144-160.*

16. Carter JH. *Determining the nearpoint addition. New Eng J Optom 1985;37:4-13.*

17. Goss DA, West RW. *Introduction to the Optics of the Eye. Boston: Butterworth-Heinemann, 2002:206-211.*

18. Goss DA. *Hypermetropia or presbyopia? Points de vue 2005;53:8-12.*

19. Morgan MW. *Accommodative changes in presbyopia and their correction. In: Hirsch MJ, Wick RE, eds. Vision of the Aging Patient. Philadelphia: Chilton, 1960:83-112.*

20. Kurtz D. *Presbyopia. In: Brookman KE. Refractive Management of Ametropia. Boston: Butterworth-Heinemann, 1996:145-179.*

21. Newman JM. *Analysis, interpretation, and prescription for the ametropias and heterophorias. In: Benjamin WJ, ed. Borish's Clinical Refraction, 2nd ed. St. Louis: Butterworth Heinemann Elsevier, 2006:963-1025.*

22. Mancil GL, Bailey IL, Brookman KE, et al. *Care of the Patient with Presbyopia, American Optometric Association Clinical Practice Guideline. St. Louis: American Optometric Association, 1998.*

23. Werner DL, Press LJ. *Clinical Pearls in Refractive Care. Boston: Butterworth-Heinemann, 2002:139-180.*

24. Sheedy JE, Shaw-McMinn PG. *Diagnosing and Treating Computer-Related Vision Problems. Amsterdam: Butterworth-Heinemann, 2003:91-113.*

25. Sheedy JE, Saladin JJ. *Exophoria at near in presbyopia. Am J Optom Physiol Opt 1975;52:474-481.*

26. Brooks CW, Borish IM. *System for Ophthalmic Dispensing, 3rd ed. St. Louis: Butterworth Heinemann Elsevier, 2007:445-449.*

27. Vodnoy BE. *Orthoptics for the advanced presbyope. Optom Weekly 1975;66:204-206.*

28. Wick B. *Vision training for presbyopic nonstrabismic patients. Am J Optom Physiol Opt 1977;54:244-247.*

29. Cohen AH, Soden R. *Effectiveness of visual therapy for convergence insufficiency for an adult population. J Am Optom Assoc 1984;55:491-494.*

30. Birnbaum MH, Soden R, Cohen AH. *Efficacy of vision therapy for convergence insufficiency in an adult male population. J Am Optom Assoc 1999;70:225-232.*

31. Scheiman M, Wick B. *Clinical Management of Binocular Vision – Heterophoric, Accommodative, and Eye Movement Disorders, 2nd ed. Philadelphia: Lippincott Williams & Wilkins, 2002:246-247.*

32. Sheedy JE. *Analysis of near oculomotor balance. Rev Optom 1979; 116:44-45.*

33. Hofstetter HW. *The zone of clear single binocular vision. Am J Optom Arch Am Acad Optom 1945;22:301-333, 361-384.*

34. Alpern M. *Types of movement. In: Davson H, ed. Muscular Mechanisms. 2nd ed. Vol 3 of The Eye. New York: Academic, 1969:65-174.*

35. Fry GA. *Basic concepts underlying graphical analysis. In: Schor CM, Ciuffreda KJ, eds. Vergence Eye Movements: Basic and Clinical Aspects. Boston: Butterworth-Heinemann, 1983:403-437.*

36. Abel CA, Hofstetter HW. *The Graphical Analysis of Clinical Optometric Findings. Los Angeles: Los Angeles College of Optometry, 1951:183-186.*

37. Gilmartin B. *The aetiology of presbyopia: a summary of the role of lenticular and extralenticular structures. Ophthal Physiol Opt 1995;15:431-437.*

38. Ciuffreda KJ. *Accommodation, the pupil, and presbyopia. In: Benjamin WJ, ed. Borish's Clinical Refraction, 2nd ed. St. Louis: Butterworth Heinemann Elsevier, 2006:93-144.*

# PRACTICE PROBLEMS

1. Given a nearpoint working distance of 40 cm and an amplitude of accommodation of 1.50 D, what add would be given on the basis of the rule: Keep half the amplitude in reserve?

2. Given a nearpoint working distance of 33.3 cm and an amplitude of accommodation of 2.50 D, what add would be given on the basis of the rule: Keep half the amplitude in reserve?

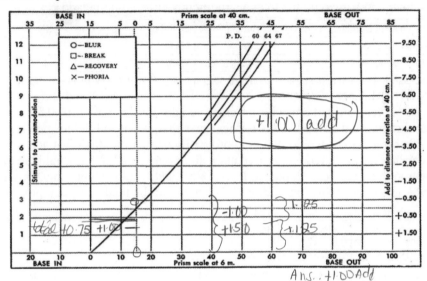

Ans.. +1.00 Add

3. Starting at a +0.75 D add over the BVA, a patient has an NRA of +1.50 D and a PRA of -1.00 D. What add would balance the NRA and PRA? Plot the NRA and PRA on the graph and note that the add that balances the NRA and PRA is at the midpoint of the range between the NRA and PRA.

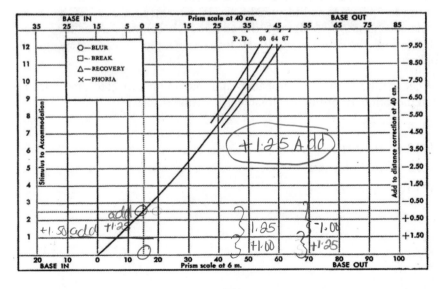

149

4. Starting at a +1.50 D add over the BVA, a patient has an NRA of +1.00 D and a PRA of -1.25 D. What add would be given on the basis of the balance of PRA and NRA at the working distance?

5. A 50 year old patient with +0.75 D sph single vision lenses for reading says that the glasses don't help as much as they used to. (a) What add would keep half the amplitude in reserve? What would the total nearpoint power be with that add? (b) What add would balance the NRA and PRA given the following findings? What would the total nearpoint power be with that add?

| Test distance/Lens | Phoria | Base-in | Base-out | NRA | PRA |
|---|---|---|---|---|---|
| Distance/ BVA | 1 exo | X/9/5 | 19/24/14 | | |
| 40 cm / BVA +0.75 | 6 exo | 17/24/12 | X/10/4 | +1.75 | -1.25 |

Subjective refraction to best visual acuity, +0.50 D sph OU. Amplitude of Acc= 3.00D
Working Distance = 40cm

6. A 53 year old patient with progressive addition lenses with +0.50 D sph for distance and +1.00 D adds for near says that he has to hold his newspaper farther out than he would like to in order to see the print. (a) What add would keep half the amplitude in reserve in the following case? What would the total nearpoint power be with that add? (b) What add would balance the NRA and PRA given the following findings? What would the total nearpoint power be with that add?

| Test distance/ Lens | Phoria | Base-in | Base-out | NRA | PRA |
|---|---|---|---|---|---|
| Distance/ BVA | 1 exo | X/10/4 | X/11/6 | | |
| 40 cm / BVA +1.75 | 12 exo | 22/25/18 | X6/2 | +0.50 | -1.00 |

Subjective refraction to best visual acuity, +0.75 D sph OU Amp. of Accomm.=+1.75
working distance = 40cm.

7. Patients HF and LV both have dissociated phorias at near of 12 Δ exo through their presbyopic adds and identical base-out vergence ranges. HF has a near associated phoria of 3Δ BI with the add and LV has zero associated phoria with the add. Which is most likely to have symptoms associated with the exophoria?

8. What are the minimum, probable, and maximum expected amplitudes of accommodation according to Hofstetter's formulas for:

  (a) a 20-year-old,

  (b) a 30-year-old,

  (c) a 40-year-old, and

  (d) a 50-year-old?

# Chapter 13
# Nonpresbyopic Accommodative Disorders

**A**ccommodative disorders in nonpresbyopic individuals can result in blurred vision, headaches, ocular discomfort, and/or other difficulties associated with near work. Accommodative dysfunction in nonpresbyopes is relatively common.[1,2] The treatments for nonpresbyopic accommodative disorders, nearpoint plus lens adds and vision therapy, are very effective in relieving ocular symptoms.[1,3-7] Probably the best first step toward an understanding of nonpresbyopic accommodative disorders is to understand the tests used in evaluating accommodative function.

## TESTS OF ACCOMMODATIVE FUNCTION
Clinical tests of accommodative function can be grouped into four categories:
1. amplitude of accommodation,
2. accommodative facility,
3. relative accommodation, and
4. tests that directly or indirectly assess lag of accommodation.

Amplitude of accommodation is a measure of the maximum amount of accommodation an individual can exert. As discussed in Chapter 3, amplitude of accommodation usually is determined by the push-up test.[8,9] Tests for accommodative facility examine the speed of accommodative changes.[10,11] The dioptric accommodative stimulus is alternated between two different levels by either a lens rock or distance procedure, as described in chapter 7. The relative accommodative tests are the plus-to-blur (or negative relative accommodation) and the minus-to-blur (or positive relative accommodation) tests.[12,13] The negative relative accommodation (NRA) and positive relative accommodation (PRA) tests were discussed in Chapter 3. Table 13.1 lists the categories of accommo-

| Table 13.1. Categories of accommodation tests and commonly used tests in each category. |
|---|
| Amplitude of accommodation |
|     • push-up test |
| Accommodative facility |
|     • lens rock |
|     • distance rock |
| Relative accommodation |
|   Negative relative accommodation |
|     • plus to blur test |
|   Positive relative accommodation |
|     • minus to blur test |
| Assessment of lag of accommodation |
|   Direct measurement of lag |
|     • MEM dynamic retinoscopy |
|     • Nott dynamic retinoscopy |
|   Indirect assessment of lag (add which yields AR=AS) |
|     • low neutral dynamic retinoscopy |
|     • binocular cross cylinder test |

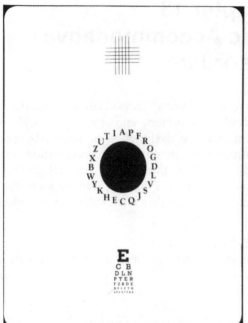

*Figure 13.1. An example of a test card that can be used for dynamic retinoscopy. The patient is directed to look at the letters just outside the aperture in the card. The examiner observes the retinoscopic reflex through the aperture in the card. The cross grid pattern at the top of the card is used for binocular cross cylinder test.*

dation tests and examples of tests in each category.

## TESTS THAT MEASURE OR ASSESS LAG OF ACCOMMODATION

The fourth category of accommodation tests includes tests that directly or indirectly assess the patient's accommodative response for a near object.[14] During accommodation for near-point viewing, the retina usually is conjugate with a point slightly behind the object of regard. In other words, for near-point targets, accommodative response usually is slightly less than the accommodative stimulus.[15-17] The amount by which the dioptric accommodative response is less than the dioptric accommodative stimulus is the *lag of accommodation*. The less common situation in which the accommodative response is greater than the accommodative stimulus is known as a *lead of accommodation*.

This category of accommodation tests can be further divided into (1) tests that measure the lag of accommodation and (2) tests in which lens power is changed to alter accommodative stimulus to the point at which dioptric accommodative stimulus and dioptric accommodative response are equal.[11] Examples of the former, in which there is a direct measure of the lag, are monocular estimation method (MEM) dynamic retinoscopy and Nott dynamic retinoscopy. Examples of the latter, in which the lag is assessed indirectly, are low neutral dynamic retinoscopy and the binocular cross-cylinder (BCC) test.

A test card with an aperture in the center usually is used for dynamic retinoscopy so that the examiner can observe the retinoscopic reflex close to the patient's visual axis through the aperture (Figure 13.1).[18] In MEM dynamic retinoscopy the amount of the lag of accommodation is estimated by judging the width, speed, and brightness of the retinoscopic reflex.[19-21] The test card and the retinoscope are placed at the same distance from the patient's spectacle plane, usually 40 cm. The patient's distance refractive correction is placed in a trial frame or the phoropter. The patient views the test card letters binocularly. With the retinoscope in plane mirror mode, with motion indicates a lag of accommodation and against motion indicates a lead of accommodation. Neutrality indicates that accommodative stimulus and accommodative response are equal. The examiner's estimate of the amount of plus power that would be required to neutralize the with motion is the estimate of the lag of accommodation. The estimate of the lag can be confirmed by very briefly placing a plus lens equal in power to the estimated lag over one eye and quickly checking to see whether neutrality is observed. The lens should be in place for a very brief period of time so that a change in accommodative response is not induced.[14,22] The average latency period for the beginning of an accommodative response is about 370 msec (a little over a third of a second),[15] so it would be very difficult to see whether neutral is present without causing a slight change in accommodation. One recommendation is to have the lens in place less than a second and then if neutrality was not present with the lens, let the patient look at the test card without the lens for at least three seconds before estimating the reflex again. Rouse et al.[22] found that MEM dynamic retinoscopy results correlate very closely with subjective optometer measurements of accommodation.

Nott[23] is credited with the development of a form of dynamic retinoscopy in which the lag of accommodation is measured by moving the retinoscope behind the plane of the test card. The test card usually is suspended from the phoropter reading rod rather than attached to the retinoscope. The patient views the test card, usually placed at 40 cm from the spectacle plane, through the distance refractive correction. A with motion observed by the examiner indicates a lag of accommodation. The examiner moves back away from the patient slowly until a neutral retinoscopic reflex is seen.[14] The dioptric accommodative stimulus is the reciprocal of the test distance in meters. If the card is at 40 cm from the spectacle plane, the accommodative stimulus is 2.50 D. The dioptric accommodative response is the reciprocal of the distance of the retinoscope from the spectacle plane in meters when neutral is observed. If neutral is noted with the retinoscope 50 cm from the spectacle plane, the accommodative response is 2.00 D. In that case, the lag of accommodation would be 0.50 D.

Low neutral dynamic retinoscopy yields the lens power with which the dioptric accommodative stimulus and dioptric accommodative response are equal.[11,24] The retinoscope and the test card are maintained at the same distance from the patient, usually 40 cm from the spectacle plane. Testing is started with the patient's distance refractive correction in place. If a lag is observed, plus lenses are added in 0.25 D steps until a neutral retinoscopic reflex is observed. The lens power added for neutrality is recorded. If, for example, the test result is +0.75 D with a 40 cm distance, then the accommodative stimulus is 0.75 D less than the 2.50 D for the test distance, or 1.75 D. Because neutral was observed at that point, the accommodative response is also 1.75 D.

Cross may have been the first to advocate adding lenses as a part of dynamic retinoscopy testing, so this is sometimes referred to as Cross dynamic retinoscopy.[24,25] Sheard proposed adding plus to the first neutral, the so-called low neutral point, as the end-point of testing.[26,27] In addition to MEM, Nott, and

**Table 13.2. Means (and standard deviations in parentheses) for MEM and Nott dynamic retinoscopy lags of accommodation for a 40 cm testing distance in various studies.**

| Study | Subjects | MEM | Nott |
|---|---|---|---|
| Rouse et al.[38] | N=721 ages, 4 to 12 yrs | OD, 0.33 D (0.35) OS, 0.35 D (0.34) | -- |
| Locke and Somers[39] | N=10 ages, 24 to 30 yrs | Examiner A, 0.50 D (0.16) Examiner B, 0.50 D (0.18) | Examiner A, 0.56 D (0.19) Examiner B, 0.63 D (0.08) |
| Jackson and Goss[40] | N=244 ages, 7.9 to 15.9 yrs | 0.23 D (0.29) | 0.29 D |
| Rosenfield et al.[41] | N=24 ages, 22.5 to 30.1 yrs | -- | 0.48 D |
| Cacho et al.[42] | N=50 ages, 15 to 35 yrs | 0.74 D (0.72) | 0.42 D (0.41) |
| Tassinari[43] | N=211 ages, 6 to 37 yrs | 0.35 D (0.34) | -- |
| Goss and Warren[44] | N=20 ages, 23 to 28 yrs | 0.56 D (0.25) | -- |

low neutral, there are other additional forms of dynamic retinoscopy that some practitioners have found to be useful.[28,29]

The binocular cross cylinder (BCC) test also yields a lens power with which dioptric accommodative stimulus and dioptric accommodative response are equal.[11,30,31] The BCC test differs from low neutral dynamic retinoscopy in that verbal responses are required from the patient, and in that the test is started with plus over the distance subjective refraction and plus is reduced to the test end-point. Details of testing procedure have been described by various authors.[20,32-35] The target that the patient views is a cross grid pattern of vertical and horizontal lines, as seen at the top of the card shown in Figure 13.1. The lamp illuminating the test card is either turned away from the card or the dimmer switch is adjusted to reduce illumination on the card. The ±0.50 D cross cylinders are put in place over both eyes with the minus cylinder axes in the vertical meridian. The cross cylinders produce an astigmatic interval so that some (more plus) lens powers will make the vertical lines darker and more distinct and some (less plus) lens powers will make the horizontal lines darker and more distinct. The test is started enough plus over the BVA to make the vertical lines more distinct (an add of +1.75 D over the BVA is usually suffi-cient for non-presbyopes). Plus is reduced until the two sets of lines are equally distinct. At that point accommodation is conjugate with the plane of the test card so that the accommodative stimulus and the accommodative response are equal. If a patient reports the horizontal lines more distinct without giving an equal response as plus is reduced, accommodative stimulus and accommoda-tive response would theoretically be equal with an add midway the add which yielded the last vertical response and the add which yielded the first horizontal response. Most authors advise recording the add which yields the first equal response, or if there is no equal response, the first horizontal response.[20,32,36]

**Table 13.3. Means (and standard deviations in parentheses) for low neutral dynamic retinoscopy for subjects viewing print letters at a 40 cm viewing distance. Values are the amount of plus added to first neutral.**

| Study | Subjects | Low neutral |
|---|---|---|
| Locke and Somers[39] | N=10; Ages, 24 to 30 yrs | Examiner A, +0.60 D (0.29) Examiner B, +0.61 D (0.21) |
| Jackson and Goss[40] | N=244; ages, 7.9 to 15.9 yrs | +0.29 D (0.38) |
| Rosenfield et al.[41] | N=24; ages, 22.5 to 30.1 yrs | +0.50 D |
| Goss and Warren[44] | N=20; ages, 23 to 28 yrs | +0.88 D (0.32) |

Some writers note that the astigmatic blur induced by the cross cylinder and the reduced contrast from the reduced illumination have variable effects on accommodation, making the BCC less useful for non-presbyopes than for presbyopes.[20,37] Dynamic retinoscopy is preferred over the BCC for assessing accommodative response in non-presbyopes. However, the BCC is deemed a useful test in both non-presbyopes and presbyopes by many clinicians.

## DYNAMIC RETINOSCOPY NORMS FOR NON-PRESBYOPES

Table 13.2 summarizes the results of several studies which gave average values for MEM. It may be noticed that there is some variability in the means from study to study. As a result, different authorities give slightly different values for normal ranges. If we take an overview of the different study results and use approximately the mean – 1 standard deviation to the mean + 1 standard deviation as the normal range, we would get a normal range of about 0 to 0.75 D lag. That range agrees with the recommendations of Rouse et al.[38] and Cooper.[45]

Results of studies on Nott dynamic retinoscopy are also given in Table 13.2. A range of about 0 to 0.75 D lag appears to be reasonable for a normal range for Nott retinoscopy also. It may be noted in Table 13.2 that two studies found similar values on MEM and Nott, but the Cacho et al.[42] found a higher average lag of MEM than on Nott. The latter result might be explained by the results of another study[46] which found similar lags on MEM and Nott for midrange lags, but higher measurements of lag on MEM than on Nott for subjects with higher lags.

Table 13.3 gives a summary of means and standard deviations for low neutral dynamic retinoscopy findings from various studies. The variability in the means of the studies represented in Table 13.3 suggests that it may be difficult to establish norms for low neutral with confidence. As discussed earlier, low neutral dynamic retinoscopy does not yield a measurement of the lag of accommodation, but rather the plus add that makes the accommodative stimulus and the accommodative response equal. As lenses are added in low neutral retinoscopy, it is expected that the accommodative response will change in response to the added lenses. In the case of a lag of accommodation, added plus will reduce the accommodative stimulus with an expected decrease in accommodative response as a result. Therefore, it is expected that the amount of plus added to reach neutral on low neutral dynamic retinoscopy would be higher than the lag of accommodation determined by MEM retinoscopy.

Norms only for this test size + distance.

Table 13.4. Summary of normal or minimum expected findings for accommodation tests. The origins of these values are described in chapters 7, 8, and 12, and in this chapter.

Amplitude of accommodation
    Minimum amplitude = 15 – (0.25)(age)
Lens rock accommodative facility (+2/-2 lenses, 20/30 letters at 40 cm)
    Monocular: minimum 11 cpm
    Binocular: minimum 10 cpm
    Monocular – Binocular: maximum 4 cpm
Morgan's minimum values for NRA and PRA:
    NRA: +1.75 D
    PRA: -1.75
Dynamic retinoscopy:
    MEM: 0 to 0.75 D lag
    Nott: 0 to 0.75 D lag
    Low neutral: 0 to +1.00 D add

For studies noted in Tables 13.2 and 13.3 that have data for both MEM and low neutral, the means for the amount of plus add on low neutral were greater than the mean lags on MEM by 0.06 D (Jackson and Goss), 0.11 D (Locke and Somers), and 0.32 D (Goss and Warren). So until more definitive studies are done, we could assume low neutral to often be about 0.25 D more plus than MEM when a lag is present, making a normal range for low neutral about 0 to +1.00 D for a 40 cm test distance in non-presbyopes. The difference between MEM and low neutral findings will be discussed further in the section below on accommodative response/accommodative stimulus functions.

Haynes[47] recommended a somewhat higher normal range of +0.50 to +1.25 D for low neutral at 40 cm (compared to his normal range of 0.44 to 0.80 D lag for MEM at 40 cm). Using a 33 cm test distance for low neutral, Whitefoot and Charman[48] found a mean ($\pm$SD) of 1.10 D ($\pm$0.58) for non-presbyopes. Table 13.4 summarizes norms for dynamic retinoscopy and other accommodation tests.

## COMPARISONS OF ACCOMMODATION TESTS

Locke and Somers[39] compared MEM retinoscopy, low neutral dynamic retinoscopy, bell retinoscopy (another form of dynamic retinoscopy), and the BCC test using two examiners and 10 young subjects. They reported that the two examiners found values that were not significantly different on the four tests. Findings obtained with MEM, low neutral, and bell dynamic retinoscopy were not significantly different from each other, but they did differ from findings obtained using the BCC test.

Wick and Hall[49] performed tests of accommodative lag, facility, and amplitude during a vision screening of schoolchildren, and found that failure on one of these tests did not effectively predict failure on the other two tests.

Jackson and Goss[40] compared the results of several accommodation tests in 244 schoolchildren. The tests included MEM, low neutral, and Nott dynamic retinoscopy and NRA, PRA, BCC, lens rock, and distance rock tests. The lens rock and distance rock accommodative facility tests correlated signifi-

**Table 13.5. Summary of findings of diagnostic significance in accommodative disorders, findings which support that diagnosis, and the treatment options.**

| | Diagnostic findings | Supporting findings | Treat-ment |
|---|---|---|---|
| Accommoda-tive insuffi-ciency | high lag of accommodation and/or low amplitude of accom-modation for age | slow on minus side of monoc-ular and binocular lens flippers; low PRA; high plus on BCC | plus add or vision therapy |
| Accommoda-tive infacility | reduced monocular and binoc-ular facility rates: slow on both minus and plus sides | NRA and PRA low; normal lag of accommodation; normal amplitude of accommodation | vision therapy |
| Accommoda-tive excess | lead of accommodation | Slow on plus side of monocular and binocular lens flippers; NRA may be low; BCC may be minus | vision therapy |

cantly with each other, but generally not significantly or highly with other tests. MEM, Nott, and low neutral, and the BCC showed significant correlations with each other, but not with most other tests.

Similar findings were reported by Allen and O'Leary[50] for 64 young adults. Various parameters of accommodative facility testing results showed statistically significant correlation coefficients with each other, but not with amplitude of accommodation or lag of accommodation. Amplitude of accommodation and lag of accommodation were not significantly correlated with each

These studies show that the results of one accommodation test correl other tests in the same category, but cannot be used to predict the re a test in one of the other categories of tests. Therefore, a complete v of accommodative function should include tests from each of the fo type categories. In other words, *a complete investigation of accommodative function should include (1) amplitude of accommodation, (2) accommodative facility, (3) NRA and PRA, and (4) some form of dynamic retinoscopy and/or the BCC test.*

## TERMS USED FOR ACCOMMODATIVE DISORDERS

There are some terms in common usage for accommodative disorders, although there is some variation in how they are defined.[1,45,51-54] *Accommodative insufficiency* is a disorder of the stimulation of accommodation. It is characterized by an abnormally low amplitude of accommodation and/or a high lag of accommodation. A total lack of accommodation in a non-presbyopic individual is called *paralysis of accommodation.* Paralysis of accommodation is a rare condition that is caused by ocular disease or trauma. A decline in accommodative ability after use of accommodation, characterized by a reduction in the amplitude of accommodation with repeated testing is *accommodative fatigue* or *ill-sustained accommodation.* Accommodative fatigue or ill-sustained accommodation is often considered to be a special case of accommodative insufficiency. Poor accommodative facility is called *accommodative infacility.* The condition in which a lead of accommodation exists is sometimes referred to as *accommodative excess.* The typical examination findings and treatments for the most common accommodative disorders are summarized in Table 13.5.

## PRESCRIPTION AND MANAGEMENT GUIDELINES

Common symptoms of accommodative insufficiency can include blur, eyestrain, headaches, and difficulties associated with reading. The key findings in accommodative insufficiency are a lag of accommodation which is higher than normal and/or an amplitude of accommodation which is lower than the minimum expected amplitude in Hofstetter's formulas. Organic causes for the reduced amplitude should be ruled out when making a diagnosis of accommodative insufficiency. In addition to low amplitude and/or high lag, supporting findings for a diagnosis of accommodative insufficiency are slowness on the minus side of monocular and binocular lens flippers, low PRA, and high plus on the BCC.

Treatments for accommodative insufficiency are plus adds and vision therapy.[1,34,45,51,52] If the lag of accommodation as determined by MEM or Nott retinoscopy is greater then 0.75 D, one way of prescribing an add is to deduct 0.25 D from the lag.[55] If the plus added for neutrality on low neutral dynamic retinoscopy is greater than 1.00 D, one way of determining the add is to deduct about 0.50 D from the test end-point. Finding the lens power that balances the NRA and PRA is another way of prescribing plus adds for nonpresbyopes,[56] just as for presbyopes, as discussed in the previous chapter. Allowing the patient to look at reading material with the proposed add in a trial frame is useful as a subjective evaluation of the add and as a demonstration to the patient.

Common symptoms of accommodative infacility include eyestrain, transient near-point blur, distance blur after near-point viewing, headaches, and reading difficulties. The key diagnostic findings in accommodative infacility are reduced monocular and binocular accommodative facility rates. Generally a large difference in quickness on plus and minus sides of the flippers is more likely to be associated with accommodative insufficiency or accommodative excess than accommodative infacility. Low NRA and low PRA findings are often found in accommodative infacility. Lag of accommodation and amplitude of accommodation are often normal. The treatment for accommodative infacility is vision therapy procedures to improve facility.[34,45,52] These procedures are usually referred to as accommodative rock. Accommodative rock training has been shown to be successful in increasing facility rates, in improving accommodative latencies and velocities, and in relieving ocular symptoms.[4-7,12,57]

Symptoms of accommodative excess can include blurred vision, eyestrain, headaches, and difficulties associated with reading and nearwork. Accommodative excess is characterized by a lead of accommodation on dynamic retinoscopy. Other findings that support a diagnosis of accommodative excess include slowness on the plus side of monocular and binocular lens flippers, low NRA, and minus on the BCC. A lead of accommodation is managed by vision therapy techniques designed to train reduction in accommodative response. A lead of accommodation may be secondary to a high exophoria. A lead sometimes occurs in exophoria because accommodative convergence is used to main-

| Patient pattern | Retinoscopy findings with varying plus add powers in diopters (Accommodative stimulus in diopters in parentheses) | | | | | | | | | |
|---|---|---|---|---|---|---|---|---|---|---|
| | 0 (2.50) | +0.25 (2.25) | +0.50 (2.00) | +0.75 (1.75) | +1.00 (1.50) | +1.25 (1.25) | +1.50 (1.00) | +1.75 (0.75) | +2.00 (0.50) | +2.25 (0.25) |
| A | 0.25W | 0.25W | 0.25W | 0.12W | N | | 0.25A | 0.25A | | |
| B | 0.25W | 0.12W | N | N | 0.12A | 0.25A | 0.50A | | | |
| C | 1.00W | 0.75W | 0.50W | 0.25W | N | | 0.25A | 0.50A | | |
| D | 1.00W | | 0.75W | | 0.50W | 0.25W | N | | | |
| E | 0.75W | 0.50W | 0.50W | 0.50W | 0.50W | 0.25W | 0.25W | 0.25W | N | 0.25A |
| F | 1.50W | 1.50W | 1.50W | 1.25W | 1.00W | 0.75W | 0.50W | 0.25W | N | 0.25A |
| G | 2.00W | 1.75W | 1.50W | 0.37W | 0.37W | 0.25W | 0.25W | N | 0.25A | |

Table 13.6. Patterns of change in accommodative response with plus adds as determined by Haynes[58] with the MEM-LN procedure. W indicates with motion on dynamic retinoscopy and A indicates against motion, so, for example, 0.25W indicates 0.25 D of with motion. N indicates a neutral retinoscopy motion.

tain fusion. If this is the case, the vision therapy program should include training to improve positive fusional vergence.

## ACCOMMODATIVE RESPONSE/ ACCOMMODATIVE STIMULUS FUNCTIONS

The estimated motion on MEM retinoscopy is an estimate of the lag (or lead) of accommodation. As discussed earlier, the lag is the amount by which the diopters of accommodative response is less than the diopters of accommodative stimulus. So if the lag is known, the accommodative response can be found by subtracting the lag from the accommodative stimulus. As MEM retinoscopy is typically performed, the patient is viewing through the BVA. This would represent the response at one accommodative stimulus level only.

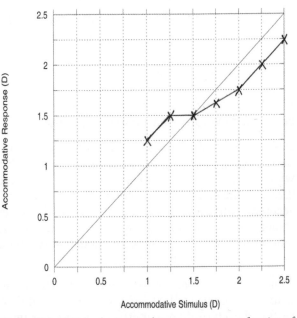

Figure 13.2. Graph of accommodative response as a function of accommodative stimulus in Haynes' case A.

On low neutral dynamic retinoscopy, plus added until a neutral reflex observed. At that point accommodative response and accommodative stim are equal. This also represents the accommodative response at only one ac

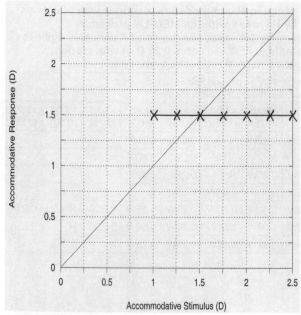

modative stimulus level. It could be helpful to the practitioner to know how patients respond to different amounts of plus add; that is, the accommodative response at other accommodative stimulus levels in addition to those obtained on MEM and low neutral retinoscopy.

Haynes[58] described a dynamic retinoscopy procedure to obtain accommodative responses at several accommodative stimuli. He called it a combined MEM-LN procedure.

*Figure 13.3. Graph of accommodative response as a function of accommodative stimulus in Haynes' case C.*

He performed MEM retinoscopy first with the BVA lenses in place, and then at each of several plus adds in 0.25 D steps until neutral and then an against motion was observed.

Haynes[58] performed his MEM-LN procedure with the test letters at 40 cm. So the accommodative stimulus was 2.50 D with the BVA in place, 2.25 D with a +0.25 D add, 2.00 D with a +0.50 D add, and so on. A with motion of 0.25 D indicated that the accommodative response was 0.25 D less than the accommodative stimulus. A neutral reflex indicated that the accommodative response and accommodative stimulus were equal. When a 0.25 D against motion was observed, the accommodative response was 0.25 D greater than the accommodative stimulus.

Table 13.6 shows patterns of findings that Haynes gave as examples of results with the combined MEM-LN procedure. He did not mention how frequently he found each of these patterns or what other types of patterns he observed. He described patterns A and B as representing "normal to superior accommodative behavior," patterns C, D, F, and G as representative of accommodative ·'sorders, and E to be a marginal case.[58] Such conclusions are consistent with
'ng at the lags of accommodation with MEM (at BVA): normal in A and B
'n both), high in C, D, F, and G (1.00, 1.00, 1.50, and 2.00 D, respec-
·marginal in E (0.75 D).

 A, the MEM as usually performed (through the BVA) was
'ow neutral was +1.00 D add. Figure 13.2 is a graph of
.onse as a function of accommodative stimulus in case

A. The MEM seen with the BVA was 0.25 D with motion, so at that point the accommodative stimulus was 2.50 D and the accommodative response was 2.25 D. With a +0.25 D add (accommodative stimulus = 2.25 D), there was a 0.25 D with motion, so the accommodative response was 2.00 D. Neutral was observed with a +1.00 D add, so accommodative stimulus and accommodative response were equal at 1.50 D. A +1.25 D add (accommodative stimulus = 1.25 D), yielded a 0.25 D against motion, so there the accommodative response was 1.50 D. These and the other points can be seen in Figure

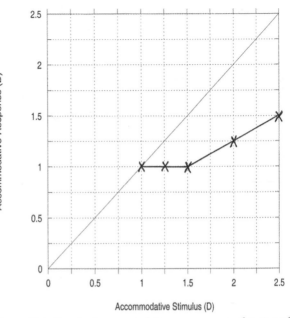

Figure 13.4. Graph of accommodative response as a function of accommodative stimulus in Haynes' case D.

13.2. The plot shows a fairly high slope from 0 add to an add of +1.00 D, indicating that this person's accommodation changed in amounts close to the powers of the plus adds. As a result, there is a notable difference between the MEM and the low neutral dioptric values.

In case C, graphed in Figure 13.3, the standard MEM was 1.00 D lag and the low neutral was +1.00 D add. In this case, the slope of the accommodative response/accommodative stimulus graph was zero, meaning that the patient did not change accommodation in response to plus adds. As a result of the zero slope, the MEM lag and the low neutral add were equal in amount.

In case D (see Figure 13.4), the standard MEM was 1.00 D lag and the low neutral was +1.50 D add. The slope was between the slopes for A and C, so the difference between MEM and low neutral was less than in case A and more than in case C.

A study of 20 young adults using Haynes' combined MEM-LN procedure confirmed the wide range of slopes suggested by Haynes' different response patterns.[44] Such results show that the difference between MEM and low neutral vary from person to person. The results also demonstrate that the response to plus adds cannot be determined based on the MEM or low neutral alone. W discussed earlier that a common way to prescribe a plus add is to deduct 0 D from the lag measured by the standard MEM through the BVA. Perl assessing how a patient responds to plus lenses could help in more confid

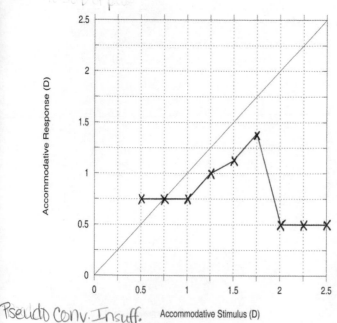

Pseudo Conv. Insuff.

*Figure 13.5. Graph of accommodative response as a function of accommodative stimulus in Haynes' case G.*

arriving at the most beneficial add power. Haynes' combined MEM-LN procedure would be one way to do this. Other authors have suggested additional methods. Tassinari[59] wrote about performing MEM as usual through the BVA and then again through an add based on the BCC test. Birnbaum[60] also mentioned performing MEM through plus adds and recommended prescribing a plus add that put the lag estimation in the 0.12 to 0.50 D range that he considered to be normal on MEM.

The adds suggested by Birnbaum's method do not always agree with the add recommended by subtracting 0.25 D from the MEM lag with the BVA. We could, for example, adapt Birnbaum's suggestion to find an add based on the first plus add that makes the accommodative response 0.25 D less than the accommodative stimulus; in other words, the first add that reduces the with motion to 0.25 D. If we use the cases in Table 13.6 from Haynes' MEM-LN method, we find that in patient C, both methods would recommend an add of +0.75 D. In patient D, subtracting 0.25 D from the lag yields a +0.75 D add, and Birnbaum's method of going to 0.25 D with motion would yield a +1.25 D add. In case F, subtraction of 0.25 D from the lag suggests a +1.25 D add, and Birnbaum's 0.25 D with motion method would suggest a +1.75 D add. For case G, subtracting 0.25 D from the lag recommends a +1.75 D add and Birnbaum's 0.25 D with method recommends a +1.25 D add.

## PSEUDO CONVERGENCE INSUFFICIENCY REVISITED

As discussed earlier, pseudo convergence insufficiency is a condition in which a high exophoria at near is secondary to accommodative insufficiency. A characteristic of pseudo convergence insufficiency is that the NPC improves with plus add. Some optometrists have also made the observation that the near phoria paradoxically decreases with a plus add in some pseudo convergence insufficiency cases. Such unexpected results could be explained by accommodative behavior like Haynes combined MEM-LN pattern G in Table 13.6. Accommodative response as a function of accommodative stimulus in case G is shown in Figure 13.5. With the BVA and with plus

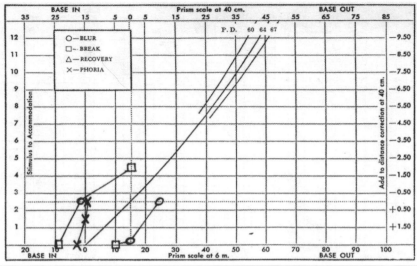

Figure 13.6. Test results and ZCSBV for patient MS.

| | Phoria | Base-in | Base-out | Plus to blur | Minus to blur |
|---|---|---|---|---|---|
| 6 m | 2 exo | X/9/4 | X/10/4 | | |
| 40 cm | 14 exo | 16/24/16 | 10/12/4 | +2.25 | -2.00 (break) |

Amplitude of accommodation = 9 D; BCC test = +1.50 D.

adds of +0.25 and +0.50 D, the accommodative response is only 0.50 D. But then at an add of +0.75 D, the accommodative response jumps up to 1.37 D. This increase in accommodative response would be associated with an increase in accommodative convergence and as a result, an improved NPC and reduced exophoria.

## ACCOMMODATION TESTS AND THE ZCSBV

The lag of accommodation and accommodative facility are not portrayed as a part of the zone of clear binocular vision (ZCSBV). As discussed earlier, the amplitude of accommodation forms the top of the ZCSBV and thus indicates its height. On the NRA and PRA tests, accommodative stimulus is changed while the convergence stimulus remains constant. So as accommodative vergence changes, there must be a compensatory change in fusional vergence in the opposite direction to maintain the same total amount of convergence. As a consequence, NRA or PRA findings may be low due to either an accommodative disorder or a vergence disorder. The NRA test often is limited by the positive fusional vergence capabilities of the patient, in which case it is plotted on the right side of the ZCSBV. If it is not limited by positive fusional vergence, it will is expected to be found on the bottom of the ZCSBV. If the PRA is found on the top of the ZCSBV, the amplitude of accommodation is its limiting factor. If the PRA is on the left side of the ZCSBV, negative fusional vergence is the limiting factor. If the NRA or PRA points are inside the boundaries of the ZCSBV, there may have been a procedural error or the patient may have a deficit in optical reflex accommodation. Such instance

163

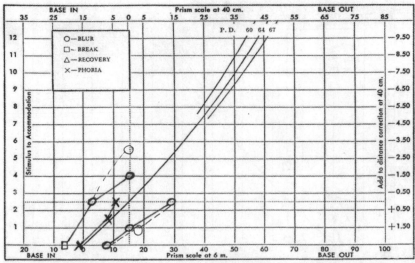

Figure 13.7. Test results and ZCSBV for patient MP.

|  | Phoria | Base-in | Base-out | Plus to blur | Minus to blur |
|---|---|---|---|---|---|
| 6 m | 2 exo | X/7/4 | 8/14/12 |  |  |
| 40 cm | 4 exo | 12/14/9 | 14/18/10 | +1.50 | -1.50 |
| 40 cm +1.00 D add | 7 exo |  |  |  |  |

the NRA and/or PRA being lower than predicted based on the vergence ranges are sometimes found in accommodative disorders.

## LACK OF SYMPTOMS DOES NOT RULE OUT AN ACCOMMODATION OR VERGENCE DISORDER

Now that we have discussed both vergence disorders and accommodative disorders, it would be a good time to emphasize that a patient may not report symptoms but still have an accommodation or vergence disorder. Symptoms may be absent simply due to an avoidance of reading or nearwork.[61] It is important, therefore, to perform thorough testing of accommodation and vergence function on all patients regardless of reported symptoms, especially in school-age children. This has perhaps been most eloquently stated by Birnbaum[62]: "patients who present with impaired accommodative and binocular findings, but without asthenopia, are generally asymptomatic either because they have developed myopia or because they avoid reading. When asthenopia is absent, many practitioners assume that existing visual problems are insignificant and do not require treatment. Recognition that patients with functional vision ~rder may be asymptomatic because they avoid or adapt leads the clinician ~ider treatment in such cases, to eliminate the need for continued avoid-~ther development of adaptive vision disorder."

RT: PATIENT MS

~ar-old female college student, complained of distance blur reading. She had worn glasses for her distance vision st them. Unaided visual acuities were 6/7.5 OD, OS, OU at distance and 20/20 OD, OS, OU at near. The cover test showed ortho at distance and exophoria at near. The subjective refraction was -0.50 D sphere OD (6/4.5), -0.50 -0.25 X 180 OS (6/4.5). Some of the examination findings are shown in Figure 13.6. The phoria findings suggest convergence insufficiency. However, the fact that the phoria line does not tilt to the right as far as the left and right sides of the ZCSBV suggests pseudo convergence insufficiency. In addition, the slightly low amplitude of accommodation for her age and the higher plus value on the BCC test suggest accommodative insufficiency. Other findings confirming the pseudo convergence insufficiency form of accommodative insufficiency were that (1) the near-point of convergence improved from 9 cm with no lenses in place to 7 cm with +0.50 D lenses in front of each eye (on repeated testing the near-point of convergence results were 9.5 cm with no lenses and 7 cm with +0.50 D lenses), and (2) with no lenses in place the lag of accommodation with Nott dynamic retinoscopy was 0.94 D. The patient reported that -0.50 D lenses in a trial frame improved distance vision and +0.50 D lenses made magazine print appear easier to read. The prescription given the patient was -0.50 D sphere OD, -0.50 -0.25 X 180 OS, +1.00 D add in progressive addition lenses.

## CASE REPORT: PATIENT MP

Patient MP, a 21-year-old male college student, complained of distance blur after near work and occasional blur at near. His spectacles were about one and half years old, and they had powers of -0.50 -0.50 X 105 OD, -0.50 -0.50 X 60 OS. His distance visual acuities with this correction were 6/6-2/6 OD, 6/6-1/6 OS, 6/6-1/6 OU, and near acuities were 20/20-1/8 OD, OS, OU. It appeared that ortho was present at distance and a slight exophoria at near when the cover test was performed with the habitual spectacles. The subjective refraction was -0.75-0.50 X 105 OD (6/4.5), -0.75 -0.50 x 75 OS (6/4.5). Some of the examination findings and the ZCSBV are given in Figure 13.7. Accommodative infacility was suggested by lens flipper testing. He could not clear either side of the +2.00/-2.00 D flippers binocularly or monocularly. He achieved only six cycles per minute with + 1.50/-1.50 D flippers binocularly and eight cycles per minute with each eye monocularly. He was instructed in accommodative facility exercises to be done at home on a daily basis. He also was scheduled for weekly clinic visits for additional training and follow-up checks. At the end of a vision therapy program his NRA and PRA had increased to + 2.50 and -3.00 D, respectively, and he had a binocular accommodative facility rate of 10 cycles per minute on +2.00/-2.00 D flippers. He reported that he no longer had occasional blurring and that he could read for up to two hours without his eyes getting tired.

## REFERENCES

1. Daum KM. Accommodative dysfunction. Doc Ophthalmol 1983;55:177-98.
2. Hokoda SC. General binocular dysfunctions in an urban optometry clinic. J Am Optom Asso 1985;56:560-562.
3. Wold RM, Pierce JR, Keddington J. Effectiveness of optometric vision therapy. J Am Optom As 1970;49:1047-1054.
4. Lui JS, Lee M, Jang J, et al. Objective assessment of accommodation orthoptics. I. Dy insufficiency. Am J Optom Physiol Opt 1979;56:285-294.

5.  Suchoff I, Petito GT. *The efficacy of visual therapy accommodative disorders and non-strabismic anomalies of binocular vision. J Am Optom Assoc 1986;57: 119-125.*

6.  Rouse MW. *Management of binocular anomalies: efficacy of vision therapy in the treatment of accommodative disorders. Am J Optom Physiol Opt 1987;64: 415-420.*

7.  Cooper J, Feldman K, Selenow A, et al. *Reduction of asthenopia after accommodative facility training. Am J Optom Physiol Opt 1987;64:430-436.*

8.  Grosvenor T. *Primary Care Optometry, 5th ed. St. Louis: Butterworth Heinemann Elsevier, 2007:120-121, 232-233.*

9.  London R. *Amplitude of accommodation. In: Eskridge JB, Amos JF, Bartlett JD, eds. Clinical Procedures in Optometry. Philadelphia: Lippincott, 1991: 69-71.*

10. Daum KM. *Accommodative facility. In: Eskridge JB, Amos JF, Bartlett JD, eds. Clinical Procedures in Optometry. Philadelphia: Lippincott, 1991 :687-697.*

11. Goss DA. *Clinical accommodation testing. Curr Opin Ophthalmol 1992;3:78-82.*

12. Grosvenor T. *Primary Care Optometry, 5th ed. St. Louis: Butterworth Heinemann Elsevier, 2007:120-121, 233-234.*

13. Carlson NB, Kurtz D. *Clinical Procedures for Ocular Examination, 3rd ed. New York: McGraw-Hill, 2004:191-192.*

14. Daum KM. *Accommodative response. In: Eskridge JB, Amos JF, Bartlett JD, eds. Clinical Procedures in Optometry. Philadelphia: Lippincott, 1991: 677-686.*

15. Ciuffreda KJ, Kenyon RV. *Accommodative vergence and accommodation in normals, amblyopes, and strabismics. In: Schor CM, Ciuffreda KJ, eds. Vergence Eye Movements: Basic and Clinical Aspects. Boston: Butterworth-Heinemann, 1983:101-173.*

16. Ciuffreda KJ. *Accommodation and its anomalies. In: Charman WN, ed. Visual Optics and Instrumentation. Boca Raton: CRC Press, 1991:231-279.*

17. Ciuffreda KJ. *Accommodation, the pupil, and presbyopia. In: Benjamin WJ, ed. Borish's Clinical Refraction, 2nd ed. St. Louis: Butterworth Heinemann Elsevier, 2006:93-144.*

18. Haynes HM. *Clinical observations with dynamic retinoscopy. Optom Weekly 1960;51:2243-2246, 2306-2309.*

19. Bieber JC. *Why nearpoint retinoscopy with children? Optom Weekly 1974;65:54-57, 78-82.*

20. Saladin JJ. *Phorometry and stereopsis. In: Benjamin WJ, ed. Borish's Clinical Refraction, 2nd ed. St. Louis: Butterworth Heinemann Elsevier, 2006:899-960.*

21. Grosvenor TP. *Primary Care Optometry, 5th ed. St. Louis: Butterworth Heinemann Elsevier, 2007:198-199.*

22. Rouse MW, London R, Allen DC. *An evaluation of the monocular estimate of dynamic retinoscopy. Am J Optom Physiol Opt 1982;59:234-239.*

23. Nott IS. *Dynamic skiametry, accommodation and convergence. Am J Physiol Opt 1925;6:490-503.*

24. Borish IM. *Clinical Refraction, 3rd ed. Boston: Butterworth-Heinemann, 1970:697-704.*

25. Cross AJ. *Dynamic Skiametry in Theory and Practice. New York: Cross Optical Co, 1911:115-123.*

26. Sheard C. *Dynamic skiametry and methods of testing the accommodation and vergence of the eyes. In: The Sheard Volume-Selected Writings in Visual and Ophthalmic Optics. Philadelphia: Chilton, 1957:125-230 (originally published as a monograph in 1920).*

27. Guyton DL, O'Connor GM. *Dynamic retinoscopy. Curr Opin Ophthalmol 1991;2:78-80.*

28. Valenti CA. *The Full Scope of Retinoscopy, revised ed. Santa Ana, CA: Optometric Extension Program, 1990.*

Birnbaum MH. *Optometric Management of Nearpoint Vision Disorders. Boston: Butterworth-inemann, 1993:168-182.*

. *Significance of fused cross cylinder test. Optom Weekly 1940;31:16-19.*

A, Afanador AJ. *The accommodative response to the near point crossed cylinder test. 1974;65: 1138-1140.*

*nalysis, 3rd ed. Chicago: Professional Press, 1965:154-156.*

*fraction, 3rd ed. Boston: Butterworth-Heinemann, 1970:839-842.*

*. Anomalies of Binocular Vision: Diagnosis and Management. St. Louis:*

35. Grosvenor TP. *Primary Care Optometry*, 5th ed. St. Louis: Butterworth Heinemann Elsevier, 2007:231-232.

36. Carlson NB, Kurtz D. *Clinical Procedures for Ocular Examination*, 3rd ed. New York: McGraw-Hill, 2004:189-190.

37. Rosenfield M. Accommodation. In: Zadnik K, ed. *The Ocular Examination: Measurements and Findings*. Philadelphia: Saunders, 1997:87-121.

38. Rouse MW, Hutter RF, Shiftlett R. A normative study of the accommodative lag in elementary school children. *Am J Optom Physiol Opt* 1984;61: 693-697.

39. Locke LC, Somers W. A comparison study of dynamic retinoscopy techniques. *Optom Vis Sci* 1989;66:540-544.

40. Jackson TW, Goss DA. Variation and correlation of clinical tests of accommodative function in a sample of school-age children. *J Am Optom Assoc* 1991;62:857-866.

41. Rosenfield M, Portello JK, Blustein GH, Jang C. Comparison of clinical techniques to assess the near accommodative response. *Optom Vis Sci* 1996;73:382-388.

42. Cacho DP, García-Munoz A, García-Bernebeu JR, López A. Comparison between MEM and Nott dynamic retinoscopy. *Optom Vis Sci* 1999;76:650-655.

43. Tassinari JT. Monocular estimate method retinoscopy: central tendency measures and relationship to refractive status and heterophoria. *Optom Vis Sci* 2002;79:708-714.

44. Goss DA, Warren DF. Use of dynamic retinoscopy to determine changes in accommodative response with varying amounts of plus add. *Indiana J Optom* 2006;9:9-14.

45. Cooper J. Accommodative dysfunction. In: Amos JF, ed. *Diagnosis and Management in Vision Care*. Boston: Butterworth-Heinemann, 1987: 431-459.

46. Goss DA, Groppel P, Dominguez L. Comparison of MEM retinoscopy and Nott retinoscopy and their interexaminer repeatabilities. *J Behav Optom* 2005;16:149-155.

47. Haynes HM. Lectures at Pacific University.

48. Whitefoot H, Charman WN. Dynamic retinoscopy and accommodation. *Ophthal Physiol Opt* 1992;12:8-17.

49. Wick B, Hall P. Relation between accommodative facility, lag, and amplitude in elementary school children. *Am J Optom Physiol Opt* 1987;64:593-598.

50. Allen PM, O'Leary DJ. Accommdation functions: co-dependency and relationship to refractive error. *Vision Res* 2006;46:491-505.

51. Daum K. Accommodative insufficiency. *Am J Optom Physiol Opt* 1983;60: 352-359.

52. Scheiman M, Wick B. *Clinical Management of Binocular Vision-Heterophoric, Accommodative, and Eye Movement Disorders*, 2nd ed. Philadelphia: Lippincott Williams & Wilkins, 2002: 334-369.

53. Duke-Elder S, Abrams D. Ophthalmic Optics and Refraction. Vol 5 in: Duke- Elder S, ed. *System of Ophthalmology*. St Louis: Mosby, 1970:451-474.

54. Somers W, Locke LC. Accommodation terminology, Reply. *Optom Vis Sci* 1990; 67:386.

55. Greenspan SB. The use of M.E.M. retinoscopy to determine near point prescriptions. *Refraction Letter* May, 1975;(21).

56. Birnbaum MH. *Optometric Management of Nearpoint Vision Disorders*. Boston: Butterworth-Heinemann, 1993: 161-167.

57. Siderov J. Improving interactive facility with vision training. *Clin Exp Optom* 1990;73:128-131.

58. Haynes HM. Clinical approaches to nearpoint power determination. *Am J Optom Physiol Opt* 1985;62:375-385.

59. Tassinari JT. Change in accommodative response and posture induced by nearpoint plus lenses per monocular estimate method retinoscopy. *J Behav Optom* 2005;16:87-93.

60. Birnbaum MH. *Optometric Management of Nearpoint Vision Disorders*. Boston: Butterworth-Heinemann, 1993:172-174.

61. Griffin JR, Grisham JD. *Binocular Anomalies: Diagnosis and Vision Therapy*, 4th ed. Amsterdam: Butterworth-Heinemann, 2002:21.

62. Birnbaum MH. *Optometric Management of Nearpoint Vision Disorders*. Boston: Butterworth-Heinemann, 1993:56.

## PRACTICE PROBLEMS

1. A 20-year-old patient has a push-up amplitude of accommodation of 7.00D. How does this compare to the minimum expected amplitude? What is the term applied to this condition? What are the potential treatments?

2. Nott retinoscopy was performed on four patients. The test distance was 40 cm. Neutrality was observed with the retinoscope at the following distances: patient SN, 50 cm; patient CD, 46 cm; patient GI, 68 cm; and patient PC, 56 cm. In each case, what are the accommodative response and the lag of accommodation? Would treatment be indicated? If so, what treatment?

3. On MEM retinoscopy you observe a with motion that you estimate to be approximately 1.25D away from neutrality. What is the lag of accommodation? Is this a normal or high lag? Does this result suggest an accommodative disorder? If so, which one?

4. Plot the accommodative response/accommodative stimulus graphs for the following findings from Haynes' combined MEM-LN procedure. What were the standard MEM and low neutral findings (i.e., MEM through the BVA and low neutral the lowest amount of plus that results in neutral)? W indicates with motion, N neutral, and A against.

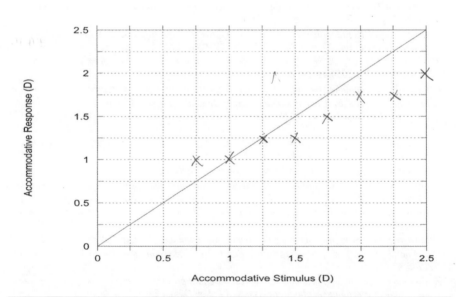

| Patient CA | | | | | | | | |
|---|---|---|---|---|---|---|---|---|
| Add (accomm. stim.) | 0 (2.50) | +0.25 (2.25) | +0.50 (2.00) | +0.75 (1.75) | +1.00 (1.50) | +1.25 (1.25) | +1.50 (1.00) | +1.75 (0.75) |
| MEM | | 0.50W | 0.50W | 0.25W | 0.25W | 0.25W | N | N | 0.25A |

AR      +2.00  +1.75  +1.75  +1.50  +1.25   |

MEM = 0.50D lag  Rt Mem = None       Birnbaum (0.25w)=+0.50 I

LN= +1.25.                LN = +1.00 Add  Birnbaum (0.50w)=no add

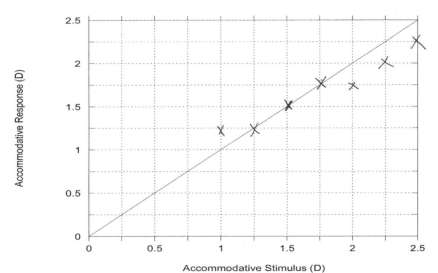

| Patient AT | | | | | | | |
|---|---|---|---|---|---|---|---|
| Add (accomm. stim.) | 0 (2.50) | +0.25 (2.25) | +0.50 (2.00) | +0.75 (1.75) | +1.00 (1.50) | +1.25 (1.25) | +1.50 (1.00) |
| MEM | 0.25W | 0.25W | 0.25W | N | N | N | 0.25A |

AR = 2.25   2.00   1.75
LN = +0.75D
MEM = +0.25D

↳ Resp is 0.25
greater than
stimulus.

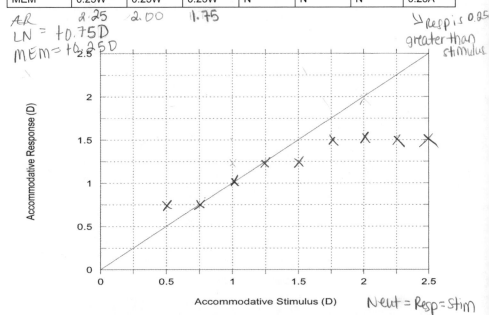

Neut = Resp = Stim

| Patient BP | | | | | | | | |
|---|---|---|---|---|---|---|---|---|
| Add (accomm. stim.) | 0 (2.50) | +0.25 (2.25) | +0.50 (2.00) | +0.75 (1.75) | +1.00 (1.50) | +1.25 (1.25) | +1.50 (1.00) | +1.75 (0.75) | +2.00 (0.50) |
| MEM | 1.00W | 0.75W | 0.50W | 0.25W | 0.25W | N | N | N | 0.25A |

RESP  +1.50  +1.50  +1.50  +1.50  +1.25

MEM = +1.00 DLag
LN = +1.25

**169** Rx MEM = +0.75
LN = +0.75

Birmbaum (0.25W)
F +0.75 add
Birbaum (0.50w)
= 0.50 add

MEM = +0.75D **add**   Birnbaum = 0.25W, +.25 **add**
LN = +1.25D add   Birnbaum = 0.50W, +0.75D add

Rx: MEM = none
LN: none

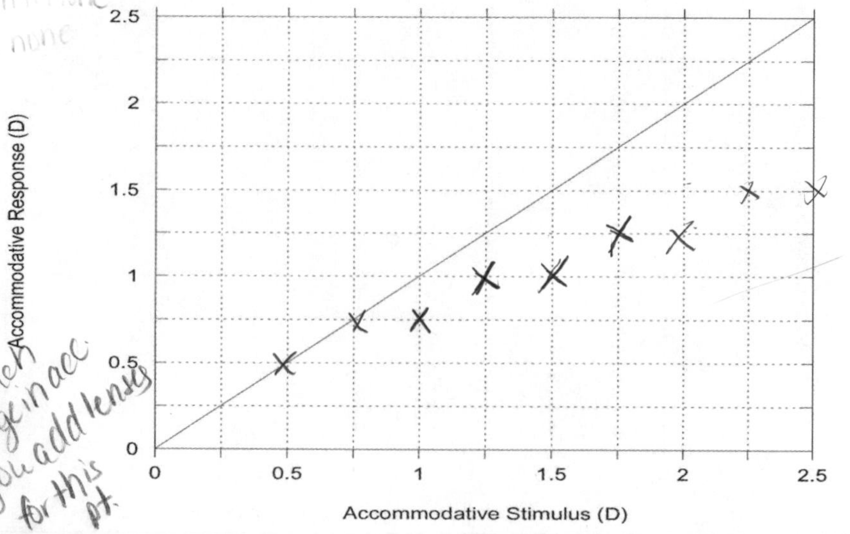

Not much change in acc as you add lenses for this pt.

**Patient OC**

| Add (accomm. stim.) | 0 (2.50) | +0.25 (2.25) | +0.50 (2.00) | +0.75 (1.75) | +1.00 (1.50) | +1.25 (1.25) | +1.50 (1.00) | +1.75 (0.75) | +2.00 (0.50) |
|---|---|---|---|---|---|---|---|---|---|
| MEM | 1.00W | 0.75W | 0.75W | 0.50W | 0.50W | 0.25W | 0.25W | N | N |

Resp:   +1.50   +1.50   +1.25   1.25   1.00   1.00   0.75   ↗ there is little change in acc.
MEM = 1.00D lag ✓   LN = +1.75D   LN+MEM close both   with lenses

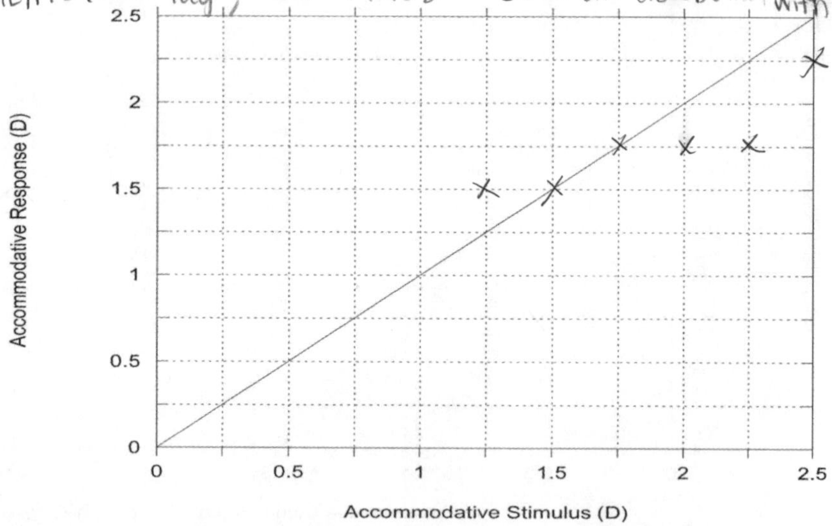

**Patient FL**

| Add (accomm. stim.) | 0 (2.50) | +0.25 (2.25) | +0.50 (2.00) | +0.75 (1.75) | +1.00 (1.50) | +1.25 (1.25) |
|---|---|---|---|---|---|---|
| MEM | 0.75W | 0.50W | 0.25W | N | N | 0.25A |

Res   +2.25   +1.75   1.75
MEM = +0.75D Lag
LN = +0.75D

Rx: MEM = none   B = (0.25W), +0.50D
LN = None   B = (0.50W), +0.25D

# Chapter 14
# Introduction to Vision Therapy for Accommodation and Convergence Disorders

Vision therapy is a treatment option available for the remediation of accommodation and vergence disorders. It can help to relieve asthenopic symptoms and can improve performance in activities such as reading which rely on efficient accommodation and vergence function. In terms of specific effects on accommodation and vergence, vision therapy can increase fusional vergence ranges, increase relative accommodation findings, and improve the latency and velocity of accommodation and vergence responses.

This chapter will provide an introduction to some basic aspects of vision therapy for the improvement of accommodation and convergence function. This chapter is not intended to be a comprehensive guide to vision therapy, but rather an overview of some of the principles involved in addressing accommodation and vergence disorders with vision therapy. Additional details on vision therapy and information on additional training procedures can be found in texts devoted largely to vision therapy.[1-6] First we will look at some common simple accommodation and vergence training procedures.

## PUSH-UP TRAINING

Push-up training is a common technique used to improve positive fusional convergence and the nearpoint of convergence. The patient brings a convenient fixation object closer in the mid-line until it feels as if the object will break into two or until it does (Figure 14.1). The patient tries to hold fusion as long as possible as the object is brought closer. This is repeated several times daily so that the patient learns to be able to bring the object closer before diplopia occurs, and the patient becomes able to do that easily. If small letters are included in the fixation object for better control of accommodation, this technique also can be used to improve the amplitude of accommodation when indicated. A disadvantage is that there is no built-in suppression control with this method. That is, there is no obvious way to make the patient aware of suppression if it is occurring. One way to check for suppression is to have the patient be aware

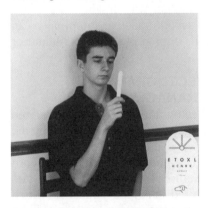

*Figure 14.1. Push-up training. The patient tries to maintain singleness of the fixation object as it is brought closer. Various targets can be used for push-up training, such as letter targets affixed to a tongue depressor, as shown here. The target used here is shown in the lower right. The addition of small letters and features aids in control of accommodation.*

of physiologic diplopia occasionally during the push-up training. Both the accommodative stimulus and the convergence stimulus increase as the fixation object is brought closer.

## BROCK STRING

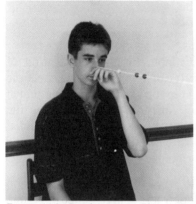

The Brock string (Figure 14.2) provides a simple, but very useful and versatile, training technique. One end of the string is tied to a chair, door knob, or other object, while the other end is held against the nose. The patient is instructed to maintain singleness of the bead being fixated. The bead is moved closer to the patient for push-up training or farther from the patient for push-away training. Both accommodative stimulus and convergence stimulus increase as the bead is brought closer. Vergence facility can be improved by having the patient alternate fixation between two or more beads.

*Figure 14.2. Brock string. The patient fixates one bead and works to maintain single vision of that bead. That bead can be moved closer to stimulate more convergence. Alternatively convergence stimulus can be varied by having the patient look from one bead to another, with the beads being separated more and more as training proceeds.*

One advantage of the Brock string is that it provides obvious suppression controls. The string should appear to be an X crossing at the fixated bead, due to physiologic diplopia. Also as a consequence of physiologic diplopia, the beads not being fixated should appear doubled. The Brock string is versatile, as, for example, it can be used for training in different fields of gaze. Another way in which the Brock string is versatile is that the convergence and accommodative stimuli also can be adjusted by training with spherical lens adds or prisms, such as with lens or prism flippers.

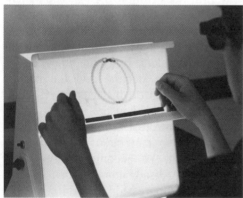

## VECTOGRAMS AND TRANAGLYPHS

Vectograms are paired polarized targets in which one is seen by the right eye and one by the left eye when polarized goggles are worn (Figure 14.3). Tranaglyphs are paired anaglyph targets in which one target is seen by the right eye and one by the left eye when a red filter is worn over one eye and a green filter over the other. Vectograms and tranaglyphs are used to train fusional vergence. Points of

*Figure 14.3. A Vectogram. One of the targets is seen by the right eye and one by the left eye when Polaroid goggles are worn. As the plastic sheets containing the targets are separated, the convergence stimulus changes.*

similarity on the targets are fused, while points of dissimilarity are used as clues that suppression is occurring.

A base-out stimulus can be induced by moving the target seen by the left eye to the right of the target seen by the right eye. This stimulates positive fusional vergence, because for single vision the lines of sight would need to cross between the patient and the target. A base-in stimulus is induced if the target seen by the left eye is moved to the left of the target seen by the right eye. Therefore, for single vision the lines of sight of the two eyes would need to cross behind the plane of the target, stimulating negative fusional vergence. In either situation, the accommodative stimulus is unchanged.

## BINOCULAR LENS ROCK
Binocular lens rock is a technique used primarily to improve accommodative facility. A pair of plus lenses and a pair of minus lenses (usually +2.00 and -2.00 D, but may be lower powers at the start of a training program) in a lens flipper bar are used to vary the accommodative stimulus. This training procedure is done by alternating between the plus and minus lenses similar to the way that lens rock accommodative facility testing is done (see chapter 7). The patient works to improve the speed and ease with which clarity of the letters can be achieved after each lens flip.

The plus lenses decrease the accommodative stimulus, while the minus lenses increase the accommodative stimulus. The convergence stimulus remains constant, so a change in accommodative convergence must be accompanied by an equal magnitude but opposite direction change in fusional vergence. Therefore, binocular lens rock training may improve fusional vergence as well as accommodative facility.

## MONOCULAR LENS ROCK
Because binocular lens rock performance may be limited by fusional vergence, a training program for accommodative facility is typically begun with monocular lens rock. This is performed in the same way as binocular lens rock, except that one eye is excluded from viewing by occlusion or some other means. Once adequate performance on monocular lens rock is achieved, the patient moves on to binocular lens rock. Because one eye is occluded, there is no convergence stimulus. Accommodative stimulus increases with the minus lens and decreases with the plus lens.

## DISTANCE ROCK
Accommodative facility training also can be done with a distance rock procedure. The patient alternates fixation between a distance target and a near target. The targets should contain letters or figures close to the patient's best corrected visual acuity. Hart charts (Figure 14.4) are examples of charts often used for this purpose. The patient clears one letter on the distance chart and then clears one letter on the near chart, alternating between them as quickly as possible. The accommodative stimulus and the convergence stimulus increase and decrease together, being at a minimum during distance fixation and maximum during near fixation.

## PRISM ROCK

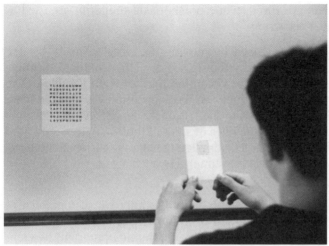

Vergence facility can be trained by prisms in a flipper bar like that used for lens rock training. There are base-out prisms on one side of the flipper and base-in prisms on the other. The patient is instructed to fuse the two images as quickly as possible after each flip from one set of prisms to the other. The accommodative stimulus is constant. The

*Figure 14.4. Distance rock training with Hart charts. On these particular charts, the letters are the same on both the distance chart and the near chart. The patient calls out one letter on the distance chart as soon as he can clear it, then one letter on the near chart, and so on back and forth between the two charts.*

base-out prisms on one side of the flipper increase the convergence stimulus, and the base-in prisms on the other side decrease the convergence stimulus.

## FREE SPACE FUSION EXERCISES

Free space fusion involves the use of two laterally separated targets, which are similar enough to be fused. Examples of free space fusion targets are displayed in Figure 14.5. Chiastopic fusion occurs by converging inside the plane of the targets so that the right eye fixates the left target and the left eye fixates the right target.[7] Orthopic fusion is achieved by converging beyond the plane of the targets so that the right eye fixates the right target and the left eye fixates the left target.[7] (Don't confuse the word orthopic with the word orthoptics, which is sometimes used as a synonym for vision therapy[8])

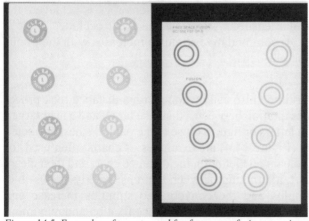

During free space fusion exercises the accommodative stimulus remains constant and depends on the distance from the spectacle plane to the target. Exercises involving chiastopic fusion are used to improve positive fusional vergence. The convergence stimulus depends on the target distance

*Figure 14.5. Examples of targets used for free space fusion exercises.*

and the amount of lateral separation of the fused targets, a greater lateral separation yielding a greater convergence stimulus. Orthopic fusion trains negative fusional vergence. On orthopic fusion widening the lateral separation of the targets decreases the convergence stimulus, thus inducing further divergence behind the plane of the target.

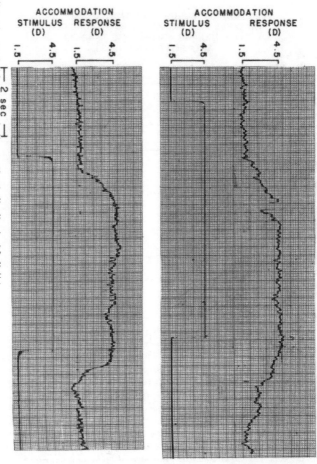

Figure 14.6. Optometer recordings demonstrating improvement in accommodation response dynamics with vision therapy. Time is on the x-axis of each trace. Accommodation in diopters is on the y-axis. The upper trace shows an accommodative response before vision therapy. The accommodative stimulus changed from 1.5 D to 4.5 D and back. The lower trace is a recording in the same subject after vision therapy. The effect of training was a decrease in latency (time between onset of stimulus and onset of response) and an increase in velocity (slope of the accommodative response; that is, the change in accommodative response per change in time). (From: Liu JS, Lee M, Jang J, et al. Objective assessment of accommodation orthoptics: dynamic insufficiency. Am J Optom Physiol Opt 1979;56:285-294 © The American Academy of Optometry, 1979)

## EFFECTIVENESS OF VISION THERAPY IN ACCOMMODATION AND VERGENCE DISORDERS

Vision therapy is highly effective in improving accommodation and vergence function in patients who are compliant with the therapy program. A large number of studies and reviews on effects of vision therapy have reported alleviation of symptoms, improvements in clinical test findings, and improvements in laboratory measures of accommodation and vergence in non-strabismic

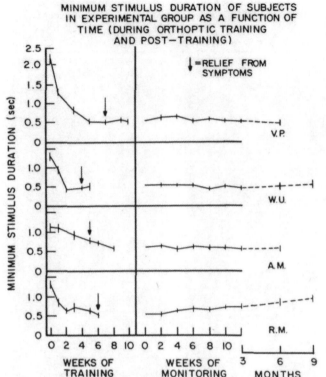

MINIMUM STIMULUS DURATION OF SUBJECTS IN EXPERIMENTAL GROUP AS A FUNCTION OF TIME (DURING ORTHOPTIC TRAINING AND POST−TRAINING)

↓ =RELIEF FROM SYMPTOMS

*Figure 14.7. Improvement in vergence response times with training in four subjects. The time required to complete a vergence response is on the y-axis and the number of weeks of training is on the x-axis. The right side of the figure shows weeks of monitoring after the completion of training on the x-axis, showing a maintenance of improvements in three of the four subjects. (From: Grisham JD, Bowman MC, Owyang LA, Chan CL. Vergence orthoptics: validity and persistence of the training effect. Optom Vis Sci 1991;68:441-451 © The American Academy of Optometry, 1991))*

accommodation and vergence disorders.[9-58] A sampling of those studies will be discussed next.

Liu et al.[16] used an objective optometer to show that the dynamics of accommodative responses improved as a result of vision therapy in three young adult subjects. Figure 14.6 shows optometer recordings before and after vision therapy. The accommodative stimulus in diopters and the accommodative response in diopters are expressed on the y-axis and time is on the x-axis. A recording before vision therapy is shown at the top of the figure and a recording after vision therapy is shown in the bottom of the figure. It may be seen that the latency of the accommodative response (time between onset of the stimulus and onset of the response) decreased with therapy and velocity of the response (slope of response as a function of time) increases with therapy. These findings were confirmed by Bobier and Sivak.[26]

Grisham et al.[45] showed that speed of vergence responses improves with vision therapy. They used an infrared eye movement monitor to objectively determine the minimum time required to complete a vergence response. This time improved for four training subjects with vergence disorders (as shown in Figure 14.7), but not in three controls who did not undergo training.

Daum[35] showed how clinical test findings changed in 179 patients with exodeviations treated with vision therapy at The Ohio State University College of Optometry. Diagnoses were convergence insufficiency in 110 patients, basic exophoria in 49 patients, and divergence excess in 18 patients. Patients with

**Table 14.1.** Mean test findings before and after vision therapy (standard deviations in parentheses) for 179 patients with exodeviations, from a study by Daum.[35] Units are prism diopters for angle of deviation and fusional vergence ranges, cm for NPC, and D for amplitude of accommodation.

| Test | N | Before therapy | After therapy | Stat. sig. of change |
|---|---|---|---|---|
| 6 m angle of deviation | 97 | 9.7 exo (10.2) | 8.6 exo (9.5) | p=0.0018 |
| 40 cm angle of deviation | 109 | 12.8 exo (7.1) | 11.5 exo (6.7) | p<0.0001 |
| ACA ratio | 96 | 4.7 (3.4) | 4.9 (3.4) | p=0.44 |
| Distance BI break | 29 | 10 (7) | 13 (9) | p=0.015 |
| Distance BI recovery | 29 | 7 (6) | 9 (7) | p=0.03 |
| Distance BO blur | 53 | 11 (6) | 15 (8) | p<0.0001 |
| Distance BO break | 53 | 15 (8) | 26 (12) | p<0.0001 |
| Distance BO recovery | 53 | 11 (8) | 20 (12) | p<0.0001 |
| 40 cm BI blur | 41 | 12 (8) | 15 (7) | p=0.014 |
| 40 cm BI break | 41 | 16 (8) | 19 (8) | p=0.05 |
| 40 cm BI recovery | 41 | 13 (7) | 15 (6) | p=0.25 |
| 40 cm BO blur | 100 | 13 (7) | 23 (12) | p<0.0001 |
| 40 cm BO break | 100 | 20 (9) | 32 (12) | p<0.0001 |
| 40 cm BO recovery | 100 | 14 (10) | 27 (12) | p<0.0001 |
| NPC | 32 | 7.8 (4.6) | 3.9 (2.6) | p<0.0001 |
| Amplitude of accommodation | 55 | 9.4 (3.0) | 11.8 (3.5) | p<0.0001 |

**Table 14.2.** Test findings before and after vision therapy (standard deviations in parentheses) for 114 patients with accommodative disorders, from a study by Daum.[24] Units are prism diopters for fusional vergence ranges and D for amplitude of accommodation.

| Test | N | Before therapy | After therapy | Stat. sig. of change |
|---|---|---|---|---|
| Near BI blur | 41 | 7 (4) | 11 (5) | p=0.0004 |
| Near BI break | 41 | 13 (6) | 15 (5) | p=0.0764 |
| Near BI recovery | 41 | 9 (6) | 11 (5) | p=0.0723 |
| Near BO blur | 64 | 12 (7) | 20 (10) | p<0.0001 |
| Near BO break | 64 | 18 (8) | 29 (11) | p<0.0001 |
| Near BO recovery | 64 | 13 (7) | 23 (11) | p<0.0001 |
| Amplitude of accommodation | 84 | 8.3 (2.7) | 11.5 (3.3) | p<0.0001 |

strabismus were not excluded from the sample, but the patient sample consisted primarily of persons without strabismus. The changes in test findings as a result of vision therapy are summarized in Table 14.1. Of the test results listed, only the ACA ratio, the BI break at distance, and the base-in recovery at near did not show statistically significant improvements. The largest changes were the increases in the base-out vergence ranges. The mean NPC after vision therapy was half of what it was before therapy. Similar to Daum's results, Brautaset and Jennings[58] found significant improvements in fusional vergence with training in convergence insufficiency, but did not find a significant change in ACA ratio.

| Table 14.3. Mean NRA and PRA before and after vision therapy in two studies. | | |
|---|---|---|
| | Sterner et al.[52] | Goss et al.[54] |
| NRA before therapy | +1.15 D | +1.75 D |
| NRA after therapy | +1.90 D | +2.42 D |
| Statistical significance of change in NRA | | p<0.0001 |
| PRA before therapy | -1.19 D | -1.67 D |
| PRA after therapy | -2.46 D | -2.84 D |
| Statistical significance of change in PRA | | p<0.0001 |

Table 14.4. Changes in symptom survey scores and test findings in children with convergence insufficiency in a study by Scheiman et al.[55] Units are cm on NPC and prism diopters on BO break. Values given are means with standard deviations in parentheses. A higher symptom score indicates a higher level of symptoms.

| | Pencil push-ups | Office-based vision therapy | Placebo vision therapy |
|---|---|---|---|
| Number of subjects | 11 | 15 | 12 |
| Symptom survey score at baseline | 29.3 (5.4) | 32.1 (7.9) | 30.7 (10.6) |
| Symptom survey score after treatment | 25.9 (7.3) | 9.5 (8.2) | 24.2 (11.9) |
| Statistical significance of change in symptom score | p=0.24 | p<0.001 | p=0.04 |
| NPC break at baseline | 14.6 (7.4) | 13.7 (7.4) | 15.5 (6.8) |
| NPC break after treatment | 9.1 (5.1) | 4.5 (3.6) | 9.3 (4.4) |
| Statistical significance of change in NPC | p=0.08 | p<0.001 | p=0.03 |
| Near BO break at baseline | 12.6 (3.2) | 12.5 (4.3) | 12.1 (3.4) |
| Near BO break after treatment | 14.25 (5.3) | 31.8 (10.0) | 19.8 (10.3) |
| Statistical significance of change in BO break | p=0.22 | p<0.001 | p=0.03 |

Daum[24] also reported changes in clinical test findings after vision therapy for accommodative disorders among patients at The Ohio State University College of Optometry. The diagnosis was accommodative insufficiency in 96 cases, accommodative infacility in 14 cases, accommodative excess in 3, and accommodative fatigue in one. Findings before and after vision therapy are summarized in Table 14.2. Improvements were observed in amplitude of accommodation and fusional vergence ranges. The results of two studies[52,54] showing improvements in NRA and PRA with vision therapy are shown in Table 14.3.

In a literature review of studies on vision therapy in convergence insufficiency, Grisham[41] compiled the results of 15 studies conducted over more than 40 years. Of a total of 1931 patients in those studies, Grisham noted an aggregate 72% cure rate and an overall 91% of patients showing either a cure or improvement.

**Table 14.5. Changes in symptom survey scores and test findings in young adults with convergence insufficiency in a study by Scheiman et al.[56] Units are cm on NPC and prism diopters on BO break. Values given are means with standard deviations in parentheses. A higher symptom score indicates a higher level of symptoms.**

| | Pencil push-ups | Office-based vision therapy | Placebo vision therapy |
|---|---|---|---|
| Number of subjects | 15 | 12 | 13 |
| Symptom survey score at baseline | 37.6 (7.7) | 36.5 (8.7) | 37.5 (11.4) |
| Symptom survey score after treatment | 26.5 (7.3) | 20.7 (10.2) | 25.2 (10.3) |
| Statistical significance of change in symptom score | p<0.001 | p<0.001 | p<0.001 |
| NPC break at baseline | 12.5 (6.6) | 12.8 (7.7) | 14.5 (7.8) |
| NPC break after treatment | 7.8 (4.1) | 5.3 (1.7) | 9.6 (4.0) |
| Statistical significance of change in NPC | p=0.001 | p=0.002 | p=0.04 |
| Near BO break at baseline | 13.6 (7.1) | 11.3 (4.3) | 11.5 (4.4) |
| Near BO break after treatment | 24.2 (12.5) | 29.7 (10.8) | 17.5 (5.7) |
| Statistical significance of change in BO break | p<0.001 | p=0.001 | p=0.003 |

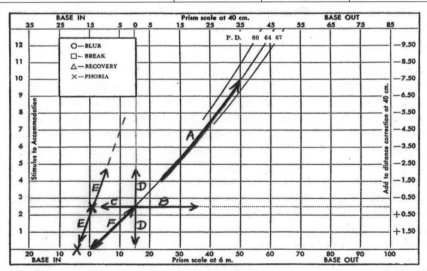

*Figure 14.8. Plots representing changes in accommodative stimulus and convergence stimulus during various vision training procedures. A, binocular push-up from 25 cm to 10 cm or pulling a Brock string bead in from 25 cm to 10 cm; B, Vectogram or Tranaglyph target at 40 cm with the plastic sheets moved to 20Δ BO on the scale; C, Vectogram or Tranaglyph target at 40 cm with the plastic sheets moved to 10Δ BI on the scale; D, binocular lens rock with +2/-2 D flippers and target at 40 cm; E, monocular lens rock with +2/-2 D flippers and target at 40 cm; F, binocular distance rock alternating fixation between targets at 6 m and 40 cm.*

In the time since the completion of that review by Grisham, Scheiman and his colleagues[55,56] have completed two studies comparing effects of pencil push-ups, office-based vision therapy, and placebo vision therapy in convergence insufficiency. The subjects were 9 to 18 years of age in one study and 19 to 30 years of age in the other study. In both studies, a 15 question symptom survey was used to assess the effect of therapy on symptoms. NPC and near BO break findings were taken before and after therapy. The office-based vision therapy group showed greater improvements in symptom survey scores, NPC, and BO break findings than the pencil push-ups group and the placebo therapy group in the study with children (Table 14.4) and in the study with young adults (Table 14.5).

## GRAPHICAL SPECIFICATION OF ACCOMMODATION AND CONVERGENCE STIMULI ON VARIOUS TRAINING PROCEDURES

One way to aid understanding of how accommodation and vergence stimuli are being changed during some of the different training procedures is to represent those changes graphically. This has been done in Figure 14.8 using the familiar accommodation and convergence graph form to represent changes in accommodation and vergence stimuli on different training techniques. A PD of 64 mm was assumed and it was assumed that the patient was viewing through BVA lenses.

Because the convergence stimulus and the accommodative stimulus are varied by changing target distance on training with the push-up method and with the Brock string, changes in convergence and accommodative stimuli change together. In Figure 14.8 the changes in stimulus levels when an object is moved from 25 cm from the spectacle plane in to 10 cm from the spectacle plane are represented by the arrow designated with the letter A.

Vectograms and Tranaglyphs have scales at the top and bottom of the plastic sheets indicating the change in convergence stimulus as the sheets are pulled apart. Those scale values can be added to the convergence stimulus for the distance from the patient to the plastic sheets. If the patient's spectacle plane is 40 cm from the vectogram and the targets are slowly separated to increase the base-out stimulus from 0 (no target separation) to 20Δ base-out, the convergence stimulus would increase from 15Δ to 35Δ, while the accommodative stimulus is unchanged. This is illustrated by arrow B in Figure 14.8. Because the accommodative stimulus is unchanged, only positive fusional vergence is stimulated. If the convergence stimulus from target separation is changed from 0 to 10Δ base-in, the total convergence stimulus would change from 15 to 5Δ (arrow C in Figure 14.8).

Arrow D in Figure 14.8 shows the change in accommodative stimulus on binocular lens rock. With a target at 40 cm and +2.00/-2.00D flippers, the accommodative stimulus alternates between 0.50 and 4.50 D, while the total convergence stimulus remains constant at 15Δ.

If a target distance of 40 cm is used with +2.00/-2.00D flippers on monocular lens rock, the accommodative stimulus changes back and forth between

0.50 and 4.50D. Because binocular fusion is prevented, there is no convergence stimulus, and the vergence position the eyes assume is the phoria position. Therefore, accommodation and convergence can be represented graphically as moving up and down the phoria line (which in this example extends from 4Δexo at distance to 14Δ exo at 40 cm), as shown with arrow E in Figure 14.8.

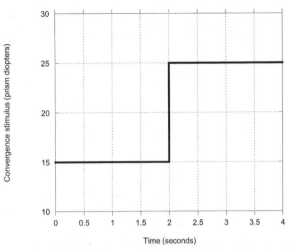

*Figure 14.9. Example of a graph of stimulus level as a function of time where there is a step change in stimulus. In this particular example, an individual with a 64 mm PD viewed an object at 40 cm for two seconds and then a 10Δ BO prism was suddenly introduced. Note that the form of the graph looks like a step.*

On binocular distance rock training, the accommodative stimulus and the convergence stimulus change together with the change in distance. With the charts placed at 6 m and 40 cm, the accommodative and convergence stimuli would be at the levels illustrated by arrow F in Figure 14.8. Arrow F is drawn as a movement back and forth between the demand line points for 6 m and 40 cm.

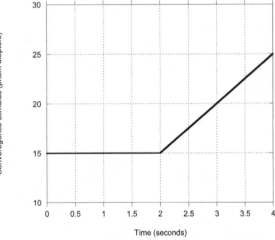

*Figure 14.10. Example of a graph of stimulus level as a function of time where there is a ramp change in stimulus. In this particular example, an individual looked at a Vectogram at 40 cm and then gradually and smoothly changed the scale setting from 0 to 10Δ BO. Note that the form of the graph looks like a ramp.*

Training procedures which change either the accommodative stimulus or the convergence stimulus while leaving the other one constant are generally more difficult than training procedures which change accommodation and convergence in the same direction. For that reason, the latter type of procedure (accommodation and vergence changing together) is generally emphasized earlier in a therapy program, and the former type of procedure (accommodation or vergence moving free of the other) is emphasized later. For procedures like

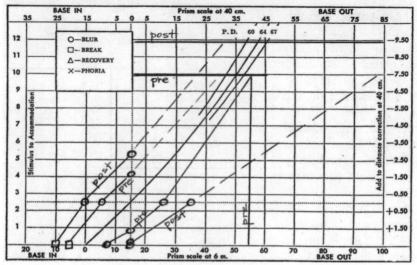

*Figure 14.11. Mean test findings before (labeled pre) and after (labeled post) vision therapy from one study.[54] The NPC improved such that the convergence amplitude increased from 54Δ to well over 100Δ. Amplitude of accommodation increased from 10.0 to 11.9 D. Vergence range blurs, NRA, and PRA also increased.*

Vectograms, Tranaglyphs, and free space fusion cards where the convergence stimulus changes and the accommodative stimulus remains constant, some blur can be allowed at first if it helps to maintain single vision. In other words, some accommodative convergence can be allowed at first to help achieve the needed total amount of convergence. However, patients should strive to learn to keep the target clear and single. In other words, they should learn to use fusional vergence without accommodative convergence.

## CHANGES IN ACCOMMODATION AND VERGENCE STIMULI AS A FUNCTION OF TIME ON VARIOUS TRAINING PROCEDURES

Figure 14.8 provided an illustration of the amounts of change in accommodation and convergence stimuli on various training procedures. It did not show how the stimuli changed with time. On some procedures, the change in stimulus is presented all at once. On other procedures, the stimulus is changed gradually. A sudden change is sometimes called a step stimulus. The reason for that terminology can be visualized in the graph of stimulus over time in Figure 14.9. A gradual change is sometimes called a ramp stimulus, from the appearance of a ramp, as shown in Figure 14.10.

When applied to changes in convergence stimuli, procedures which introduce step changes in stimulus are sometimes referred to as jump vergences. An example would be prism rock. Procedures which yield ramp changes in convergence stimulus are sometimes called smooth vergences. Slowly pulling the Vectogram sheets apart would represent a smooth vergence. The Brock string can be used for either smooth vergences or jump vergences. Fixating on one bead and moving it slowly toward the patient would be a smooth vergence. Changing fixation between beads at different distances would be a jump vergence.

## SEQUENCING OF PROCEDURES IN A VISION THERAPY PROGRAM

An important aspect of designing a vision therapy program is to plan the sequence in which the patient will work on various procedures. Some of the principles involved in sequencing procedures are as follows:

1. Start the therapy program by emphasizing the direction of deficiency. For example, in exophoria, start with working on the base-out vergences. Or in accommodative insufficiency, start with work on stimulation of accommodation. Later in the therapy program, work should be done in both directions.

2. Start with less challenging tasks that the patient can achieve and work toward good performance on difficult procedures. Other factors being equal, smooth vergences tend to be easier than jump vergences, so jump vergences are usually done later. Procedures in which accommodation and convergence stimuli change together (e.g., distance rock, Brock string) are easier than procedures in which either the accommodative stimulus or the convergence stimulus changes and the other is constant (e.g., binocular lens rock, Vectograms, free space fusion). Also targets which are larger with more peripheral features are generally easier for fusional vergence training than smaller more central targets.

3. When training fusional vergence on procedures where the accommodative stimulus remains constant, such as free space fusion cards, some blur can be allowed if it aids fusion, but the patient should work toward achieving clear and single vision.

4. Increases in the magnitudes of accommodation and vergence findings are emphasized more in the early phases of a therapy program. Quickness and ease of accommodation and vergence responses are emphasized later in the therapy program.

Textbooks on vision therapy should be consulted for further information on sequencing of training procedures and on the planning and organization of vision therapy.

## GRAPHICAL REPRESENTATION OF VISION THERAPY RESULTS

Several authors[59-63] have described the plotting of accommodation and vergence data to aid in planning vision therapy and in portraying vision therapy results. Because a graph can summarize a large amount of data, it can be a convenient way of illustrating improvements in accommodation and vergence with vision therapy in case reports or in aggregate data. Figure 14.11 shows how this can be done using mean test data before and after vision therapy from one study.

## REFERENCES

1. Rosner J, Rosner J. Vision Therapy in a Primary-Care Practice. New York: Professional Press, 1988.
2. Richman JE, Cron MT. Guide to Vision Therapy. South Bend, IN: Bernell Corp, 1988.
3. Birnbaum MH. Optometric Management of Nearpoint Vision Disorders. Boston: Butterworth-Heinemann, 1993:281-393.

4. Press LJ, ed. *Applied Concepts in Vision Therapy*. Santa Ana, CA: Optometric Extension Program Foundation, 2008.

5. Griffin JR, Grisham JD. *Binocular Anomalies-Procedures for Vision Therapy*, 4th ed. Amsterdam: Butterworth-Heinemann, 2002.

6. Scheiman M, Wick B. *Clinical Management of Binocular Vision-Heterophoric, Accommodative, and Eye Movement Disorders*, 2nd ed. Philadelphia: Lippincott Williams & Wilkins, 2002: 121-369.

7. Hofstetter HW, Griffin JR, Berman MS, Everson RW. *Dictionary of Visual Science and Related Clinical Terms*, 5th ed. Boston: Butterworth-Heinemann, 2000:209.

8. Hofstetter HW, Griffin JR, Berman MS, Everson RW. *Dictionary of Visual Science and Related Clinical Terms*, 5th ed. Boston: Butterworth-Heinemann, 2000:369.

9. Hoffman L, Cohen AH, Feuer G. Effectiveness of non-strabismus optometric vision training in a private practice. *Am J Optom Arch Am Acad Optom* 1973;50:813-816.

10. Wick B. Vision training for presbyopic nonstrabismic patients. *Am J Optom Physiol Opt* 1977;54:244-247.

11. Cooper J, Duckman R. Convergence insufficiency: incidence, diagnosis, and treatment. *J Am Optom Assoc* 1978;49:673-680.

12. Wold RM, Pierce JR, Keddington J. Effectiveness of optometric vision therapy. *J Am Optom Assoc* 1978;49:1047-1054.

13. Vaegan. Convergence and divergence show large and sustained improvement after short isometric exercise. *Am J Optom Physiol Opt* 1979;56:23-33.

14. Vaegan, McMonnies C. Clinical vergence training. *Aust J Optom* 1979;62:28-36.

15. Weisz CL. Clinical therapy for accommodative responses: transfer effects upon performance. *J Am Optom Assoc* 1979;50:209-216.

16. Liu JS, Lee M, Jang J, Ciuffreda KJ, Wong JH, Grisham JD, Stark L. Objective assessment of accommodation orthoptics: dynamic insufficiency. *Am J Optom Physiol Opt* 1979;56:285-294.

17. Cooper J, Feldman J. Operant conditioning of fusional convergence ranges using random dot stereograms. *Am J Optom Physiol Opt* 1980;57:205-213.

18. Dalziel CC. Effect of vision training on patients who fail Sheard's criterion. *Am J Optom Physiol Opt* 1981;58:21-23.

19. Goodson RA, Rahe AJ. Visual training effects on normal vision. *Am J Optom Physiol Opt* 1981;58:787-791.

20. Pantano FM. Orthoptic treatment of convergence insufficiency: A two-year follow-up report. *Am Orthoptic J* 1982;32:73-80.

21. Daum KM. The course and effect of visual training on the vergence system. *Am J Optom Physiol Opt* 1982;59:223-227.

22. Kertesz AE. The effectiveness of wide-angle fusional stimulation in the treatment of convergence insufficiency. *Invest Ophthalmol Vis Sci* 1982;22:690-693.

23. North RV, Henson DB. Effect of orthoptics upon the ability of patients to adapt to prism-induced heterophoria. *Am J Optom Physiol Opt* 1982;59:983-986.

24. Daum KM. Accommodative dysfunction. *Doc Ophthalmol* 1983;55:177-198.

25. Daum KM. Accommodative insufficiency. *Am J Optom Physiol Opt* 1983;60:352-359.

26. Bobier WR, Sivak JG. Orthoptic treatment of subjects showing slow accommodative responses. *Am J Optom Physiol Opt* 1983;60:678-687.

27. Daum KM. A comparison of the results of tonic and phasic vergence training. *Am J Optom Physiol Opt* 1983;60:769-775.

28. Cooper J, Selenow A, Ciuffreda KJ, Feldman J, Faverty J, Hokoda SC, Silver J. Reduction of asthenopia in patients with convergence insufficiency after fusional vergence training. *Am J Optom Physiol Opt* 1983;60:982-989.

29. Daum KM. Accommodative dysfunction. *Doc Ophthalmol* 1983;55:177-198.

30. Daum KM. Divergence excess: characteristics and results of treatment with orthoptics. *Ophthalmic Physiol Opt* 1984;4:15-24.

31. Daum KM. Convergence insufficiency. *Am J Optom Physiol Opt* 1984;61:16-22.

32. Daum KM. Equal exodeviations: characteristics and results of treatment with orthoptics. *Aust J Optom* 1984;67:53-59.

33. Cohen AH, Soden R. *Effectiveness of visual therapy for convergence insufficiencies for an adult population. J Am Optom Assoc* 1984;55:491-494.

34. American Optometric Association. *Position statement on vision therapy. J Am Optom Assoc* 1985;56:782-783.

35. Daum KM. *Characteristics of exodeviations: II. Changes with treatment with orthoptics. Am J Optom Physiol Opt* 1986;63:244-251.

36. Suchoff IB, Petito GT. *The efficacy of vision therapy. J Am Optom Assoc* 1986;57:119-125.

37. Griffin JR. *Efficacy of vision therapy for non-strabismic vergence anomalies. Am J Optom Physiol Opt* 1987;64:411-414.

38. Rouse MW. *Management of binocular anomalies: Efficacy of vision therapy in the treatment of accommodative disorders. Am J Optom Physiol Opt* 1987;64:415-420.

39. Cooper J, Feldman J, Selenow A, Fair R, Buccerio F, MacDonald D, Levy M. *Reduction of asthenopia after accommodative facility training. Am J Optom Physiol Opt* 1987;64:430-436.

40. Cohen AH, Lowe SE, Steele GT, Suchoff IB, Gottlieb DD, Trevorrow TL. *The efficacy of optometric vision therapy. J Am Optom Assoc* 1988;59:95-105.

41. Grisham JD. *Vision therapy results for convergence insufficiency: a literature review. Am J Optom Physiol Opt* 1988;65:448-454.

42. Cooper J. *Review of computerized orthoptics with specific regard to convergence insufficiency. Am J Optom Physiol Opt* 1988;65:455-463.

43. Mazow ML, France TD, Finkleman S, Frank J, Jenkins P. *Acute accommodative and convergence insufficiency. Tr Am Ophthalmol Soc* 1989;87:158-173.

44. Siderov J. *Improving interactive facility with vision training. Clin Exp Optom* 1990;73:128-131.

45. Grisham JD. *Vergence orthoptics: validity and persistence of the training effect. Am J Optom Physiol Opt* 1991;68:441-451.

46. Lane KA, Maples WC. *Parents' satisfaction with vision therapy. J Behav Optom* 1995;6:151-153.

47. Ficarra AP, Berman J, Rosenfield M, Portello JK. *Vision training: predictive factors for success in visual therapy for patients with convergence excess. J Optom Vis Dev* 1996;27:213-219.

48. Gallaway M, Scheiman M. *The efficacy of vision therapy for convergence excess. J Am Optom Assoc* 1997;68:81-86.

49. Sterner B, Abrahamsson M, Sjöström A. *Accommodative facility training with a long term follow up in a sample of school aged children showing accommodative dysfunction. Doc Ophthalmol* 1999;99:93-101.

50. Birnbaum MH, Soden R, Cohen AH. *Efficacy of vision therapy for convergence insufficiency in an adult male population. J Am Optom Assoc* 1999;70:225-232.

51. American Academy of Optometry American Optometric Association Joint Statement. *Vision Therapy: Information for Health Care and Other Allied Professionals. Optom Vis Sci* 1999;76:739-740.

52. Sterner B, Abrahamsson M, Sjöström A. *The effects of accommodative facility training on a group of children with impaired relative accommodation – a comparison between dioptric treatment and sham treatment. Ophthal Physiol Opt* 2001; 21:470-476.

53. Ciuffreda KJ. *The scientific basis for and efficacy of optometric vision therapy in nonstrabismic accommodative and vergence disorders. Optom* 2002;73:735-762.

54. Goss DA, Strand K, Poloncak J. *Effect of vision therapy on clinical test results in accommodative dysfunction. J Optom Vis Dev* 2003;34:61-63.

55. Scheiman M, Mitchell GL, Cotter S, et al. *A randomized clinical trial of treatments for convergence insufficiency in children. Arch Ophthalmol* 2005;123:14-24.

56. Scheiman M, Mitchell GL, Cotter S, et al. *A randomized clinical trial of vision therapy/orthoptics versus pencil push-ups for the treatment of convergence insufficiency in young adults. Optom Vis Sci* 2005;82:583-593.

57. Aziz S, Cleary M, Stewart HK, Weir CR. *Are orthoptic exercises an effective treatment for convergence and fusion deficiencies? Strabismus* 2006;14:183-189.

58. Brautaset RL, Jennings AJM. *Effects of orthoptic treatment on the CA/C and AC/A ratios in convergence insufficiency. Invest Ophthalmol Vis Sci* 2006;47:2876-2880.

59. Hofstetter HW. *Orthoptics specification by a graphical method. Am J Optom Arch Am Acad Optom* 1949;26:439-444.

60. Flom MC. *The use of accommodative convergence relationship in prescribing orthoptics. California Optometrist* 1953;21:72-75.

61. Schapero M. *The characteristics of ten basic visual training problems. Am J Optom Arch Am Acad Optom* 1955;32:333-342.

62. Heath GG. *The use of graphic analysis in visual training. Am J Optom Arch Am Acad Optom* 1959;36:337-350.

63. Borish IM. *Clinical Refraction, 3rd ed. Boston: Butterworth-Heinemann,* 1970:917-923.

# Chapter 15
# Vertical Imbalances

Vertical imbalances, as well as horizontal imbalances, may be a cause of visual complaints. The person with a vertical phoria may complain of a pulling sensation, headaches, asthenopia, skipping lines or losing place when reading, and/or a diplopia in which the images are one above the other or diagonal to each other.

Any vertical movement on the cover test should be recorded. However, it should be noted that the minimum eye movement that can be seen by an observer under ideal conditions is about two prism diopters.[1-3] von Noorden[4] suggested that the minimum eye movement that can be seen with the conditions under which the cover test is usually performed is three to four prism diopters. Because small vertical phorias can be clinically significant and the amount of eye movement that can be observed on the cover test is limited, *the absence of a vertical movement on the cover test does not rule out a vertical imbalance.* Some other additional method of testing for vertical dissociated phoria should be done on every patient along with the cover test. In addition to the von Graefe technique in the phoropter, the dissociated phoria can be taken by means of the modified Thorington test, the Maddox rod test, the stereoscope, or other methods.[5]

If the vertical dissociated phoria is not zero, the vertical associated phoria (the vertical prism which reduces the vertical fixation disparity to zero) should be tested. Because accommodative convergence does not affect vertical phorias, spherical lens adds are not used to treat a primary vertical imbalance. The treatment of choice for vertical imbalances is vertical prism. A less commonly used option is vision therapy.

In cases of high refractive error, it is important that there be no tilt of the phoropter or of the spectacles, so that a vertical phoria is not induced by the lenses. One way to solve this problem in the phoropter is to align the patient so that the target is seen through the pinholes and then to repeat the phoria.

The vertical fusional amplitudes can be used as a check on the dissociated vertical phoria. The following formula can be used to see if the vertical dissociated phoria and vertical fusional vergence ranges yield consistent results:

(Base-down to break - Base-up to break)/2 = Predicted vertical phoria

If the resultant correcting prism value is positive, base-down is suggested; if negative, base-up is suggested. The vertical phoria may differ from the prediction from the vertical fusional amplitude imbalance as a result of the lateral vergence difference during the two types of measurement. If so, the imbalance between the vertical fusional ranges may be the more important test result, according to Borish.[6]

Diagnol or vertical diplopia = vertical imbalance.

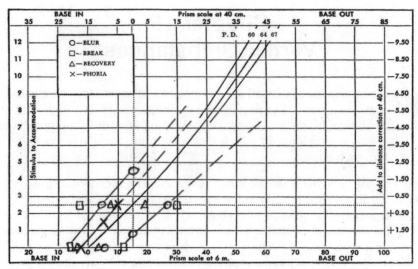

*Figure 15.1. Example of test findings in symptomatic vertical phoria.*

| | Phoria | Base-in | Base-out | Plus to blur | Minus to blur |
|---|---|---|---|---|---|
| Distance | 2 exo | X/5/3 | 6/12/4 | | |
| 40 cm | 5 exo | 10/18/8 | 12/15/4 | +1.75 | -2.00 |
| 40 cm +1.00 D add | 9 exo | | | | |

*von Graefe vertical dissociated phorias: distance, 3Δ BU OS; near, 3Δ BU OS; Near vertical vergence ranges: left supravergence, 1/-2; left infravergence, 7/4; Associated phorias: distance, 2ΔBU OS; near, 2Δ BU OS.*

The names typically used for vertical fusional ranges are supravergence and infravergence indicating the direction of movement of the eye in response to the manipulation of prism over that eye. For example, increasing base-down prism over the left eye induces left supravergence and increasing base-up prism over the left eye induces left infravergence. It is expected that left supravergence will be equal or close to right infravergence and left infravergence will be equal or close to right supravergence.

Some clinicians recommend vision therapy to try to provide comfortable binocular vision to patients with vertical phorias, even though the prescription of some prism may be necessary after the completion of the training program. Wick and Scheiman[7,8] described a training program for vertical phorias in which horizontal vergence training, vertical vergence training, and antisuppression training are combined.

Vertical prism adaptation has been described by many investigators.[9-15] Patients with effective prism adaptation are usually asymptomatic. In general, vertical prism should not be prescribed for asymptomatic patients even if the vertical dissociated phoria is not zero because such patients may be those with good prism adaptation ability. A test which can be used to rule out significant vertical prism adaptation is to measure vertical dissociated phorias before and immediately after wearing vertical correcting prism for thirty minutes. A

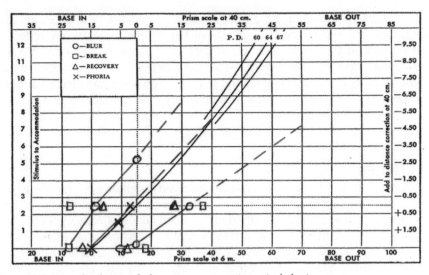

*Figure 15.2. Example of testing findings in asymptomatic vertical phoria.*

|  | Phoria | Base-in | Base-out | Plus to blur | Minus to blur |
|---|---|---|---|---|---|
| Distance | 0 | X/8/4 | 10/18/12 |  |  |
| 40 cm | 2 exo | 14/22/12 | 17/22/12 | +2.25 | -2.75 |
| 40 cm +1.00 D add | 9 exo |  |  |  |  |

*von Graefe vertical dissociated phorias: distance, 2Δ BD OS; near, 2Δ BD OS; Associated phorias: distance, 0; near, 0.*

significant increase in vertical phoria suggests the presence of prism adaptation and unlikely usefulness of prism prescription.[16]

Although vertical fixation disparity curves are not used as commonly as horizontal fixation disparity curves, they can be plotted using an instrument such as the Disparometer or the Saladin card. Vertical fixation disparity also can be determined with the Wesson fixation disparity card by rotating the card 90 degrees so that the fixation disparity lines are horizontal. Most vertical fixation disparity curves are best fitted by a straight line.[17]

The vertical associated phoria is the vertical prism that reduces the vertical fixation disparity to zero. It can be measured with devices such as the Mallett unit, Bernell lantern associated phoria target, AO vectographic slide, or Borish card. *There seems to be unanimous opinion that the vertical associated phoria is the best way to prescribe vertical prism.*[8,12,18-24] If the vertical associated phoria is zero, no prism prescription is indicated. A prism prescription equal to the associated phoria, even as little as one or sometimes one-half prism diopter, often will be effective in relieving the symptoms of vertical phorias. Rutstein and Eskridge[17] suggested that in prescribing vertical prism, it is important to measure associated phorias at distance and near with the patient viewing straight ahead and in down-gaze.

Borish[6] presented a subjective technique for evaluating the acceptance of vertical prism. The technique consists of having the patient view letters of best visual acuity at both distance and near, with the proposed prism in a trial frame, and requesting the patient to indicate whether there is an improvement in visual acuity or a subjective feeling of relief. The prism can then be oriented in other directions and the steps repeated to test the possibility of the prism simply having a placebo effect. If the prism is subjectively agreeable to the patient only with the base oriented the same as in the original measurement, it should be prescribed.

## EXAMPLES

An example of test findings in symptomatic vertical phoria is given in Figure 15.1. The von Graefe vertical dissociated phorias are 3Δ right hyper at both distance and 40 cm. The direction of imbalance in the vertical vergence ranges is consistent with the dissociated phoria results. Vertical associated phorias are 2Δ BU OS at distance and near. It may be noted that the lateral phorias are within normal ranges, but lateral fusional vergence findings are low or borderline. A vertical prism prescription based on the associated phoria should be helpful in reducing symptoms.

Figure 15.2 presents findings in an example of asymptomtic vertical phoria. Dissociated phoria testing yields 2Δ left hyper, but the vertical associated phorias are zero. It may also be observed that the lateral fusional vergence ranges are within Morgan's normal ranges. No vertical prism prescription would be indicated in this case.

## SUMMARY

(1) A vertical imbalance should be corrected with prism:

    (a) whenever it is accompanied by significant ocular symptoms,

    (b) when the testing techniques give consistent results,

    (c) when the dissociated vertical phoria is found with an imbalance in the vertical fusional vergence ranges and, in particular, with a vertical fixation disparity in the same direction, and

    (d) when there is an absence of significant prism adaptation.

(2) Associated phorias should be used as the basis for prescribing vertical prism power.

## REFERENCES

1. Ludvigh E. Amount of eye movement objectively perceptible to the unaided eye. Am J Ophthalmol 1949;32:649-650.
2. Romano PE, von Noorden GK. Limitations of cover test in detecting strabismus. Am J Ophthalmol 1971;72:10-12.
3. Fogt N, Baughman BJ, Good G. The effect of experience on the detection of small eye movements. Optom Vis Sci 2000;77:670-674.
4. von Noorden GK. Burian-von Noorden's Binocular Vision and Ocular Motility: Theory and Management of Strabismus, 2nd ed. St. Louis: Mosby, 1980:187.

5.  Daum KM. *Heterophoria and heterotropia. In: Eskridge JB, Amos JF, Bartlett JD, eds. Clinical Procedures in Optometry.* Philadelphia: Lippincott, 1991:72-90.

6.  Borish IM. *Clinical Refraction, 3rd ed.* Chicago: Professional Press, 1970:872-873.

7.  Wick B. *Vision therapy for cyclovertical heterophoria. In: London R, ed. Ocular Vertical and Cyclovertical Deviations.* Problems in Optometry 1992;4:652-666.

8.  Scheiman M, Wick B. *Clinical Management of Binocular Vision - Heterophoric, Accommodative, and Eye Movement Disorders, 2nd ed.* Philadelphia: Lippincott, 2002:392-425.

9.  Ellerbrock V, Fry GA. *The after-effect induced by vertical divergence.* Am J Optom Arch Am Acad Optom 1941; 18:450-454.

10. Ellerbrock VJ. *Tonicity induced by fusional movements.* Am J Optom Arch Am Acad Optom 1950;27:8-20.

11. Carter DB. *Effects of prolonged wearing of prism.* Am J Optom Arch Am Acad Optom 1963;40:265-273.

12. Sheedy JE. *Fixation Disparity Curves.* Columbus, OH: Vision Analysis, 1979:7-8.

13. Henson DB; North R. *Adaptation to prism-induced heterophoria.* Am J Optom Physiol Opt 1980;57:129-137.

14. Rutstein RP, Eskridge JB. *Clinical evaluation of vertical fixation disparity. Part III. Adaptation to vertical prism.* Am J Optom Physiol Opt 1985;62:585-590.

15. Eskridge JB. *Vertical muscle adaptation. In: London R, ed. Ocular Vertical and Cyclovertical Deviations.* Problems in Optometry 1992;4:622-628.

16. Daum KM, McCormack GL. *Fusion and binocularity. In: Benjamin WJ, ed. Borish's Clinical refraction, 2nd ed.* St. Louis: Butterworth Heinemann Elsevier, 2006:145-191.

17. Rutstein RP, Eskridge JB. *Clinical evaluation of vertical fixation disparity. Part one.* Am J Optom Physiol Opt 1983;60:688-693.

18. Mallett RFJ. *Fixation disparity in clinical practice.* Aust J Optom 1969;52: 97-109.

19. Grosvenor T. *Clinical use of fixation disparity.* Optom Weekly 1975;66: 1224-1228.

20. Eskridge JB, Rutstein RP. *Clinical evaluation of vertical fixation disparity. Part IV. Slope and adaptation to vertical prism of vertical heterophoria patients.* Am J Optom Physiol Opt 1986;63:662-667.

21. Rutstein RP, Eskridge JB. *Studies in vertical fixation disparity.* Am J Optom Physiol Opt 1986;63:639-644.

22. Amos JF, Rutstein RP. *Vertical deviations. In: Amos JF, ed. Diagnosis and Management in Vision Care.* Boston: Butterworth-Heinemann, 1987: 515-583.

23. Cotter SA, Frantz KA. *Prescribing prism for vertical deviations. In: London R, ed. Ocular Vertical and Cyclovertical Deviations.* Problems in Optometry 1992;4:629-645.

24. Wick B. *Prescribing prism for patients with vertical heterophoria. In: Cotter, SA, ed. Clinical Uses of Prism-A Spectrum of Applications - Mosby's Optometric Problem Solving Series.* St. Louis: Mosby-Year Book; 1995:149-175.

## OTHER SUGGESTED READING

London R, ed. *Ocular Vertical and Cyclovertical Deviations.* Problems in Optometry 1992;4:541-683.

# Chapter 16
# Additional Concepts and
# Considerations in Case Analysis

One of the most interesting areas of optometry and vision science is the study of accommodation and convergence. So far we have only scratched the surface of this subject. This chapter examines some additional elements of this topic that have clinical import. We will also discuss a number of clinical implications of accommodation and convergence function and related concerns. Some of the concepts discussed in this chapter, such as CAC ratios, PCT ratios, and dark focus, are not regular features of case analysis today, but it is possible that they might be incorporated into clinical care in the future.

## CONVERGENCE ACCOMMODATION

Convergence accommodation is the accommodation induced by or associated with convergence.[1] Convergence accommodation is sometimes called disparity-induced accommodation, because it is accommodation associated with fusional vergence, which is also known as disparity vergence.[2] The required conditions for the measurement of convergence accommodation are binocular fusion, the lack or diminution of blur cues to accommodation, and stimulation of vergence by base-in prism or base-out prism. An increase in vergence, as stimulated by base-out prism, causes an increase in accommodation, and a decrease in vergence, as stimulated by base-in prism, is associated with a decrease in accommodation.

A CAC ratio can be calculated by finding the amount of convergence accommodation elicited by a given amount of convergence. The CAC ratio is the ratio of change in convergence accommodation (CA) to change in convergence (C). The CAC ratio is not usually determined clinically, but it could be measured by doing the binocular cross-cylinder test through different amounts of prism or by performing Nott or monocular estimation method dynamic retinoscopy at different prism settings while the patient views a target that does not contain an adequate stimulus for the control of optical reflex accommodation.[3-6]

An example of a clinically derived CAC ratio is given in Figure 16.1. With a 6Δ base-in prism in place, the binocular cross-cylinder end-point is +1.00D over the subjective refraction to best visual acuity. The test was done at 40 cm and the base-in prism reduced the convergence stimulus by 6Δ, so the convergence stimulus for this point is 15Δ - 6Δ = 9Δ. The accommodative stimulus is 2.50 D - 1.00 D = 1.50 D. So the point for this finding is plotted on the graph at 9Δ on the x-axis and 1.50 D on the y-axis. That point and two other points are plotted on the graph in Figure 15.1. Accommodation changed 0.25 D for each 6Δ change in convergence. Therefore, the slope of the line, the CAC ratio, is 0.04 D/Δ:

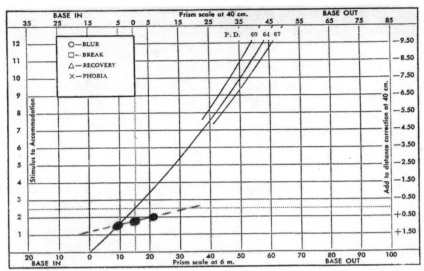

*Figure 16.1 xample of the plot of findings used in the clinical derivation of a CAC ratio. The points plotted with circles are from the following data obtained using a 40 cm test distance.*

| Prism Setting | Convergence Stimulus (in Δ) | Binocular cross cylinder results (add over the subjective refraction) | Accommodative Stimulus (in D) |
|---|---|---|---|
| 6Δ base-in | 15 − 6 = 9 | +1.00 D | 2.50 − 1.00 = 1.50 |
| 0 | 15 | +0.75 D | 2.50 − 0.75 = 1.75 |
| 6Δ base-out | 15 + 6 = 21 | +0.50 D | 2.50 − 0.50 = 2.00 |

$$\text{CAC ratio} = (0.25\ \text{D}) / (6\ \Delta) = 0.04\ \text{D}/\Delta$$

Daum et al.[5] reported a mean CAC ratio of 0.06 D/Δ. The mean slope of the convergence accommodation line (CAC ratio) is less than the mean slope of the phoria line (inverse of the ACA ratio).[5,6]

One way that convergence accommodation has been classically explained is that the convergence occurring during the elicitation of the convergence accommodation curve is simply a combination of accommodative convergence and fusional convergence. Because there is no stimulus to accommodation present, accommodative convergence can be used along with fusional convergence without inducing a blur. To clarify this concept, Fry[7] called accommodative convergence "triad convergence" to indicate that accommodation, accommodative convergence, and pupil constriction occur together. Convergence accommodation, then according to Fry, is the accommodation that occurs with triad convergence, and the convergence occurring under these conditions is a combination of triad convergence and fusional convergence, no accommodation being associated with fusional convergence. A diagram illustrating Fry's concept is given in Figure 16.2.

More recently, convergence accommodation has been described as occurring due to a direct neurological link from to accommodation from the neural element controlling vergence.[8-13] A change in accommodation induces a change

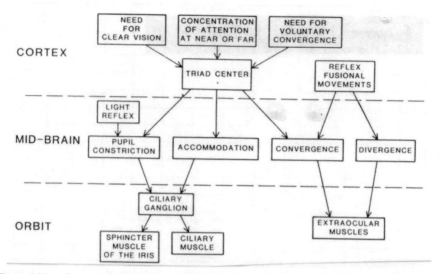

*Figure 16.2. A diagram illustrating the neural mechanisms proposed by Fry for accommodation and vergence. (Reprinted with permission from Fry GA. Basic concepts underlying graphical analysis. In: Schor CM, Ciuffreda KJ, eds. Vergence Eye Movements: Basic and Clinical Aspects. Boston: Butterworth-Heinemann, 1983:403-437.)*

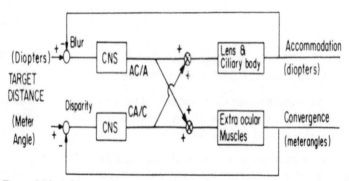

*Figure 16.3. A diagram illustrating the mechanisms for interaction of accommodation and convergence from Schor. (Reprinted with permission from Schor CM. Models of mutual interaction between accommodation and convergence. Am J Optom Physiol Opt 1985;62:369-374.)*

in accommodative convergence, and a change in convergence in response to retinal disparity induces a change in convergence accommodation. A diagram proposed by Schor[11] to illustrate the dual interaction of accommodation and convergence is shown in Figure 16.3.

As a consequence of convergence accommodation, patients with esophoria at near often have high lags of accommodation.[14] The negative fusional convergence they exert to compensate for the esophoria is associated with a decrease in accommodation. Computer modeling shows that lag of accommodation is expected to increase as CAC increases if ACA is normal or high and lag of accommodation will increase as ACA increases if CAC is normal or high.[13]

## PRISM ADAPTATION

The phenomenon responsible for a shift in phorias after binocular viewing through prisms is prism adaptation. Viewing through base-in prism causes an exo shift and base-out prism causes an eso shift. The use of fusional vergence induces prism adaptation. Because prism adaptation is elicited by the use of fusional vergence, Alpern[15] called it *fusional aftereffect*, and because its time course is slower than fusional vergence but it helps to maintain fusion, Schor[10] called it *slow fusional vergence*. It also has been called *vergence adaptation*.

In most individuals, adaptation to base-out prism is greater than adaptation to base-in prism. For this reason, some practitioners recommend taking base-in fusional vergence amplitudes before base-out. There is general agreement that phorias should be measured before fusional amplitudes so that the effect of prism adaptation on the phorias will be minimized.

There are considerable differences in the extent to which prism adaptation is present in different individuals. Prism adaptation is beneficial because it replaces fusional vergence effort. Persons who exhibit a great deal of vergence adaptation are generally asymptomatic.

Studies by Rosenfield et al.[16] and by Rainey[17] suggest that vergence adaptation causes shifts in dissociated phorias through a change in tonic vergence without a change in the ACA ratio. Thus in terms of the ZCSBV, the change associated with vergence adaptation would be a change in lateral position of the zone.

## DRUG EFFECTS ON THE ACA RATIO AND VERGENCE FUNCTION

Some drugs will temporarily change the ACA ratio by their effects on accommodation or on the central nervous system. Drugs which affect the ciliary muscle will alter the ACA ratio due to their effects on accommodation. For example, parasympathomimetic (cholingergic) drugs allow a given level of innervation to the ciliary muscle to yield a greater dioptric amount of accommodation. Stimulation of the near triad then produces relatively easier accommodation than before drug application. Accommodative convergence is unaffected. Thus, the ACA ratio is reduced as long as the drug is active.

Parasympatholytic (anti-cholinergic) drugs have a cycloplegic effect; that is, they reduce ciliary muscle activity. When innervation to accommodation and accommodative convergence occurs after application of a parasympatholytic drug, accommodative convergence occurs as usual, but accommodation is reduced. As a result, the ACA ratio increases dramatically. The time course of the ACA ratio change is directly related to the time course of the cycloplegic effect of the drugs.[15] A consequence of this effect is that all accommodation and vergence testing should be completed before instillation of a mydriatic or cycloplegic agent.

A drug with well-known central nervous system effects on the ACA ratio is ethyl alcohol,[18] which causes a dose-related reduction in the ACA ratio as well as an increase in tonic convergence and a reduction in fusional vergence amplitudes. As the level of intoxication increases, the ability to retain single vision decreases, because distance esophoria increases, near-point exophoria increases, and fusional reserves decrease.

The effects of caffeine on vergence have also been studied.[19] Distance dissociated phoria moves in the eso direction after ingestion of caffeine and the response ACA ratio decreases. The increase in tonic vergence is enough that the near phoria may also shift toward eso even though the ACA ratio decreases.

## PROXIMAL ACCOMMODATION AND PROXIMAL CONVERGENCE
The change in convergence associated with a change in viewing distance is composed of changes in accommodative convergence, proximal convergence, and fusional convergence. Each of these components is important in the total vergence response.[20] Likewise, accommodation responds to proximity cues or awareness of nearness in addition to optical defocus. The former is often called *proximal accommodation*, and the latter is referred to as *optical reflex accommodation*.

Because proximity cues are important in accommodation and convergence responses, many clinicians will emphasize the awareness of changes of perceived distance and size during vision training programs. For instance, the SILO response will be brought to the patient's attention. The SILO response is the appearance of a target getting smaller and closer associated with convergence occurring in response to increasing base-out prism, and the appearance of a target getting larger and farther away during divergence stimulated by increasing base-in prism. The amount of proximal convergence occurring with a given change in test distance can be changed with vision training.[21,22]

The ratio of change in proximal convergence to change in test distance is often referred to as the PCT ratio,[22] which is measured in prism diopters per diopter. One method that has been used to derive PCT ratios is to subtract the gradient ACA ratio (which does not include changes in distance) from the calculated ACA ratio (which does involve changes in distance). If we use Morgan's norms for the determination of a PCT ratio, one finds

PCT ratio = calculated ACA - gradient ACA

PCT ratio = 5.2 $\Delta$/D - 4 $\Delta$/D

PCT ratio = 1.2 $\Delta$/D

Average calculated and gradient ACA ratios can be used to find the mean PCT ratio for a group of individuals, but a serious drawback of this method for one individual is that any measurement error in any of the three involved phorias will significantly affect the resultant PCT ratio. Another potential clinical method for the determination of a PCT ratio is to do a distance dissociated phoria through the subjective refraction and a 40 cm dissociated phoria through a +2.50 D add. Assuming that the accommodative responses are the same during both phoria measurements, the formula for the PCT ratio in prism diopters per diopter would be:

PCT ratio = [(conv. stim. for 40 cm)+(40 cm phoria with +2.50 D add)-(dist. phoria)] / 2.50 D

If the accommodative responses are the same, the change in vergence position is due to proximal vergence. Adding the convergence stimulus for 40 cm to the dissociated phoria at 40 cm with a +2.50 D add gives the vergence position of the eyes compared to parallelism of the lines of sight. Then the distance dissociated phoria is subtracted to determine how much the eyes converged. The denominator is 2.50 D representing the near distance of 40 cm. To take an example, if the distance phoria is 1Δ exo and the near phoria with +2.50 D add is 12Δ exo for a person with a 64 mm PD, the PCT ratio would be:

PCT ratio = [(15Δ) + (-12 Δ) - (-1 Δ)] / 2.50 D

PCT ratio = 4Δ / 2.50 D

PCT ratio = 1.6 Δ/D

A method for deriving a PCT ratio under binocular conditions similar to the one just discussed for dissociated conditions involves plotting a fixation disparity curve (FDC) at distance with the patient viewing through the subjective refraction and another FDC curve at 40 cm with the patient viewing through a +2.50 D add. This method involves finding the x-intercepts on the fixation disparity curves. The formula for the PCT ratio would be:

PCT ratio = [(conv. stim. for 40 cm)+(40 cm x-int. with +2.50 D add)-(dist. x-int.)] / 2.50 D

Using that FDC method, Wick[23] found a mean PCT ratio of 4.2 Δ/D for 20 young adults, and Joubert and Bedell[24] found a mean PCT ratio of 2.9 Δ/D for 18 adult subjects. With a similar fixation disparity method, Ogle and Martens[25] reported an average PCT ratio of 1.5 Δ/D for 104 subjects.

PCT ratios measured under binocular conditions, such as with the FDC method, tend to be higher than those measured under dissociated conditions.[23,24] This seems logical because stereopsis would contribute to an awareness of nearness. Mean PCT ratios reported in the literature measured under dissociated conditions have varied from 0.7 to 2.0 Δ/D.[22]

Rosenfield et al.[26] reported that proximal accommodation and proximal convergence are constant at a very low level for targets at or beyond 3 m, and that both proximal accommodation and proximal convergence change linearly with target distance expressed in diopters or meter angles for objects closer than 3 m. (The meter angle is an angular unit for convergence in which one meter angle is a reciprocal meter. It is usually measured from the spectacle plane. Diopters and meter angles are thus equal in magnitude for a given target distance.)

## DARK FOCUS AND DARK VERGENCE
When sufficient cues for optical reflex accommodation are not present, such as in darkness or in empty visual field, accommodation focuses for an intermediate distance. The amount of accommodation occurring in darkness is known

as the *dark focus*. Leibowitz and Owens[27] found a mean dark focus of 1.52D (SD = 0.77D) in 220 college students. This accommodation in darkness is responsible for the phenomenon known as *night myopia*.[28-30]

A potential clinical method for measuring the dark focus is performing retinoscopy in a dark room. Results from retinoscopy done in a dark room have been reported to correlate with laboratory measurements of dark focus.[31,32] Clinical determination of dark focus may aid in prescribing lenses for patients bothered by night myopia, such as when driving at night.[30,33]

The vergence position of the eyes in darkness also has been studied; this often is referred to as *dark vergence*. The dark vergence position can be predicted by adding the amount of accommodative convergence expected to occur with the dark focus (determined by multiplying the dioptric dark focus by the ACA ratio) to the distance phoria.[34,35] As we have discussed, the distance phoria is the physiologic position of rest of the eyes when accommodation is at a zero level. Thus, dark vergence is determined by the physiologic position of rest of vergence and the accommodative convergence that is associated with the accommodation that occurs in the dark.

The dioptric dark focus level for a given individual is relatively stable over time.[36,37] However, dark focus increases temporarily after near fixation and dark focus decreases after distance fixation.[38-42] This shift in dark focus in the direction of the fixation distance is an accommodative adaptation, analogous to prism adaptation in the vergence system.

Accommodation is controlled by the opposing actions of the parasympathetic and sympathetic divisions of the autonomic nervous system.[43,44] Experimentation and a review of the literature led Gilmartin and Hogan[45,46] to conclude that variability in dark focus is due to variability in parasympathetic rather than sympathetic ciliary muscle tone.

## RELATING NORMALCY OF TONIC VERGENCE AND ACA RATIOS TO VERGENCE CASE TYPES

The distance dissociated phoria can be viewed as a measure of tonic vergence. We can think of the vergence case types in terms of the relationship of tonic vergence and ACA ratio as shown in Table 16.1. In convergence insufficiency, tonic vergence is normal and the ACA ratio is low. In convergence excess, tonic vergence is normal and the ACA ratio is high. Tonic vergence has a leptokurtic frequency distribution with the vast majority of individuals having normal tonic vergence. Thus, convergence insufficiency and convergence excess are the most common vergence disorders.

Basic exophoria and basic esophoria are normal ACA ratio conditions with low and high tonic vergence, respectively. In Table 16.1, two entries do not fit exactly into the way that we have defined the vergence disorders, the low tonic vergence, low ACA ratio case and the high tonic vergence, high ACA ratio case. We have used normalcy of distance and near phorias (along with supporting findings) to define the vergence disorders. Most practitioners would probably

| Table 16.1. Classification of vergence disorder by normalcy of tonic vergence and ACA ratio. | | | |
|---|---|---|---|
| ACA Ratio | Tonic vergence – *distance fixation* | | |
| | Low (> 2Δ exo) | Normal (ortho to 2Δ exo) | High (eso) |
| Low | (Convergence insufficiency)* | Convergence insufficiency | Divergence insufficiency |
| Normal | Basic exo | Normal | Basic eso |
| High | Divergence excess | Convergence excess | (Convergence excess)* |

*see text for explanation*

classify the high tonic vergence, high ACA ratio case as convergence excess. However, such patients may have difficulty at distance as well as at near. In terms of treatment, this case can be viewed as a combination of basic eso (high tonic vergence) and convergence excess (high ACA ratio). So, in some cases, both base-out prism and near plus add may incorporated into the treatment. Likewise, most practitioners would probably classify the low tonic vergence, low ACA ratio case as convergence insufficiency. This case combines elements of basic exophoria (low tonic vergence) and convergence insufficiency (low ACA ratio). The best treatment in such cases is vision therapy, just as in both basic exo and convergence insufficiency.

## USE OF AN ENGINEERING MODEL TO DESCRIBE RELATIONSHIP OF ACCOMMODATIVE AND VERGENCE STIMULI TO RESPONSES

Diagrams borrowing on engineering concepts have sometimes been used to sketch accommodation and vergence function from the stimuli to the responses and to illustrate the interactions of accommodation and vergence. Such a diagram in elementary form was used to illustrate the concept of convergence accommodation in Figure 16.3. A more comprehensive diagram is shown in Figure 16.4, taken from Hung et al.[47] AS represents a blur stimulus to accommodation. Depth of focus, the DSP or dead space operator for accommodation, and accommodative controller gain (ACG) determine how much optical reflex accommodation occurs in response to the blur stimulus. ADAPT represents adaptation feeding back on the accommodative controller gain. DS is a distance stimulus which through the perceived distance (PDG) elicits proximal accommodation and proximal vergence. The total accommodative response (AR) is determined by the sum of optical reflex accommodation, proximal accommodation from the accommodative proximal gain (APG), convergence accommodation (CA), and the basic tonus in the accommodative system (ABIAS).

VS represents a retinal disparity stimulus to fusional vergence. Panum's fusional area (DSP) and the vergence controller gain (VCG) determine how much vergence occurs in response to retinal disparity. Note that the output of VCG feeds back via adaptation to VCG. In other words, the use of fusional vergence causes prism adaptation. Prism adaptation then by feeding back on VCG reduces the amount of fusional vergence necessary, showing why

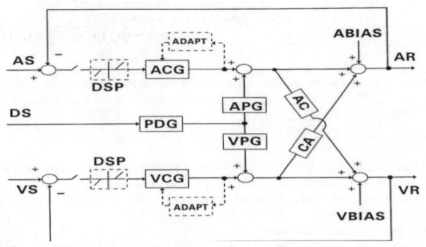

Figure 16.4. An engineering model of the accommodation and vergence systems. The acronyms and abbreviations used in the diagram are as follows:

*ABIAS* = basic tonus in the accommodative system;

*AC* = accommodative convergence;

*ACG* = accommodative controller gain (how much the accommodative system responds to a given change in accommodative stimulus);

*ADAPT* = adaptation (accommodative adaptation in the accommodative system and vergence adaptation of prism adaptation in the vergence system);

*APG* = accommodative proximal gain (how much the accommodative system responds to a given proximity stimulus);

*AR* = accommodative response;

*AS* = accommodative stimulus (specifically here from blur);

*CA* = convergence accommodation;

*DS* = distance stimulus (distance of the object being viewed from the subject);

*DSP* = dead space operator (a span over which the system may not respond, depth of focus in the accommodative system and Panum's fusional area in the vergence system);

*PDG* = perceived distance gain (subjectively perceived estimate of the distance of the object from the subject);

*VBIAS* = tonic vergence;

*VCG* = vergence controller gain (how much fusional vergence occurs in response to a given retinal disparity stimulus);

*VPG* = vergence proximal gain (how much the vergence system responds to a given proximity stimulus);

*VR* = vergence response;

*VS* = vergence stimulus (specifically here retinal disparity).

*(Reprinted with permission from Hung GK, Ciuffreda KJ, Rosenfield M. Proximal contribution to a linear static model of accommodation and vergence. Ophthal Physiol Opt 1996;16:31-41.)*

prism adaptation is valuable to the patient in reducing strain on fusional vergence. VPG represents how much proximal vergence occurs in response to the perceived distance. The total vergence response (VR) is the sum of the fusional vergence from VCG, proximal vergence from VPG, accommodative convergence (AC), and tonic vergence (VBIAS).

## A NOTE ON POTENTIAL SOURCES OF ASTHENOPIA

In investigating the potential sources of asthenopia, we can say that of the Maddox components of convergence, asthenopia is related to stress on fusional convergence. The usefulness of clinical guidelines such as Sheard's criterion or of fixation disparity data is attributable to the fact that they are related to the stress on fusional convergence. Because poor accommodation skills can cause ocular discomfort, the clinician should examine all areas of accommodative function in patients with asthenopia.

Asthenopia also can result from uncorrected refractive conditions, such as hyperopia, astigmatism, and anisometropia and, in some cases, from the consequences of correcting a refractive error, such as in correction-induced aniseikonia. Birnbaum[48,49] also has proposed a physiologic mechanism by which stress and psychological factors may alter accommodation and vergence function and thus play a role in contributing to asthenopia.

Vertical oculomotor imbalances are another potential source of asthenopia. Examination of the patient with asthenopia includes comprehensive evaluation of horizontal and vertical vergence, accommodation, and refractive error. If problems in those areas are ruled out, an additional contributor to asthenopic symptoms, particularly during reading and near work, is dysfunction of version eye movements, which is discussed in chapter 18.

## A NOTE ON ACCOMMODATION AND VERGENCE FUNCTION IN OCCUPATIONAL, EDUCATIONAL, AND RECREATIONAL PERFORMANCE

Good accommodation and vergence function is important for optimum performance in learning, work, and recreation. The tests and analyses discussed in this book can be used to find and remediate accommodation and vergence disorders which can interfere in these areas. Visual skills, such as accommodation, vergence, and eye movements are associated with reading ability,[50-57] and improvement in those skills can be of benefit for patients having difficulty reading.[58]

Eyestrain and discomfort associated with computer use is a common patient presenting complaint.[59,60] A careful analysis of accommodation and vergence is an important part of the investigation of such complaints. It also has been observed that accommodation and vergence are important in sports performance. There is much helpful literature available on visual skills and related considerations in reading, computer use, and sports.[61-76]

## REPEATABILITY AND COMPARISONS OF PHORIA AND FUSIONAL VERGENCE TESTS

Ways to evaluate how good clinical tests are include the repeatability of the tests and how closely they compare to established tests. A synonym for repeatability is reliability. A metric often used to describe repeatability is the 95% limits of agreement or 95% confidence interval, the calculated range in which 95 of 100 repeated measurements are likely to fall. More difficult to determine is validity, which is a determination of how well the test measures what it purports to measure. A way that is often used to assess validity is to compare the results of a given test to the results obtained with an established or standard test.

Studies have found the modified Thorington phoria test to be more repeatable than the von Graefe phoria test, which in turn is more repeatable than the Maddox rod phoria test.[77,78] One study found the Howell phoria card to have better repeatability than the von Graefe test, but not as good as the modified Thorington test.[79] The 95% limits of agreement for the modified Thorington at near have been reported at about $\pm 2$ to $\pm 3$ $\Delta$.[78,79] The 95% limits of agreement reported for the von Graefe test at near are $\pm 2.5$ to $\pm 5$ $\Delta$.[77,79] Distance dissociated phoria measurements are more repeatable than near dissociated phoria measurements.[77] Daum's[80] suggestion that lateral phoria measurements are "... accurate within 3 to 5 prism diopters" appears reasonable for near phorias.

Some studies have found a mean near phoria which is 1 to 2 $\Delta$ more exo with the von Graefe test than with the modified Thorington,[78,81,82] but one study found mean values which were very close on the two tests.[79] The standard deviations are greater and the ranges of values are wider on the von Graefe test at near than on the modified Thorington at near.[78,79] Higher phoria values are sometimes found on the von Graefe test than on the modified Thorington test.

The mean near phoria on the Maddox rod test tends to be more exo than the von Graefe test mean.[83] The likely explanation for this is that accommodation is not as well controlled with the Maddox rod test because the objects seen by the patient during the Maddox rod test are a white light and a red line as opposed to letters. Because accommodation is not controlled, the lag of accommodation increases resulting in less accommodative convergence and thus a more divergent dissociated phoria. At distance, the Maddox rod often yields a more esophoria than the von Graefe, again because accommodation is not well controlled. On a distance phoria, if accommodation is not controlled, accommodation will increase resulting in more accommodative convergence and then a more convergent dissociated phoria.

The 95% limits of agreement for the alternating cover test in which the examiner neutralizes the observed eye movement with prism has been reported to be $\pm 3.6$ $\Delta$.[84] The repeatability is slightly better for a subjective form of the cover test in which patient perceived target movement is neutralized with prism.[84] The minimum amount of eye movement that can be observed under ideal conditions averages about 2 $\Delta$.[85-87] von Noorden[88] suggested that with the usual less than ideal conditions under which the cover test is performed in the clinical setting, the limit may be more in the neighborhood of 3 to 4 $\Delta$. As a result, small phorias can sometimes be interpreted as ortho on the cover test.

One study found the 95% confidence intervals for phoropter mounted rotary prism fusional vergence ranges to be between 2 and 2.5 $\Delta$ for distance BI break, distance BI recovery, and near BI recovery; between 3 and 4 $\Delta$ for near

BI break and near BO break; between 4 and 5 Δ for distance BO blur, distance BO recovery, and near BI blur; and 5 and 5.5 Δ for distance BO break, near BO blur, and near BO recovery.[89] Thus base-in fusional vergence ranges are somewhat more repeatable than base-out ranges. Another study found 95% confidence intervals of 1.7 Δ for BI break and 6.8 Δ for BO break using hand-held rotary prisms.[90] Fusional vergence ranges measured with prism bars have been reported to be comparable to objective measures of fusional vergence ranges.[91]

## PERFORMANCE TESTS

After deriving a tentative lens or prism prescription, many practitioners will check that prescription in a trial frame. The prescription can be evaluated by simply asking the patient about subjective observations of clarity and comfort. But the prescription can also be checked by what may be referred to as performance tests. That is, the examiner can see if the performance on a given test or procedure is improved by the tentative prescription. Some of the tests which can be used in this way include visual acuity, ranges of clear and comfortable vision, near point of convergence, pursuit and saccadic eye movements, stereopsis, and hand-eye coordination activities.[92] Advantages of such performance tests are that they provide tangible results which can be demonstrated to the patient, they can provide more objective confirmation to the examiner than simply the subjective report of the patient, and they may represent a more natural visual environment than some tests, particularly tests in the phoropter. It has been suggested that more use can be made of stereopsis as a barometer of binocular vision function.[93]

## DEPTH OF FOCUS EFFECTS ON THE ZONE OF CLEAR SINGLE BINOCULAR VISION

Depth of focus makes clear vision possible even when there is a (small) lag or lead of accommodation. A blur during fusional vergence testing occurs when accommodation has shifted the depth of field such that the object of regard is no longer within it. If we plotted a ZCSBV with accommodative response values rather than stimulus values, the base-out blur points would be shifted up by an amount limited by the depth of focus, because accommodative convergence is being used. Likewise, the base-in blur points would be shifted down because accommodation decreases.

When the dioptric stimulus to accommodation equals zero, presumably accommodation is already relaxed. This situation has two effects on the ZCSBV. First, it explains why a break without a blur can be expected on the base-in fusional vergence measurement at distance. If a blur is obtained on this test, the patient may have been under-plussed or over-minused on the refraction. Second, the situation may make the ZCSBV narrower at the zero stimulus to accommodation level than at other accommodation levels. Thus, depth of focus can contribute to a fanning-out of the ZCSBV, just as proximal convergence (discussed in Chapter 4) does.

Tests of accommodation (negative relative accommodation, positive relative accommodation, and amplitude) also are influenced by the depth of focus. For a person with a large depth of focus (such as from a small pupil diameter), the negative relative accommodation may extend below the bottom of the graph. For a patient with a moderate to large pupil diameter, if the negative relative accommodation point extends substantially below the zero stimulus to accommodation line (negative relative accommodation at 40 cm greater than approximately 3.00D), the suspicion is of too much minus or not enough plus on the refraction. Depth of focus also explains why an amplitude of accommodation greater than zero is obtained for an individual with absolute presbyopia.

## COMMENTS ON USES AND VARIOUS ASPECTS OF THE GRAPH

Now that you are an accomplished plotter of optometric findings, it might be useful to review the first few chapters to better understand the construction of graphs, the scales on the graphs, the basis for the plotting of various findings, and so on. As indicated earlier, the scale at the bottom of the graph is an absolute scale, with 0 indicating parallelism of the lines of sight, values to the left of 0 indicating divergence from parallelism, and values to the right of 0 indicating various levels of convergence of the lines of sight. From this, we can think of the positions of the lines of sight as being in space rather than as being merely points marked on a paper. We can determine how much the eyes converge or diverge during any given test. For example, if an individual with a 64 mm PD measures $8\Delta$ exophoria at 40 cm, the eyes are actually converged $7\Delta$ during that test: $15 + (-8) = 7$.

A graphical display of data can be a very effective means of recognizing patterns in the relationships of variables. We have used the accommodation and convergence graph in helping to learn about fundamental accommodation and convergence concepts, to assess the consistency of test findings for individual patients, and to aid in the confirmation of vergence disorder case types. Because the graph shows the relationship of accommodation and vergence, it has several potential uses, which Hofstetter[94] listed as follows:

1. The interrelationships of accommodation and convergence can be evaluated readily.

2. The interdependence of various findings becomes obvious.

3. Prediction of test findings other than those investigated during the examination is possible.

4. Erroneous findings can be detected.

5. Conventional rules for the prescription of lenses and prisms can be easily applied to the graph.

6. In orthoptics, a guide for determining diagnosis, therapy, and prognosis can be provided.

7. In case reports, a large body of data can be pictorially summarized.

8. An effective teaching aid can be provided.

One of the potential uses of the graph (no. 3 in Hofstetter's list) is the prediction of test results. The demand line represents the accommodative stimulus and the convergence stimulus for objects at various distances when the patient is looking through lenses equal in power to the subjective refraction. When lens power is varied from the subjective refraction, the accommodative stimulus changes but the convergence stimulus remains the same for a given distance. Thus, to predict performance through various adds, one simply moves straight up (for minus spherical lens changes) or straight down (for plus) from the demand line point for the test distance in question and observes the relationship of the ZCSBV to this point. This procedure can be used to confirm observations about the patient's status without the spherical correction as well as to help in deciding whether to use an add or an alteration in lens power in the spectacle lenses prescribed.

Chapter 3 discussed the five geometric properties of the ZCSBV and their clinical correlates. The slope of the ZCSBV is correlated with the inverse of the ACA ratio. The ACA ratio represents the amount of accommodative convergence (AC) occurring with a given amount of accommodation (A). Convergence is given on the x-axis and accommodation on the y-axis, so the ACA ratio can be calculated as $\Delta x/\Delta y$ ($\Delta$ here indicating change in rather than prism diopters). This is what is done in many laboratory studies of response ACAs: several phorias are plotted at intermediate accommodative stimulus levels, and the slope of the phoria line is calculated. Clinically, we can easily do much the same thing. If several phorias are plotted, we can draw a best-fitting straight line through them by visual inspection and calculate the inverse of the slope using the scale values on the graph. In addition, any two phorias, regardless of the lens powers or distances used, can be employed to calculate ACA ratios:

$\Delta x$ = (convergence stimulus #1 + phoria #1) − (convergence stimulus #2 + phoria #2)

$\Delta y$ = stimulus to accommodation #1 − stimulus to accommodation #2

ACA ratio = $\Delta x / \Delta y$

The formulas for calculated and gradient ACA ratios are simplifications of this formula. The phoria line is generally fairly linear. Some non-linearity may exist at minimum and maximum accommodation levels, and some non-linearity may appear in clinically derived phoria lines as a result of poorly controlled accommodation on some phorias or as a result of proximal convergence when both test distance and lens power are varied.

## ALTERNATIVE FORMS OF THE GRAPH
The clinical graph for accommodation and convergence data has been presented in different forms on occasion. One variation is the use of the spectacle plane rather than the ocular centers of rotation for computation of convergence values. The demand line then becomes linear. Sometimes different units have been used for convergence, as for example, degrees, centrads, or meter angles.[95] A centrad is 0.01 radians. A radian is the angle subtended when a line is moved through an arc equal to its length. Because the circumference

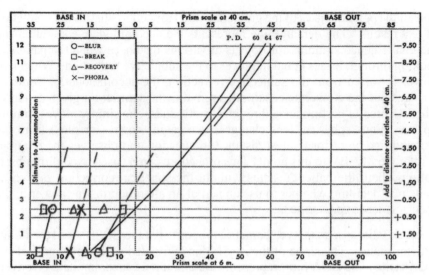

*Figure 16.5. An example of graphical display of test data in strabismus.*

|  | Phoria/Tropia | Base-in | Base-out |
|---|---|---|---|
| 6 m | 8Δ exophoria | X/18/10 | 2/6/-2 |
| 40 cm | 17Δ exotropia | 27/30/20 | X/-4/-10 |

of a circle is equal to 2(pi) times its radius, there are 2(pi) radians in a circle, and therefore, 1 radian is about 57.3 degrees. One centrad would thus be about 0.573 degrees. Prism diopters and centrads are approximately equal for small angles. A prism diopter is a linear separation of 1 cm at a distance of 1 m. A centrad is the angle subtended by an *arc* of 1 cm at a distance of 1 m.

Meter angles can be converted into prism diopters by multiplying the number of meter angles by the PD in cm. If meter angles are used for convergence and convergence is referenced to the spectacle plane rather than the centers of rotation of the eyes, the demand line becomes a 1:1 line, with the number of meter angles of convergence stimulus equaling the number of diopters of accommodative stimulus for each fixation distance. Sometimes accommodation is represented on the x-axis and convergence on the y-axis.[6,96]

## THE GRAPH IN STRABISMUS
Even though it is rarely done, clinical findings could also be portrayed graphically in strabismic cases. In everyday vision it is likely that a strabismus occurs at distances at which the demand line does not lie within the lateral limits of the ZCSBV. In the artificial conditions of the phoropter, most patients will give up clear vision to retain single vision (and thus will report a blur before a break).

An example of strabismus findings is given in Figure 16.5. The symbols used in this figure are the same as those used previously. The magnitude of a tropia is marked with an X, as is the magnitude of a phoria. The line through these points is called the phoria-tropia line when both phorias and tropias are repre-

Table 16.2. Mean rates of childhood myopia progression in diopters per year as a function of nearpoint phoria from two studies.
(Standard deviations were given in the Roberts and Banford paper.
Higher exophoria was greater than 4Δ exo in the Roberts and Banford study and greater than 6Δ exo in the Goss study.)

|  | Roberts and Banford[109] | | Goss[110] | | |
|---|---|---|---|---|---|
|  | N | Mean | N | Mean | SD |
| Higher exophoria | 76 | -0.43 | 67 | -0.45 | 0.27 |
| Ortho and low exo | 105 | -0.39 | 110 | -0.39 | 0.25 |
| Esophoria | 167 | -0.48 | 77 | -0.50 | 0.32 |

Table 16.3. Mean rates of childhood myopia progression in diopters per year for single vision lens (SV) wearers, bifocal lens (BF) wearers, or progressive addition lens (PAL) wearers in different studies as a function of nearpoint phoria.

|  | Ortho & exo, SV | Ortho & exo, BF or PAL* | Eso, SV | Eso, BF or PAL* |
|---|---|---|---|---|
| Roberts and Banford (1967)[9] | -0.41 (n=181) | -0.38 (n=17) | -0.48 (n=167) | -0.28 (n=65) |
| Goss and Uyesugi (1995)[12] | -0.42 (n=103) | -0.44 (n=55) | -0.59 (n=52) | -0.33 (n=66) |
| Fulk and Cyert (1996)[13] | X | X | -0.57 (n=14) | -0.39 (n=14) |
| Fulk et al. (2000)[14] | X | X | -0.50 (n=39) | -0.40 (n=36) |
| Edwards et al. (2002)[15] | -0.63 (n=112) | -0.59* (n=100) | -0.63 (n=21) | -0.45* (n=21) |
| Brown et al. (2002)[16] | -0.59 (n=18) | -0.42* (n=20) | -0.65 (n=14) | -0.29* (n=16) |
| Gwiazda et al. (2004), higher lag subjects[17] | -0.52 (n=85) | -0.45* (n=72) | -0.57 (n=34) | -0.36* (n=42) |
| Gwiazda et al. (2004), lower lag subjects[17] | -0.50 (n=60) | -0.42* (n=65) | -0.38 (n=55) | -0.41* (n=55) |

sented or the tropia line when only tropias are represented. In the findings in Figure 16.5, an exophoria is noted at distance, whereas an exotropia is noted at 40 cm. To estimate the distance within which a strabismus is manifest, one can find the point at which the demand line crosses outside the blur or blur-break line. In this example, the point is approximately at the 1.25D stimulus to accommodation level. Converting this to a distance one gets approximately 80 cm, suggesting that this individual is likely to manifest a tropia anywhere inside about 80 cm.

Strabismus is frequently accompanied by various sensory anomalies. One of these anomalies is suppression. If the suppression is deep, the patient may have a total lack of sensory fusion, which results in an absence of fusional amplitude (motor fusion). In such cases one cannot plot a ZCSBV. However, the tropia line can still be plotted and an ACA ratio can still be calculated. In fact, determination of the ACA ratio is an important part of strabismus diagnosis. The ACA ratio and the graph can be used to predict the effect of minus adds (exotropes) or plus adds (esotropes) on the amount of the lateral tropia at a given distance.

Another sensory anomaly that may accompany strabismus is anomalous retinal correspondence, which is present when the amount of tropia measured objectively (objective angle of strabismus) differs significantly from the amount of tropia measured subjectively (subjective angle of strabismus). The difference between the objective angle and the subjective angle is the angle of anomaly. In anomalous retinal correspondence, both an objective tropia line and a subjective tropia line could be plotted. The distance between them on the graph represents the angle of anomaly. In the normal condition, called normal retinal correspondence, the subjective angle is equal to the objective angle within the limits of clinical measurement errors.

## ZONE OF ZERO ASSOCIATED PHORIA
Using an associated phoria target, there is often a range of prism powers over which fixation disparity is zero. Godio and Rutstein[97-100] constructed what they referred to as a zone of zero associated phoria (ZZAP). They found that it tended to parallel the lateral limits of the zone of clear single binocular vision (ZCSBV), but the ZZAP was narrower than the ZCSBV. In 201 asymptomatic subjects, they found that the width of the ZZAP at distance averaged 2.9Δ BI (SD=2.2) to 3.5Δ BO (SD=3.4). At near, the width of the ZZAP averaged 6.3Δ BI to 7.0Δ BO (SD=6.3).[97] They suggested that the ZZAP might be helpful as a complement to standard dissociated phoria and fusional vergence range findings.[99]

## RELATION OF MYOPIA ONSET AND PROGRESSION TO ACCOMMODATION AND VERGENCE FUNCTION
The results of a large number of studies suggest a relationship of refractive error development to nearpoint accommodation and vergence function.[101-104] Myopes as a group tend to have less dark focus accommodation, less optical reflex accommodation, and less proximally induced accommodation than emmetropes as a group. Emmetropic children who become myopic tend to have a more convergent near dissociated phoria, a more convergent midpoint of the lateral width of the ZCSBV, and a lower PRA than emmetropic children who remain emmetropic.[105-108] Children who are becoming myopic show a convergent shift in near dissociated phoria which averages about 3 to 4Δ over a two to two and a half year period of time beginning before the onset of myopia and continuing after its onset.[108]

Two studies determined mean rates of childhood myopia progression in diopters per year for different levels of nearpoint dissociated phoria.[109,110] Myopia progression rates were lowest in patients with ortho and low exo at near (Table 16.2).

Over the years many clinicians have prescribed bifocal lenses to try to slow childhood myopia progression. Papers in the literature have reported varying levels of success.[111] However, a consistent finding of such studies is that plus adds for near reduce progression rates more in patients with esophoria at near, than in patients with ortho and exophoria. This was first reported by Roberts and Banford.[109] Results from several studies[109,112-117] are summarized in Table 16.3.

Various theories of myopia etiology invoke a connection with accommodation. One theory suggests that the use of accommodation induces mechanical changes in the eye leading to axial elongation of the eye and myopia. That theory is several decades old. Perhaps its strongest advocate was Francis Young.[118-120] Another prominent theory is the defocus theory, which suggests that a high lag of accommodation when doing near work leads to axial elongation and myopia. In the defocus theory, the defocus from the lag provides a signal to ocular growth to move the retina posteriorly closer to the best focused image. The first descriptions of the defocus theory appeared in print in the 1980s and 1990s.[121-128] Other theories suggest a role in myopia etiology for the transient shifts toward increased accommodation after intensive near work. As more is learned about the relationship of accommodation and convergence function to refractive development, it may be possible to design accommodation and vergence treatment regimens that will play an important role in refractive development.

## REFERENCES

1. Balsam MD, Fry GA. Convergence accommodation. Am J Optom Arch Am Acad Optom 1959;36:567-575.

2. Rosenfield M, Gilmartin B. Disparity-induced accommodation in late-onset myopia. Ophthal Physiol Opt 1988;8:353-355.

3. Schor CM, Narayan V. Graphical analysis of prism adaptation, convergence accommodation, and accommodative convergence. Am J Optom Physiol Opt 1982;59:774-784.

4. Tsuetaki TX, Schor CM. Clinical method for measuring adaptation of tonic accommodation and vergence accommodation. Am J Optom Physiol Opt 1987; 64:437-449.

5. Daum KM, Rutstein RP, Houston G IV, Clore HA, Corliss DA. Evaluation of a new criterion of binocularity. Optom Vis Sci 1989;66:218-228.

6. Goss DA. Pratt system of clinical analysis of accommodation and convergence. Optom Vis Sci 1989;66:805-806.

7. Fry GA. Basic concepts underlying graphical analysis. In: Schor CM, Ciuffreda KJ, eds. Vergence Eye Movements: Basic and Clinical Aspects. Boston: Butterworth-Heinemann, 1983:403-437.

8. Semmlow JL. Oculomotor responses to near stimuli: the near triad. In: Zuber BL, ed. Models of Oculomotor Behavior and Control. Boca Raton: CRC Press, 1981:161-191.

9. Semmlow JL. Hung GK. The near response: theories of control. In: Schor CM, Ciuffreda KJ, eds. Vergence Eye Movements: Basic and Clinical Aspects. Boston: Butterworth-Heinemann, 1983: 175-195.

10. Schor CM. Fixation disparity and vergence adaptation. In: Schor CM, Ciuffreda KJ, eds. Vergence Eye Movements: Basic and Clinical Aspects. Boston: Butterworth- Heinemann, 1983:465-516.

11. Schor CM. Models of mutual interaction between accommodation and convergence. Am J Optom Physiol Opt 1985;62:369-374.

12. Saladin JJ. Phorometry and stereopsis. In: Benjamin WJ, ed. Borish's Clinical Refraction, 2nd ed. St. Louis: Butterworth Heinemann Elsevier, 2006:899-960.

13. Schor C. The influence of interactions between accommodation and convergence on the lag of accommodation. Ophthal Physiol Opt 1999;19:134-150.

14. Goss DA, Rainey BB. Relationship of accommodative response and nearpoint phoria in a sample of myopic children. Optom Vis Sci 1999;76:292-294.

15. Alpern M. Types of movement. In: Davson H, ed. Muscular Mechanisms. 2nd ed. Vol 3 of The Eye. New York: Academic, 1969:65-174.

16. Rosenfield M, Rappon JM, Carrel MF. Vergence adaptation and the clinical AC/A ratio. Ophthal Physiol Opt 2000;20:207-211.

17. Rainey BB. The effect of prism adaptation on the response AC/A ratio. Ophthal Physiol Opt 2000;20:199-206.

18. Hogan RE, Linfield PB. The effects of moderate doses of ethanol on heterophoria and other aspects of binocular vision. Ophthal Physiol Opt 1983;3: 21-31.

19. Zhai H, Goss DA, Hammond RW. The effect of caffeine on the accommodative response/accommodative stimulus function and on the response AC/A ratio. Current Eye Res 1993;12:489-499.

20. North RV, Henson DB, Smith TJ. Influence of proximal, accommodative and disparity stimuli upon the vergence system. Ophthal Physiol Opt 1993; 13:239-243.

21. Mannen DL. Bannon MJ, Septon RD. Effects of base-out training on proximal convergence. Am J Optom Physiol Opt 1981;58:1187-1193.

22. Hokoda SC, Ciuffreda KJ. Theoretical and clinical importance of proximal vergence and accommodation. In: Schor CM, Ciuffreda KJ, eds. Vergence Eye Movements: Basic and Clinical Aspects. Boston: Butterworth-Heinemann, 1983:75-97.

23. Wick B. Clinical factors in proximal vergence. Am J Optom Physiol Opt 1985;62:1-18.

24. Joubert C, Bedell HE. Proximal vergence and perceived distance. Optom Vis Sci 1990;67:29-35.

25. Ogle KN, Martens TG. On the accommodative convergence and the proximal convergence. Arch Ophthalmol 1957;57:702-715.

26. Rosenfield M, Ciuffreda KJ, Hung GK. The linearity of proximally induced accommodation and vergence. Invest Ophthalmol Vis Sci 1991;32: 2985-2991.

27. Leibowitz HW, Owens DA. New evidence for the intermediate position of relaxed accommodation. Doc Ophthalmol 1978;46: 133- 147.

28. Leibowitz HW, Owens DA. Night myopia and the intermediate dark focus of accommodation. J Opt Soc Am 1975;65:1121-1128.

29. Hope GM, Rubin Ml. Night myopia. Surv Ophthalmol 1984;29:129-136.

30. Goss DA, Eskridge JB. Myopia. In: Amos JF, ed. Diagnosis and Management in Vision Care. Boston: Butterworth-Heinemann, 1987:121-171.

31. Owens DA, Mohindra L Held R. Near retinoscopy and the effectiveness of a retinoscope beam as an accommodative stimulus. Invest Ophthalmol Vis Sci 1980; 18:942-949.

32. Bullimore MA, Gilmartin B, Hogan RE. Objective and subjective measurement of tonic accommodation. Ophthal Physiol Opt 1986;6:57-62.

33. Owens DA, Leibowitz HW. Night myopia: cause and a possible basis for amelioration. Am J Optom Physiol Opt 1976;53:709-717.

34. Wolf KS, Bedell HE, Pedersen SB. Relations between accommodation and vergence in darkness. Optom Vis Sci 1990;67:89-93.

35. Rosenfield M, Ciuffreda KJ. Distance heterophoria and tonic vergence. Optom Vis Sci 1990;67:667-669.

36. Miller RJ. Temporal stability of the dark focus of accommodation. Am J Optom Physiol Opt 1978;55:447-450.

37. Owens RL, Higgins KE. Long-term stability of the dark focus of accommodation. Am J Optom Physiol Opt 1983;60:32-38.

38. Ebenholtz SM. Accommodative hysteresis: relation to resting focus. Am J Optom Physiol Opt 1985;62:755-762.

39. Ebenholtz SM. Long-term endurance of adaptive shifts in tonic accommodation. Ophthal Physiol Opt 1988;8:427-431.

40. McBrien NA, Millodot M. Differences in adaptation of tonic accommodation with refractive state. Invest Ophthalmol Vis Sci 1988;29:460-469.

41. Gilmartin B, Bullimore M. Adaptation of tonic accommodation to sustained visual tasks in emmetropia and late-onset myopia. Optom Vis Sci 1991;68: 22-26.

42. Ong E, Ciuffreda KJ. Accommodation, Nearwork and Myopia. Santa Ana, CA: Optometric Extension Program, 1997:97-142.

43. Cogan DC. Accommodation and the autonomic nervous system. Arch Ophthalmol 1937; 18:739-766.

44. Stephens KG. *Effect of the sympathetic nervous system on accommodation. Am J Optom Physiol Opt 1985;62:402-406.*

45. Gilmartin B, Hogan RE. *The relationship between tonic accommodation and ciliary muscle innervation. Invest Ophthalmol Vis Sci 1985;26:1024-1028.*

46. Gilmartin B. *A review of the role of sympathetic innervation of the ciliary muscle in ocular accommodation. Ophthal Physiol Opt 1986;6:23-37.*

47. Hung GK, Ciuffreda KJ, Rosenfield M. *Proximal contribution to a linear static model of accommodation and vergence. Ophthal Physiol Opt 1996;16:31-41.*

48. Birnbaum MH. *Nearpoint visual stress: a physiological model. J Am Optom Assoc 1984;55:825-835.*

49. Birnbaum MH. *Nearpoint visual stress: clinical implications. J Am Optom Assoc 1985;56:480-490.*

50. Pavlidis GT. *Eye movement differences between dyslexia, normal, and retarded readers while sequentially fixating digits. Am J Optom Physiol Opt 1985;62:820-832.*

51. Grisham JD, Simons HD. *Refractive error and the reading process: a literature analysis. J Am Optom Assoc 1986;57:44-55.*

52. Simons HD, Grisham JD. *Binocular anomalies and reading problems. J Am Optom Assoc 1987;58:578-587.*

53. Simons HD, Gassler PA. *Vision anomalies and reading skill: a meta-analysis of the literature. Am J Optom Physiol Opt 1988;65:893-904.*

54. Simons HD. *An analysis of the role of vision anomalies in reading interference. Optom Vis Sci 1993;70:369-373.*

55. Garzia RP, Franzel AS. *Refractive status, binocular vision, and reading achievement. In: Garzia RP, ed. Vision and Reading. St. Louis: Mosby, 1996:111-131.*

56. Richman JE, Garzia RP. *Eye movements and reading. In: Garzia RP, ed. Vision and Reading. St. Louis: Mosby, 1996:133-148.*

57. Bowan MD. *Learning disabilities, dyslexia, and vision: A subject review, a rebuttal, literature review, and commentary. Optom 2002;73:553-570.*

58. Bonilla-Warford N, Allison C. *A review of the efficacy of oculomotor vision therapy in improving reading skills. J Optom Vis Dev 2004;35:108-115.*

59. Sheedy JE, Parsons SD. *The Video Display Terminal Clinic: clinical report. Optom Vis Sci 1990;67:622-626.*

60. Sheedy JE. *Vision problems at video display terminals: a survey of optometrists. J Am Optom Assoc 1992;63:687-692.*

61. Solan HA. *Learning disabilities. In: Rosenbloom AA, Morgan MW, eds. Principles and Practice of Pediatric Optometry. Philadelphia: Lippincott, 1990:486-517.*

62. Grisham JD, Simons H. *Perspectives on reading disabilities. In: Rosenbloom AA, Morgan MW, eds. Principles and Practice of Pediatric Optometry. Philadelphia: Lippincott, 1990:518-559.*

63. Press LJ. *Vision and school performance. In: Press LJ, Moore BD, eds. Clinical Pediatric Optometry. Boston: Butterworth-Heinemann, 1993:81-92.*

64. Birnbaum MH. *Optometric Management of Nearpoint Vision Disorders. Boston: Butterworth-Heinemann, 1993:257-280.*

65. Scheiman MM, Rouse MW, eds. *Optometric Management of Learning-Related Vision Problems, 2nd ed. St. Louis: Mosby, 2006.*

66. Garzia RP, ed. *Vision and Reading. St. Louis: Mosby, 1996.*

67. Griffin JR, Christenson GN, Wesson MD, Erickson GB. *Optometric Management of Reading Dysfunction. Boston: Butterworth-Heinemann, 1997.*

68. Garzia RP, Borsting EJ, Nicholson SB, et al. *Care of the Patient with Learning Related Vision Problems. St. Louis: American Optometric Association, 2000.*

69. Scheiman M, Wick B. *Clinical Management of Binocular Vision – Heterophoric, Accommodative, and Eye Movement Disorders, 2nd ed. Philadelphia: Lippincott Williams & Wilkins, 2002:550-572, 596-620.*

70. Sheedy JE. *Video display terminals: solving the vision problems. In: Sheedy JE, ed. Environmental Optics. Problems in Optometry. Philadelphia: Lippincott, 1990; 2(1):1-16.*

71. Sheedy JE. *Video display terminals: solving the environmental problems.* In: Sheedy JE, ed. *Environmental Optics. Problems in Optometry.* Philadelphia: Lippincott, 1990; 2(1):17-31.

72. Pitts DG. *Visual display terminals: visual problems and solutions.* In: Pitts DG, Kleinstein RN, eds. *Environmental Vision: Interactions of the Eye, Vision, and the Environment.* Boston: Butterworth-Heinemann, 1993:333-349.

73. Sheedy JE, Shaw-McMinn PG. *Diagnosing and Treating Computer-Related Vision Problems.* Amsterdam: Butterworth-Heinemann, 2003.

74. Classé JG, ed. *Sports Vision. Optometry Clinics.* Norwalk, CT: Appleton & Lange, 1993; 3(1).

75. Reichow AW, Stoner MW, eds. *Sports Vision.* Santa Ana, CA: Optometric Extension Program, 1993.

76. Loran DFC, MacEwen CJ. *Sports Vision.* Oxford: Butterworth-Heinemann, 1995.

77. Schroeder TL, Rainey BB, Goss DA, Grosvenor TP. *Reliability of and comparisons among methods of measuring dissociated phorias. Optom Vis Sci* 1996;73:389-397.

78. Rainey BB, Schroeder TL, Goss DA, Grosvenor TP. *Inter-examiner repeatability of heterophoria tests. Optom Vis Sci* 1998;75:719-726.

79. Wong EPF, Fricke TR, Dinardo C. *Interexaminer repeatability of a new, modified Prentice card compared with established phoria tests. Optom Vis Sci* 2002;79:370-375.

80. Daum KM. *Heterophoria and heterotropia.* In: Eskridge JB, Amos JF, Bartlett JD, eds. *Clinical Procedures in Optometry.* Philadelphia: Lippincott, 1991:72-90.

81. Hirsch MJ, Bing LB. *The effect of testing method on values obtained for phoria at forty centimeters. Am J Optom Physiol Opt* 1948;25:407-416.

82. Hirsch MJ. *Clinical investigation of a method of testing phoria at forty centimeters. Am J Optom Physiol Opt* 1948;25:492-495.

83. Scobee RG, Green EL. *Tests for heterophoria – reliability of tests, comparisons between tests, and effect of changing testing conditions. Trans Am Acad Ophthalmol Otolaryngol* 1947;51:179-197.

84. Rainey BB, Schroeder TL, Goss DA, Grosvenor TP. *Reliability of and comparisons among three variations of the alternating cover test. Ophthal Physiol Opt* 1998;18:430-437.

85. Ludvigh E. *Amount of eye movement objectively perceptible to the unaided eye. Am J Ophthalmol* 1949;32:649-650.

86. Romano PE, von Noorden GK. *Limitations of cover test in detecting strabismus. Am J Ophthalmol* 1971;72:10-12.

87. Fogt N, Baughman BJ, Good G. *The effect of experience on the detection of small eye movements. Optom Vis Sci* 2000;77:670-674.

88. von Noorden GK. *Burian-von Noorden's Binocular Vision and Ocular Motility: Theory and Management of Strabismus, 2nd ed.* St. Louis: Mosby, 1980:187.

89. Penisten DK, Hofstetter HW, Goss DA. *Reliability of rotary prism fusional vergence ranges. Optom* 2001;72:117-122.

90. Brozek J, Simonson E, Bushard WJ, et al. *Effects of practice and the consistency of repeated measurements of accommodation and vergence. Am J Ophthalmol* 1948;31:191-198.

91. Wesson MD, Masin LC, Boyles ST. *Objective testing of vergence ranges. J Am Optom Assoc* 1995;66:338-342.

92. Apell RJ. *Performance test battery: A very useful tool for prescribing lenses. J Behav Optom* 1996;7:7-10.

93. Saladin JJ. *Stereopsis from a performance perspective. Optom Vis Sci* 2005;82:186-205.

94. Hofstetter HW. *The graphical analysis of clinical optometric findings.* In: *Transactions of the International Ophthalmic Optical Congress 1961.* London: Lockwood, 1962:456-460.

95. Hofstetter HW. *Graphical analysis.* In: Schor CM, Ciuffreda KJ, eds. *Vergence Eye Movements: Basic and Clinical Aspects.* Boston: Butterworth-Heinemann, 1983:439-464.

96. Hofstetter HW. *A revised schematic for the graphic analysis of the accommodation-convergence relationship. Can J Optom* 1968;30:49-52.

97. Godio LB, Rutstein RP. *The range of zero-associated phoria in an asymptomatic clinical population. Am J Optom Physiol Opt* 1981;58:445-450.

98. Godio LB, Rutstein RP. *Clinical comparison of the zone of clear single binocular vision with the zone of zero-associated phoria. Am J Optom Physiol Opt* 1981;58:1194-1198.

99. Godio LB. Rutstein RP. Common clinical configuration of the zone of zero-associated phoria. Am J Optom Physiol Opt 1983;60:514-518.

100. Rutstein RP, Godio LB. Zone of zero-associated phoria in patients with convergence insufficiency. Am J Optom Physiol Opt 1983;60:582-585.

101. Birnbaum MH. Optometric Management of Nearpoint Vision Disorders. Boston: Butterworth-Heinemann, 1993: 11-32.

102. Ong E, Ciuffreda KJ. Accommodation, Nearwork and Myopia. Santa Ana, CA: Optometric Extension Program, 1997.

103. Rosenfield M, Gilmartin B, eds. Myopia and Nearwork. Oxford: Butterworth-Heinemann, 1998.

104. Goss DA. Relation of nearpoint esophoria to the onset and progression of myopia in children. J Optom Vis Dev 1999;30:25-32.

105. Goss DA. Clinical accommodation and heterophoria findings preceding juvenile onset of myopia. Optom Vis Sci 1991;68:110-116.

106. Drobe B, de Saint-André R. The pre-myopic syndrome. Ophthal Physiol Opt 1995;15:375-378.

107. Goss DA, Jackson TW. Clinical findings before the onset of myopia in youth. 2. Zone of clear single binocular vision. Optom Vis Sci 1996;73:263-268.

108. Goss DA, Jackson TW. Clinical findings before the onset of myopia in youth. 3. Heterophoria. Optom Vis Sci 1996;73:269-278.

109. Roberts WL, Banford RD. evaluation of bifocal correction technique in juvenile myopia. Optom Weekly 1967;58(38):25-28,31; 58(39):21-30; 58(40):23-28; 58(41):27-34; 58(43):19-24,26.

110. Goss DA. Variables related to the rate of childhood myopia progression. Optom Vis Sci 1990;67:631-636.

111. Grosvenor T, Goss DA. Clinical Management of Myopia. Boston: Butterworth-Heinemann, 1999:113-128.

112. Goss DA, Uyesugi EF. Effectivness of bifocal control of childhood myopia progression as a function of near point phoria and binocular cross-cylinder. J Optom Vis Dev 1995;26:12-17.

113. Fulk GW, Cyert LA. Can bifocals slow myopia progression? J Am Optom Assoc 1996;67:749-754.

114. Fulk GW, Cyert LA, Parker DE. A randomized trial of the effect of single-vision vs. bifocal lenses on myopia progression in children with esophoria. Optom Vis Sci 2000;77:395-401.

115. Edwards MH, Li RW-H, Lam CS-Y, et al. The Hong Kong progressive lens myopia control study: Study design and main findings. Invest Ophthalmol Vis Sci 2002;43:2852-2858.

116. Brown B, Edwards MH, Leung JTM. Is esophoria a factor in slowing of myopia by progressive lenses? Optom Vis Sci 2002;79:638-642.

117. Gwiazda JE, Hyman L, Norton TT, et al. Accommodation and related risk factors associated with myopia progression and their interaction with treatment in COMET children. Invest Ophthalmol Vis Sci 2004;45:2143-2151.

118. Young FA. The nature and control of myopia. J Am Optom Assoc 1977;48:451-457.

119. Young FA. Primate myopia. Am J Optom Physiol Opt 1981;58:560-566.

120. Young FA, Leary GA. Accommodation and vitreous chamber pressure: a proposed mechanism for myopia. In: Grosvenor T, Flom MC, eds. Refractive Anomalies: Research and Clinical Applications. Boston: Butterworth-Heinemann, 1991:301-309.

121. Raviola E, Wiesel TN. An animal model of myopia. N Eng J Med 1985;312:1609-1615.

122. Wickham MG. Growth as a factor in the etiology of juvenile-onset myopia. In: Goss DA, Edmondson LL, Bezan DL, eds. Proceedings of the 1986 Northeastern State University Symposium on Theoretical and Clinical Optometry. Tahlequah, OK: Northeastern State University, 1986:117-137.

123. Goss DA. Retinal image-mediated ocular growth as a possible etiological factor in juvenile-onset myopia. In: Vision Science Symposium: A Tribute to Gordon G. Heath. Bloomington: Indiana University, 1988:165-183.

124. Smith EL III. Experimentally induced refractive anomalies in mammals. In: Grosvenor T, Flom MC, eds. Refractive Anomalies: Research and Clinical Applications. Boston: Butterworth-Heinemann, 1991:246-267.

125. Wallman J. *Retinal factors in myopia and emmetropization: clues from research on chicks.* In: Grosvenor T, Flom MC, eds. *Refractive Anomalies: Research and Clinical Applications.* Boston: Butterworth-Heinemann, 1991:268-286.

126. Gwiazda J, Thorn F, Bauer J, Held R. *Myopic children show insufficient accommodative response to blur.* Invest Ophthalmol Vis Sci 1993;34:690-694.

127. Goss DA, Zhai H. *Clinical and laboratory investigations of the relationship of accommodation and convergence function with refractive error – a literature review.* Doc Ophthalmol 1994;86:349-380.

128. Goss DA, Wickham MG. *Retinal-image mediated ocular growth as a mechanism for juvenile onset myopia and emmetropization – a literature review.* Doc Ophthalmol 1995;90:341-375.

## OTHER SUGGESTED READING

Ciuffreda KJ, Tannen B. *Eye Movement Basics for the Clinician.* St. Louis: Mosby, 1995:127-160.

Schor CM, Ciuffreda KJ, eds. *Vergence Eye Movements: Basic and Clinical Aspects.* Boston: Butterworth-Heinemann, 1983.

Hung GK. *Models of Oculomotor Control.* River Edge, NJ: World Scientific, 2001.

## PRACTICE PROBLEMS

1. A binocular cross cylinder test has an endpoint at an add of +0.50 D. The test is repeated with 6Δ base-in, and the endpoint is +1.00 D. What is the CAC ratio?

2. MEM dynamic retinoscopy is performed using a target without sufficient blur cues for accommodation. The lag of accommodation is 1.00 D. When this is repeated with 6Δ base-out, the lag is 0.75 D. What is the CAC ratio?

3. What is the PCT ratio if the calculated ACA ratio is 4.7 Δ/D and the gradient ACA ratio is 3 Δ/D?

4. A patient with a 64 mm PD has a distance dissociated phoria with BVA of 2Δ exo, a 40 cm dissociated phoria with BVA of 4Δ exo, and a 40 cm dissociated phoria with a +1.00 D add of 8Δ exo. What is the PCT ratio?

5. An individual with a 64 mm PD has a distance dissociated phoria of 2Δ exo and a 40 cm dissociated phoria with a +2.50 D add of 14Δ exo. What is the PCT ratio?

# Chapter 17
# Other Systems of Case Analysis

**G**oing back to a statement made in the first paragraph of the first chapter of this book, we noted that in order to effectively diagnose accommodation and vergence disorders it is necessary to use a comprehensive battery of accommodation and vergence tests, along with a systematic method of analyzing those test findings. As observed by Schmitt,[1] "no clinical test in isolation is all that informative….only when clinical data are compared within the framework of a rational model is it possible for the practitioner to construct a performance profile which can reflect how well an individual patient may perform visually."

Previous chapters in this book have described a system in which test findings are compared to norms and the pattern of results establishes a case type. Previous chapters have also cited some of the literature supporting the scientific background and clinical effectiveness of such an approach. This is a normative analysis system similar to those described by other authors.[2-9] Normative analysis is the term often applied to a system of case analysis in which accommodation and vergence findings are compared to their corresponding norms, and then the pattern of which tests are normal and which are abnormal indicates the type of accommodation and vergence disorder.

In the late 19th century and early 20th century, many practitioners were not well educated in the nature, science, and complexities of accommodation and vergence function. To make standardized and efficient case analysis possible, methods of analysis were presented as fairly mechanistic and formalized processes. So for example, OEP analysis (which will be discussed below) was developed in the first half of the 20th century and presented a series of analytical steps and attendant prescription mandates. Various rules of thumb, including some we have discussed earlier, such as Sheard's criterion and Percival's criterion, introduced in about the same era, could also be applied in a mechanistic fashion.

The development of Morgan's system of normative analysis (which will also be discussed below) represented somewhat of a departure in that groups of tests could be evaluated and the practitioner could base prescription decisions on general principles rather than on formalized recommendations. A general normative analysis approach of this type, enhanced by the advancement of knowledge in the intervening years, is used by the majority of practitioners today. The approach presented in this book is essentially a form of normative analysis incorporating principles of accommodation and vergence test norms, of rules of thumb as informative guidelines rather than formal rules, of the zone of clear single binocular vision as a teaching tool and means for evaluating the consistency of test findings, and of fixation disparity and associated phoria analysis. Scheiman and Wick[10] have referred to normative analysis

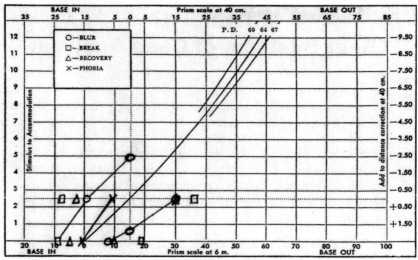
*Figure 17.1. Plot of the OEP expecteds.*

which incorporates and synthesizes principles from various analysis systems and from the scientific study of accommodation and vergence function as integrative analysis.

There are many rules of thumb and systems of analysis proposed throughout the years in addition to the ones covered so far in this text. Some of these were discussed by Borish.[11] A few specialized unique systems of analysis will be described below. As you read about these various systems of case analysis, note that they generally require a constellation of test findings be taken to establish a pattern of correlated test findings which then suggests a particular syndrome or case type.

## OPTOMETRIC EXTENSION PROGRAM ANALYSIS

The Optometric Extension Program (OEP) is an organization that was formed in the 1920s. The analysis system usually referred to as OEP analysis was developed by Skeffington, Lesser, and their colleagues.[12-14] The developers and followers of OEP analysis made some philosophical assumptions concerning accommodation and convergence disorders.[15-17] One of these is that anomalous clinical findings are the result of nearpoint stress. Prism is not a treatment option of OEP analysis, because a prism prescription is viewed as treating a symptom rather than treating the underlying disorder.[17] In many clinical analysis systems, vergence problems are talked about partially in terms of the demand on fusional vergence and the fusional vergence reserve. Thus eyestrain can result from the pattern of a high demand and/or a low reserve. The OEP philosophy as originally expounded by Skeffington and colleagues differs in its viewpoint. It views an anomalous pattern of clinical findings as developing in response to the stresses of near point vision activity. Plus adds and vision therapy are viewed as methods of relieving near point stress.

Skeffington suggested that the stress response to sustained near work leads the individual to converge closer than the plane of accommodation. This in

216

**Table 17.1. The Optometric Extension Program (OEP) test numbers and expecteds. The near tests are performed with a test distance of 16 inches with the exception of test no. 19.**

| Test number | Test description | Expecteds |
|---|---|---|
| 1 | Ophthalmoscopy | |
| 2 | Ophthalmometry (keratometry) | |
| 3 | Habitual lateral phoria at distance | 0.5 exo |
| 13A | Habitual lateral phoria at near | 6 exo |
| 4 | Distance retinoscopy | |
| 5 | Dynamic retinoscopy at 20 inches (50 cm) | |
| 6 | Dynamic retinoscopy at 40 inches (1 m) | |
| 7 | Subjective refraction: maximum plus to 20/20 minus visual acuity | |
| 7A | Subjective refraction: maximum plus to best distance visual acuity | |
| 8 | Lateral phoria at distance through #7 finding | 0.5 exo |
| 9 | Base-out to first blur at distance | 7 to 9 |
| 10 | Base-out to break and recovery at distance | 19/10 minimum |
| 11 | Base-in to break and recovery at distance | 9/5 minimum |
| 12 | Vertical phoria and vertical fusional vergence ranges at distance | Ortho, ranges equal |
| 13B | Lateral phoria at near through #7 finding | 6 exo |
| 14A | Unfused (monocular) cross cylinder | |
| 15A | Lateral phoria through #14A finding | |
| 14B | Fused (binocular) cross cylinder | |
| 15B | Lateral phoria at near through #14B finding | |
| 16A | Base-out to blur out at near | 15 |
| 16B | Base-out to break and recovery at near | 21/15 minimum |
| 17A | Base-in to blur out at near | 14 |
| 17B | Base-in to break and recovery at near | 22/18 minimum |
| 18 | Vertical phoria and vertical fusional vergence ranges at near | ortho, ranges equal |
| 19 | Analytical amplitude (minus to blur of 0.62 m or J4 letters with card at 13 inches) | |
| 20 | Minus to blur out | -2.25 to -2.50 |
| 21 | Plus to blur out | +1.75 to +2.00 |

turn can lead to negative adaptations, such as inefficient reading performance, development of refractive error, or avoidance of near work. The use of plus lenses for near work can allow the individual to converge to a point closer than the plane of accommodation and avoid resultant maladaptive changes.[18]

OEP analysis incorporates test results from a standardized testing routine. In the OEP testing routine, tests are assigned numbers. The OEP literature often uses these test numbers instead of the names of the tests. The OEP test numbers and expecteds are given in Table 17.1. The OEP expecteds are graphed in Figure 17.1. It may be noted that the OEP expecteds are very similar to Morgan's mean values. They are all within one or two prism diopters of Morgan's means except the near phoria and the base-in and base-out recoveries at near. The plus to blur and minus to blur are essentially the same in the OEP expecteds and Morgan's mean values.

The OEP analysis procedure begins with determining the case type. The case type is identified as A, B1, B2, or C through a procedure called "checking, chaining, and typing." These steps are (1) check: determine whether findings are high or low by comparing them with the expecteds; (2) chain: list the test numbers in a particular sequence above a horizontal line if they are high and below the line if they are low; and (3) type: use the "informative sequence" from checking and chaining to determine the case type. The characteristic patterns of high and low findings for each of the case types are as follows:

A:

$$\frac{}{\text{4 -11 -13B -17B}}$$

B1:

$$\frac{5}{\text{9-11-16B}}$$

B2:

$$\frac{5}{\text{9-11-17B}}$$

C:

$$\frac{\text{15A}}{\text{5 -10 -16B}}$$

The vast majority of cases are either B1 or B2 cases. Convergence insufficiency, pseudoconvergence insufficiency, and basic exo cases are usually typed B1, and convergence excess cases are usually typed B2. The remainder of the tests in the informative sequence are used to identify seven subtypes or "deteriorations" of B cases.

A series of rules are then applied to determine the lens prescription. The maximum plus prescribed for distance is the #7 finding, which is the point in the subjective refraction at which plus has been reduced to the level at which the patient can read most of the 20/20 line. The maximum plus prescribed for near is based on a formula that includes the #14B, #15B, and #19 test results. In B1 cases, full maximum plus is recommended for distance and near. In B2 cases, the directive is to prescribe the full plus at near but cut plus at distance. In C cases, the mandate is to cut plus at distance and near.

B type cases are more likely to benefit from plus adds for near than are C type cases, the C type case being viewed as an uncharacteristic response to stress from near work.[17] Flax[19] suggested that B2 individuals were more likely to prefer full minus or reduced plus at distance than B1 individuals because the processing style of the former may be more dependent on critical form vision.

In OEP analysis the #16A, #17A, #20, and #21 findings are referred to as "equilibrium findings." Calculations are done to determine what these tests would yield if started at different levels of plus. An OEP directive is that the plus prescribed should not be so much that the equilibrium findings would be reversed from the habitual. In other words, if the #21 with the habitual correction is greater in magnitude than the #20, the plus prescribed should not be so high that the #20 becomes greater in magnitude than the #21.

**Table 17.2. Grouping of tests suggested by Morgan.**

| Group | Tests |
|-------|-------|
| A | 40 cm base-in blur, break, and recovery<br>40 cm minus to blur<br>Amplitude of accommodation<br>Distance base-in break and recovery |
| B | 40 cm base-out blur, break, and recovery<br>40 cm plus to blur<br>Distance base-out blur, break, and recovery |
| C | Gradient ACA ratio<br>Distance phoria<br>40 cm phoria<br>Calculated ACA ratio |

Some findings also are used to establish a stage of embeddedness of a vision problem. There are directives concerning lens acceptance at different stages of embeddedness, with nonembedded cases thought to be more likely to accept plus lens application. Further information on OEP testing and analysis can be obtained from various sources.[14-26] In addition to the test numbering and analysis system, OEP literature sometimes uses a unique terminology in which physiological functions are described by a behavioral outcome correlate. For example, accommodation is part of a process referred to as identification and convergence is part of a process called centering.[27] Although the formal OEP analysis procedure is not commonly used today, there are many advocates for the importance of the underlying concepts.

## MORGAN'S NORMATIVE ANALYSIS

In chapter 7, we discussed the norms developed by Meredith Morgan. In order to examine the relationship between different test findings, Morgan calculated coefficients of correlation of phoria, vergence range, and relative accommodation test findings with each other.[28-30] On the basis of the signs and magnitudes of the correlation coefficients, he placed each finding in one of three groups, which he labeled groups A, B, and C. (Table 17.2).

Most patients fit into one of three categories: (1) group A and B findings normal, (2) group A findings low and group B findings high, or (3) group A findings high and group B findings low. Morgan suggested that when group A findings were low (usually in esophoria), the treatment options were plus adds, base-out prism, or vision therapy. In cases with low group B findings (typical of exophoria), he suggested treatment options included base-in prism, vision therapy, and minus adds. Whether prism, vision therapy, or adds are applied,

**Table 17.3. Haynes normative data for vergence amplitude, posture, ranges, and response time. The test numbers are from the OEP test numbering system. PE is probable error, 0.6745 x SD.**

| Test | Mean | PE |
|---|---|---|
| NPC break | 6.4 cm | 1.8 |
| NPC recovery | 10.2 cm | 4.3 |
| #8 (phoria at distance) | 0.5Δ exo | 1.7 |
| #13B (phoria at 40 cm) | 4.0Δ exo | 3.5 |
| Phoria at 25 cm | 6.5Δ exo | 4.0 |
| #9 (base-out to blur at distance) | 8Δ | 3.0 |
| Base-out to blur out at distance | 12 | 3.0 |
| #10 break | 19 | 4.6 |
| #10 recovery | 9 | 3.0 |
| #11 break | 8 | 2.2 |
| #11 recovery | 3.5 | 1.8 |
| #10 recovery - #8 | 9 | 3.0 |
| #11 recovery - #8 | 3 | 1.8 |
| #11 recovery - #10 recovery | 12 | 2.8 |
| #11 break - #10 break | 28 | 4.0 |
| Base-out to blur at 40 cm | 13 | 4.0 |
| #16A (base-out to blur out at 40 cm) | 16 | 4.0 |
| #16B break | 19 | 4.7 |
| #16B recovery | 9 | 4.0 |
| Base-in to blur at 40 cm | 11 | 3.0 |
| #17A (base-in to blur out at 40 cm) | 14 | 3.0 |
| #17B break | 20 | 2.8 |
| #17B recovery | 12 | 2.9 |
| #16B recovery - #13B | 11 | 4.0 |
| #17B recovery - #13B | 8 | 3.3 |
| #17B recovery - #16B recovery | 22 | 4.0 |
| #17B break - #16B break | 38 | 5.0 |
| BI blur at 40 cm - BO blur at 40 cm | 23 | 5.0 |
| #17A - #16A (BI blur out – BO blur out) | 30 | 6.0 |
| Vergence facility, 0 to 8Δ BO | 23 cpm | 5.0 |
| Vergence facility, 0 to 8Δ BI | 18 cpm | 5.0 |

Morgan further proposed, depends on the results of the group C tests, the age of the patient, and the professional judgment of the practitioner.

## HAYNES' NORMATIVE ANALYSIS

Harold M. Haynes developed a unique system of normative analysis which he taught to several decades of students at Pacific University College of Optometry. Unfortunately it appears that he never published the system. The following discussion of Haynes' analysis system comes from my class notes, along with notes provided by Stuart Mann and Scott Cooper. The application of this system does not result in a diagnosis, but rather provides accom-

| Test | Mean | PE |
|---|---|---|
| Table 17.4. Haynes normative data for accommodative posture, ranges, and response time. The test numbers are from the OEP test numbering system. PE is probable error, 0.6745 x SD. | | |
| #14A (monoc. cross cylinder at 40 cm) | +1.25 D | 0.37 |
| Monocular cross-cylinder at 25 cm | +2.00 | 0.50 |
| #14B (binoc. cross cylinder at 40 cm) | +1.00 | 0.37 |
| Binocular cross cylinder at 25 cm | +1.62 | 0.50 |
| MEM dynamic retinoscopy, 40 cm | +0.62 | 0.18 |
| Low neutral dynamic retinoscopy, 40 cm | +0.87 | 0.37 |
| Minus to blur | 2.50 | 0.87 |
| #20 (minus to blur out) | 3.50 | 1.00 |
| Minus to blur recovery | 2.62 | 1.00 |
| #20 - recovery | 0.87 | 0.62 |
| #20 - #21 | 6.00 | 1.12 |
| Minus to blur recovery - #14B | 4.50 | 1.12 |
| Plus to blur | 1.87 | 0.37 |
| #21 (plus to blur out) | 2.37 | 0.50 |
| Plus to blur recovery | 1.87 | 0.37 |
| #21 - recovery | 0.50 | 0.37 |
| Plus to blur recov. - minus to blur recov. | 5.25 | 1.12 |
| Plus to blur recovery - #14B | 1.00 | 0.37 |
| #19 net | 4.25 | 1.25 |
| #5 - #4 | 1.12 | 0.37 |
| Accomm. facility, 0 to +2.00 D | 21 cpm | 5.0 |
| Accomm. facility, 0 to -2.00 D | 21 cpm | 5.0 |

modative index (Ai) and convergence index (Ci) scores which can be used to describe the magnitude of the problem, to relate examination results to severity of symptoms, to quantify changes with treatment, or to demonstrate changes over time.

Haynes established norms based on examinations of 15 to 35 year olds. He expressed the norms in terms of the mean and the probable error. The probable error (PE) is equal to 0.6745 times the standard deviation. One probable error either side of the mean would represent the central 50% of a normal distribution. The norms in Haynes' analysis are given in Tables 17.3 (vergence tests) and 17.4 (accommodation tests).

In this analysis system, normal is considered to be within 1 PE either side of the mean. For some tests, called type I tests by Haynes, results higher than the normal range were considered superior performance and results lower than the normal range were considered inferior or abnormal. Type I tests include relative accommodation tests (plus and minus to blur), near point of convergence (NPC), and fusional vergence ranges. On type II tests, results outside of the normal range were considered abnormal regardless of whether they were

Table 17.5. Points assigned to each test depending on the number of probable errors (PE) it was away from the mean in the Haynes normative analysis system. Type I or one-tailed tests are relative accommodation tests, NPC, and fusional vergence ranges. Type II or two-tailed tests are cross cylinder tests, MEM and low neutral dynamic retinoscopy, and phorias.

| | Type I tests | Type II tests |
|---|---|---|
| More than 3 PE below mean | 0 (inferior) | 0 (hypo) |
| -2 to -3 PE from mean | 1 (inferior) | 1 (hypo) |
| -1 to -2 from mean | 2 (inferior) | 2 (hypo) |
| -1 to +1 PE from mean | 3 (normal) | 3 (normal) |
| +1 to +2 from mean | 4 (superior) | 2 (hyper) |
| +2 to +3 from mean | 4 (superior) | 1 (hyper) |
| More than 3 PE above mean | 4 (superior) | 0 (hyper) |

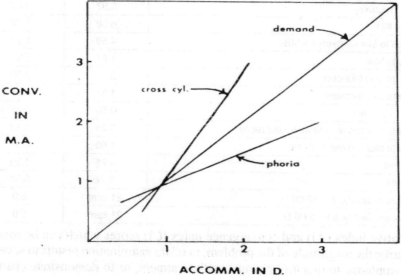

*Figure 17.2. Average phoria and BCC data from Pratt plotted on the coordinates he used. (Reprinted with permission from Goss DA. Pratt system of clinical analysis of accommodation and convergence. Optom Vis Sci 1989;66:805-806.)*

higher or lower than the normal range. Type II tests include cross cylinder tests, MEM and low neutral dynamic retinoscopy, and phorias.

Haynes assigned points to each test depending on how many probable errors it was away from the mean. The points assigned are summarized in Table 17.5. To derive an accommodative index score (Ai), the number of points for each accommodative test were summed and divided by the number of tests, and that number was then multiplied by 10. Similarly, for a convergence index (Ci) score, the points assigned for convergence tests were added up, divided by the number of tests, and multiplied by 10. The formula for the index scores is thus:

Index score = 10 [($\sum$ point scores)/(number of tests)]

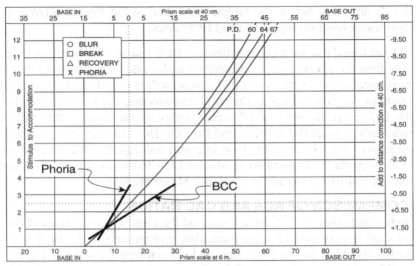

*Figure 17.3. Average phoria and BCC data from Pratt plotted on the more familiar graph form. (Reprinted with permission from Goss DA. Pratt system of clinical analysis of accommodation and convergence. Optom Vis Sci 1989;66:805-806.)*

A normal index score would be 30. Deviation from 30 would indicate the severity of a problem or the level of superiority of performance. Haynes suggested that index scores less than 25 could indicate potential vision therapy cases. An improved index score with time would indicate improved performance but not necessarily a change in diagnosis.

## PRATT'S PLOTTING OF PHORIA AND BINOCULAR CROSS-CYLINDER LINES

Various investigators[31-33] have discussed systems for plotting ACA and CAC lines and for using this information for clinical analysis. Laboratory accommodative convergence and disparity-induced accommodation data have been plotted on graphs similar to our clinical accommodation and convergence graph.[34,35] Pratt was perhaps the first to use such plots of accommodative convergence and convergence accommodation for clinical analysis.[36]

Pratt plotted phoria, binocular cross-cylinder (BCC), fusional vergence range, and relative accommodation data with accommodation in diopters on the x-axis and convergence in meter angles on the y-axis. He measured phorias at 40 cm with various plus and minus adds, and did the BCC test at 40 cm through different base-in and base-out prism settings. The average data derived by Pratt for phorias and BCC tests are plotted in Figure 17.2 on coordinates like he used and in Figure 17.3 on the more familiar graph form.[36] The phoria and BCC lines cross at about the 1 D point on the demand line on the average. The lateral placements and slopes of the phoria and BCC lines vary from patient to patient, but the BCC line always has a steeper slope when convergence is on the y-axis (Figure 17.2) and the phoria line has the steeper slope when accommodation is on the y-axis (Figure 17.3). Points plotted for stimulus levels above or below the ranges illustrated in the figures often introduced non-linearities into the phoria and BCC lines.

If Pratt found that for a given patient the BCC line was farther from the demand line than the phoria line, he prescribed a plus add. The power of the plus add was equal to the displacement in diopters on the x-axis from the 2.5 meter angle point on the demand line to the point that was midway between the phoria and BCC lines at the level of 2.5 meter angles on the y-axis. If the phoria line was farther from the demand line than the BCC line, Pratt prescribed a base in prism. The power of the base in prism was equal to the distance on the y-axis from the 2.5 D point on the demand line to the point midway between the phoria and BCC lines at the level of 2.5D on the x-axis.

## COMPARISON OF ACA AND CAC RATIOS

Schor and others[31-33,37-43] have discussed the clinical implications of the model of dual interactions of accommodation and convergence. In this model, if either the ACA or the CAC ratio is high without the other being low, there will be a binocular disorder. Take, for example, a case in which the ACA ratio is high, as in convergence excess, and the CAC ratio is average. As a result of the high ACA ratio, negative fusional vergence is required. The convergence accommodation change associated with negative fusional vergence is a decrease in accommodation. If the CAC ratio is not low, there will then need to be an increase in optical reflex accommodation to compensate for the decrease from convergence accommodation. This accommodation produces accommodative convergence and so on, back and forth between accommodative convergence and convergence accommodation.

The stopping point of these interactions leaves accommodation and vergence errors in the form of lag of accommodation and fixation disparity, respectively. Schor and Narayan[31] recommended correcting these errors with spherical lens adds (for convergence accommodation errors) or with prism (for accommodative convergence errors). The prism prescription should be equal to the associated phoria.

Schor and colleagues[31,37,38,41,42] include prism adaptation and accommodative adaptation in this model. Adaptation serves to reduce the interactions of accommodation and vergence. As prism adaptation replaces fusional vergence over a period of seconds or minutes, the amount of convergence accommodation is reduced. Likewise, accommodative adaptation reduces the lag of accommodation. Some vision training procedures may serve to improve the prism adaptation capabilities of an individual and are thus recommended in cases of accommodation and vergence interaction disorders.

Daum et al.[33] reported a study assessing a diagnostic criterion similar to Sheard's criterion, but based on the interaction model. They presented a graphical method and a formula for determining the fusional demand under binocular conditions. They determined a CAC ratio with Nott retinoscopy with the target at 40 cm using varying amounts of prism to change the level of convergence. An example of their graph is shown in Figure 17.4. The ACA

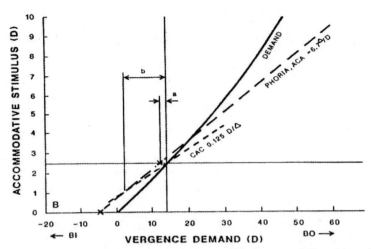

*Figure 17.4. An example of the plot of ACA and CAC lines used by Daum et al. The subject whose data are portrayed here had a distance dissociated phoria of 4Δ exo and a near dissociated phoria of 2Δ exo. The letter a represents the magnitude of the near dissociated phoria. The letter b represents the magnitude of the vergence imbalance predicted by interactions of accommodative convergence and convergence accommodation. (Reprinted with permission from Daum KM, Rutstein RP, Houston G IV, Clore KA, Corliss DA. Evaluation of a new criterion of binocularity. Optom Vis Sci 1989;66:218-229 © The American Academy of Optometry, 1989.*

line was drawn through the phoria points. The CAC line was plotted with a slope equal to the CAC ratio through the 40 cm demand line point. The lateral displacement of the intersection of these lines from the demand line point for 40 cm represented the demand on vergence under binocular conditions due to the interactions of accommodative convergence and convergence accommodation. The formula for the demand on vergence under binocular conditions (DV) is:

$$DV = (CR - (AR \times ACA)) / (1 - (ACA \times CAC))$$

where CR is the convergence response from both accommodative convergence and fusional convergence, AR is the accommodative response from both blur-driven accommodation and convergence accommodation, ACA is the ACA ratio, and CAC is the CAC ratio. DV was then used as the demand value in the classical Sheard's criterion formula. It may be noted that if both ACA and CAC ratio are high, there would be increased demand on vergence.

Daum et al.[33] examined 100 subjects to test the effectiveness of this new criterion in distinguishing symptomatic from asymptomatic individuals. The new criterion correctly distinguished six subjects more than the classical Sheard's criterion, but stepwise discriminant analysis did not show superiority of the calculated fusional demand or the new criterion over the near phoria or the classical Sheard's criterion value. Daum et al.[33] suggested that further development of the procedure is needed.

## REFERENCES

1.   Schmitt E. Viewpoint: Is there an identity crisis in optometry? J Behav Optom 2004;15:49-50.
2.   Grisham JD. Treatment of binocular dysfunctions. In: Schor CM, Ciuffreda KJ, eds. Vergence Eye Movements: Basic and Clinical Aspects. Boston: Butterworth-Heinemann, 1983:605-646.

3. Cooper J. Accommodative dysfunction. In: Amos JF, ed. Diagnosis and Management in Vision Care. Boston: Butterworths, 1987:431-459.

4. Wick BC. Horizontal deviations. In: Amos JF, ed. Diagnosis and Management in Vision Care. Boston: Butterworth-Heinemann, 1987:461-513.

5. Saladin JJ. Horizontal prism prescription. In: Cotter SA, ed. Clinical Uses of Prism - A Spectrum of Applications - Mosby's Optometric Problem Solving Series. St Louis: Mosby-Year Book, 1995:109-147.

6. Rutstein RP, Daum KM. Anomalies of Binocular Vision: Diagnosis & Management. St. Louis: Mosby, 1998:61-94, 147-188.

7. Griffin JR, Grisham JD. Binocular Anomalies: Diagnosis and Vision Therapy, 4th ed. Amsterdam: Butterworth-Heinemann, 2002:40-57, 69-100.

8. Scheiman M, Wick B. Clinical Management of Binocular Vision - Heterophoric, Accommodative, and Eye Movement Disorders, 2nd ed. Philadelphia: Lippincott Williams & Wilkins, 2002:223-369.

9. Grosvenor TP. Primary Care Optometry, 5th ed. St. Louis: Butterworth Heinemann Elsevier, 2007:224-239, 257-268.

10. Scheiman M, Wick B. Clinical Management of Binocular Vision - Heterophoric, Accommodative, and Eye Movement Disorders, 2nd ed. Philadelphia: Lippincott Williams & Wilkins, 2002:59-61.

11. Borish IM. Clinical Refraction, 3rd ed. Chicago: Professional Press, 1970:861-937.

12. Skeffington AM. Differential Diagnosis in Ocular Examination. Chicago: A.J. Cox, 1931.

13. Lesser SK. Fundamentals of Procedure and Analysis in Optometric Examination, 3rd ed. Fort Worth, TX: S.K. Lesser, 1934.

14. Birnbaum MH. Optometric Management of Nearpoint Vision Disorders. Boston: Butterworth-Heinemann, 1993:33-71.

15. Manas L. Visual Analysis, 3rd ed. Chicago: Professional Press, 1965.

16. Margach CB. Introduction to Functional Optometry. Duncan, OK: Optometric Extension Program Foundation, 1979.

17. Birnbaum MH. Optometric Management of Nearpoint Vision Disorders. Boston: Butterworth-Heinemann, 1993:121-160.

18. Flax N. Functional case analysis: an interpretation of the Skeffington model. Am J Optom Physiol Opt 1985;62:365-368.

19. Flax N. A current look at the OEP B1 and B2 case typings. In: Selected Works of Nathan Flax, volume 1. Santa Ana, CA: Optometric Extension Program, 2007:12-15.

20. Dvorine I. Theory and Practice of Analytical Refraction and Orthoptics. Baltimore: French-Bray, 1948.

21. Lesser SK. Introduction to Modern Analytical Optometry, rev. ed. Duncan, OK: Optometric Extension Program, 1969.

22. Slade GC. Modern Clinical Optometry-A Guide and Review. Duncan, OK: Optometric Extension Program, 1972.

23. Pheiffer CH. Analytical Analysis of A.M. Skeffington and Associates. Duncan, OK: Optometric Extension Program Foundation, 1981.

24. Schmitt EP. The Interpretation and Significance of the Embedded and Non-embedded Syndromes in Behavioral Optometric Case Analysis. Santa Ana, CA: Optometric Extension Program, 1993.

25. Schmitt EP. Guidelines for Clinical Testing, Lens Prescribing, and Vision Care. Santa Ana, CA: Optometric Extension Program, 1996.

26. Schmitt EP. The Skeffington Perspective of the Behavioral Model of Optometric Data Analysis and Vision Care. Bloomington, IN: Authorhouse, 2006.

27. Kraskin RA. The use & misuse of language: centering & identification. J Behav Optom 2003;14:87-93.

28. Morgan MW. The clinical aspects of accommodation and convergence. Am J Optom Arch Am Acad Optom 1944;21:301-313.

29. Morgan MW. Analysis of clinical data. Am J Optom Arch Am Acad Optom 1944;21:477-491.

30. Morgan MW. The analysis of clinical data. Optom Weekly 1964;55():27-34; 55():23-25.

31. Schor CM, Narayan B. Graphical analysis of prism adaptation, convergence accommodation, and accommodative convergence. Am J Optom Physiol Opt 1982;59:774-784.

32. Wick B, London R. Analysis of binocular visual function using tests made under binocular conditions. Am J Optom Physiol Opt 1987;64:227-240.

33. Daum KM, Rutstein RP, Houston G IV, Clore KA, Corliss DA. Evaluation of a new criterion of binocularity. Optom Vis Sci 1989;66:218-228.
34. Fincham EF, Walton J. The reciprocal actions of accommodation and convergence. J Physiol 1957;137:488-508.
35. Balsam MH, Fry GA. Convergence accommodation. Am J Optom Arch Am Acad Optom 1959;36:567-575.
36. Goss DA. Pratt system of clinical analysis of accommodation and convergence. Optom Vis Sci 1989;66:805-806.
37. Schor CM. Fixation disparity and vergence adaptation. In: Schor CM, Ciuffreda KJ, eds. Vergence Eye Movements: Basic and Clinical Aspects. Boston: Butterworth-Heinemann, 1983:465-516.
38. Schor CM. Analysis of tonic and accommodative vergence disorders of binocular vision. Am J Optom Physiol Opt 1983;60:1-14.
39. Wick B. Clinical factors in proximal vergence. Am J Optom Physiol Opt 1985;62:1-18.
40. Saladin JJ. Interpretation of divergent oculomotor imbalance through control system analysis. Am J Optom Physiol Opt 1988;65:439-447.
41. Schor C. Influence of accommodative and vergence adaptation on binocular motor disorders. Am J Optom Physiol Opt 1988;65:464-475.
42. Schor C, Horner D. Adaptive disorders of accommodation and vergence in binocular dysfunction. Ophthal Physiol Opt 1989;9:264-268.
43. Scheiman M, Wick B. Clinical Management of Binocular Vision-Heterophoric, Accommodative, and Eye Movement Disorders, 2nd ed. Philadelphia: Lippincott Williams & Wilkins, 2002:451-470.

# Chapter 18
# Oculomotor Dysfunction

Oculomotor dysfunction is a term used to describe reduced efficiency of version eye movements. This chapter provides a brief overview of oculomotor dysfunction. Although this condition does not fall within the scope of the title of this book, it can produce symptoms similar to accommodation and vergence disorders, including difficulty with nearpoint activities. So far the only type of eye movements we have talked about are vergence eye movements, the type of eye movements in which the lines of sight of the two eyes are moving in opposite directions. In both convergence, with the lines of sight of the two eyes moving toward each other, and divergence, with the lines of sight moving away from each other, the eyes are rotating in opposite directions.

Version eye movements are eye movements in which the eyes rotate in the same direction, both to the left or both to the right when considering eye movements in the horizontal meridian. Saccades and pursuits are two types of versions. Saccades are version eye movements which rotate the eyes to shift fixation from one object to another. Saccades are very high velocity eye movements compared to other types of eye movements. Pursuits are version eye movements which rotate the eyes to maintain fixation on a moving object. Pursuit velocities generally match the velocity of the moving object up to a limit. Maximum pursuit velocities are much slower than saccades – on the order of one-tenth the velocity of saccades. If pursuits cannot keep up with a moving target, saccades will be interposed to catch up to the target.

Oculomotor dysfunction is below normal saccade and/or pursuit function. Impairment of saccades and pursuits can also occur as a result of various drugs, neurological diseases, and neuromuscular diseases. Lists and tables in reference books can be consulted for the sources of such impairment.[1-4] The term functional oculomotor dysfunction is sometimes used to clearly distinguish oculomotor dysfunction from drug or disease induced abnormalities of eye movements.

Symptoms of oculomotor dysfunction can be manifested during reading such as in loss of place, head movement, need to use a finger to keep one's place, reduced reading speed, or poor comprehension. Poor sports performance, such as difficulty following the flight of a ball, may also be associated with oculomotor dysfunction. Oculomotor dysfunction can be a primary condition, or it can be secondary to uncorrected refractive error, vergence disorders, or accommodative problems. For example, Sohrab-Jam[5] found that when nearpoint plus adds were applied as indicated by dynamic retinoscopy, there were improvements in eye movements during a reading task.

## EYE MOVEMENTS DURING READING

The eye movements which occur during reading are saccades. In the reading of English and other languages read from left to right, saccades move the lines of sight across a line from left to right. There are fixation pauses between the saccades. It is during these fixation pauses that a span of letters is perceived. When the end of a line is reached, a saccade moves the lines of sight right to left and slightly down to the beginning of the next line. Occasionally in the midst of a line, a saccade from right to left will occur moving the lines of sight back to letters which had already been scanned. These movements from right to left in the midst of a line are called regressions.

Skilled readers exhibit shorter periods of time during the fixation pauses, have fewer regressions, and may have fewer fixation pauses per line.[6,7] There are developmental trends in these characteristics, with children showing improvement as their reading skill increases. These characteristics are also affected by the difficulty of the reading material.

## CLINICAL TESTS

A number of tests have been used to assess efficiency or functionality of eye movements. These tests should be distinguished from tests which determine whether there is a full range of motion of the extraocular muscles. Tests which assess the efficiency of function of saccades and pursuits can be grouped into three categories: (1) direct observation methods, (2) visual-verbal naming tests, and (3) electronic techniques.

The direct observation testing method for saccades involves instructing the patient to look back and forth on command between objects held by the examiner. The examiner observes the saccades which occur in response to each command. For direct observation of pursuits, the patient follows an object moved by the examiner. Obviously such tests may vary widely in testing procedures, interpretation, and recording scales. A specific direct observation testing procedure which has been gaining popularity is the NSUCO Oculomotor Test.[2] Testing procedures have been standardized and the specific observations which indicate given scores on the test have been outlined. Patients are scored using an ordinal scale from 1 to 5 on ability, accuracy, head movement, and body movement during saccades and pursuits. The repeatability of the test has been studied and age norms for children have been established.[8] Details on the performance and interpretation of the test are available in a monograph by Maples,[9] who developed the test.

Visual-verbal naming tests are tests in which the patient gives verbal responses based on what they see on standardized charts. It appears that the first visual verbal naming test for saccades was the Pierce Saccade Test, which is no longer commercially available. A very similar test based on the Pierce test is the King-Devick Test.[10] On the King-Devick Test there are three charts, each with eight horizontal rows of numbers. There are five unevenly spaced numbers in each row. There are horizontal lines connecting the numbers on each row on the first chart, but not on the second and third charts. The vertical spacing between rows decreases from charts 1 and 2 to chart 3. Thus difficulty increases from chart 1 to chart 3. The patient is timed on each chart and the number of errors made when calling out the numbers is recorded. There are age norms for times and errors for children 6 to 14 years of age.

Another visual-verbal test for saccades is the Developmental Eye Movement (DEM) Test.[11] This test was developed because of the observation that performance on the King-Devick test was dependent upon the automaticity of number naming as well as on eye movement ability. Number naming is considered to be factored out on the DEM test by having patient first read vertical columns of numbers. Then their time and error performance on horizontal rows is compared to their performance on the vertical columns.

A test which can be considered to be a visual-verbal test of pursuits is the Groffman Visual Tracing test.[12] On this test, there are five letters, A through E, at the top of the page and five numbers, 1 through 5, at the bottom of the page. Each letter is connected with one number by way of five curved continuous intersecting lines which appear to be in a tangled pattern. The patient's task is to follow the line from each letter to the corresponding number without using a finger or a pointer as a guide. The patient is timed for each letter, and scoring depends on the time and whether the correct number was reported. Norms are given for ages from 7 years to 12 years and over.

Electronic instruments for the assessment of eye movements typically operate based on infrared reflections from the eye. An example of commercially available electronic instruments is the Visagraph.[13-15] This instrument is particularly designed to assess eye movements during reading, providing a trace of eye position as a function of time for each eye, and yields several numerical values, such as the numbers of fixations and regressions, and average span of recognition.

## TREATMENT

If oculomotor dysfunction which is not secondary to uncorrected refractive error or any accommodation or vergence disorder is diagnosed, eye movement skills can be improved through vision therapy.[16] Various studies have shown that vision therapy for oculomotor dysfunction leads to improved reading speed and improved efficiency of eye movements during reading.[16-19] There are numerous training techniques used in vision therapy for oculomotor dysfunction. The various training procedures include workbooks, computer programs, various instruments, projector or blackboard exercises, and other procedures.[20-24]

## REFERENCES

1. Ciuffreda KJ, Tannen B. Eye Movement Basics for the Clinician. St. Louis: Mosby, 1995:55,93.
2. Maples WC. Oculomotor dysfunctions: classification of saccadic and pursuit deficiencies. In: Press LJ, ed. Applied Concepts in Vision Therapy. St. Louis: Mosby, 1997:120-136.
3. Leigh RJ, Zee DS. The Neurology of Eye Movements, 3rd ed. New York: Oxford University Press, 1999:562-563.

4.  Scheiman M, Wick B. *Clinical Management of Binocular Vision – Heterophoric, Accommodative, and Eye Movement Disorders*, 2nd ed. Philadelphia: Lippincott Williams & Wilkins, 2002:377-380.

5.  Sohrab-Jam G. Eye movement patterns and reading performance in poor readers: immediate effects of convex lenses indicated by book retinoscopy. *Am J Optom Physiol Opt* 1976;53:720-726.

6.  Ciuffreda KJ, Tannen B. *Eye Movement Basics for the Clinician*. St. Louis: Mosby, 1995:161-173.

7.  Scheiman M, Wick B. *Clinical Management of Binocular Vision – Heterophoric, Accommodative, and Eye Movement Disorders*, 2nd ed. Philadelphia: Lippincott Williams & Wilkins, 2002:370-371.

8.  Maples WC, Atchley J, Ficklin T. Northeastern State University College of Optometry's oculomotor norms. *J Behav Optom* 1992;3:143-150.

9.  Maples WC. *NSUCO Oculomotor Test*. Santa Ana, CA: Optometric Extension Program, 1995.

10. Lieberman S, Cohen AH, Rubin J. NYSOA K-D test. *J Am Optom Assoc* 1983;54:631-637.

11. Garzia RP, Richman JE, Nicholson SB, Gaines CS. A new visual-verbal saccade test: the Developmental Eye Movement test (DEM). *J Am Optom Assoc* 1990;61:124-135.

12. Groffman S. Visual tracing. *J Am Optom Assoc* 1966;37:139-141.

13. Maino D. The Visagraph: eye movement recording system. In: Press LJ, ed. *Computers and Vision Therapy Programs*. Santa Ana, CA: Optometric Extension Program, 1992: 71-74.

14. Colby D, Laukkanen HR, Yolton RL. Use of the Taylor Visagraph II system to evaluate eye movements made during reading. *J Am Optom Assoc* 1998;69:22-32.

15. Ciuffreda MA, Ciuffreda KJ, Santos D. Visagraph baseline analysis and procedural guidelines. *J Behav Optom* 2003;14:60-64.

16. Scheiman M, Wick B. *Clinical Management of Binocular Vision – Heterophoric, Accommodative, and Eye Movement Disorders*, 2nd ed. Philadelphia: Lippincott Williams & Wilkins, 2002:372-374.

17. Rounds BB, Manley CW, Norris RH. The effect of oculomotor training on reading efficiency. *J Am Optom Assoc* 1991;62:92-99.

18. Solan HA, Feldman J, Tujak L. Developing visual and reading efficiency in older adults. *Optom Vis Sci* 1995;72:139-145.

19. Ciuffreda KJ, Tannen B. *Eye Movement Basics for the Clinician*. St. Louis: Mosby, 1995:177-180.

20. Vogel GL. Saccadic eye movements: theory, testing, and therapy. *J Behav Optom* 1995;6:3-12.

21. Maples WC. Ocular motility therapy. In: Press LJ, ed. *Applied Concepts in Vision Therapy*. St. Louis: Mosby, 1997:246-262.

22. Griffin JR, Christenson GN, Wesson MD, Erickson GB. *Optometric Management of Reading Dysfunction*. Boston: Butterworth-Heinemann, 1997:174-176.

23. Griffin JR, Grisham JD. *Binocular Anomalies: Diagnosis and Vision Therapy*, 4th ed. Amsterdam: Butterworth-Heinemann, 2002:527-533.

24. Scheiman M, Wick B. *Clinical Management of Binocular Vision – Heterophoric, Accommodative, and Eye Movement Disorders*, 2nd ed. Philadelphia: Lippincott Williams & Wilkins, 2002:380-389.

# Chapter 19
# Historical and Biographical Notes

Many of the tests and guidelines discussed in this book are named for their originators. The developers of various ideas presented in this book have often been mentioned in conjunction with the discussion of those ideas. With the belief that it is important to honor individuals who were contributors to our field of study and with the thought that readers may wish to know something about the persons behind the names, this chapter will present brief biographical sketches as memorials to some of the persons who made contributions from which we benefit. They will be discussed in alphabetical order.

## ANDREW JAY CROSS (1855-1925)

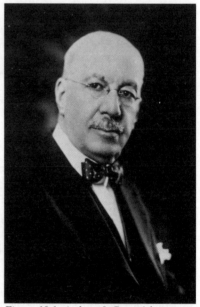

Andrew J. Cross worked as an optometrist in various cities in the Western and Eastern United States from 1876 until 1889, when he established a practice in New York city.[1] It was after that move that he became heavily involved in the efforts to professionalize optometry and to establish optometry licensure laws. Writing in 1929, Arrington[1] observed that Cross "came to be known as the Grand Old Man of Optometry, - an appellation which he richly earned; for it will hardly be disputed that no single man gave of himself more fully and freely to the cause of optometry, and none had more valuable gifts to give." In 1898, Cross became president of the New York State Society of Optometrists. In 1900-1901, he was president of the American Association of Opticians, the organization that became the American Optometric Association.[2]

*Figure 19.1. Andrew J. Cross (photo courtesy of International Library, Archives, and Museum of Optometry, St. Louis).*

Cross is well known for his role in the development of dynamic retinoscopy. He wrote two books on the theory and application of dynamic retinoscopy: *A System of Ocular Skiametry – Including Such Portions of Optometry as are Pertinent to the Use of the "Shadow Test" with the Plane Mirror* (1903) and *Dynamic Skiametry in Theory and Practice – Embracing its Association with Static Skiametry and with Those Optometric Methods Wherein the Correlation of Accommodation and Convergence Must Be Considered* (1911). Cross also worked on the invention of a monocentric bifocal lens.[1] Cross was an instructor in the optometry school at Columbia University from 1911 to 1924. According to Arrington,[1] Cross "had a genius for expounding optical theories and facts in a way that made them simple to grasp, and study under him was a pleasure."

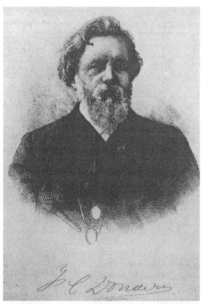

*Figure 19.2. Frans Cornelis Donders (reprinted by permission from Duke-Elder S, Abrams D. Ophthalmic Optics and Refraction, vol. 5 in: Duke-Elder S, ed. System of Ophthalmology. St. Louis: Mosby, 1970:254).*

## FRANS CORNELIS DONDERS (1818-1889)

Frans Cornelis Donders was born in Tilburg, Holland. He attended medical school in Utrecht, Holland from 1835 to 1840. He passed examinations for the doctor of medicine degree from Leiden University. After service as a military medical officer, in 1842, he started a long career in teaching, research, journal editing, and medical practice in Utrecht. Most of the more than 340 publications by Donders were on ophthalmology and physiology.[3] They included a widely used physiology textbook.

After publishing a series of papers on refractive errors, Donders was asked by the New Sydenham Society of London to write a book on the topic.[4] The 635-page *On the Anomalies of Accommodation and Refraction of the Eye* was published in English in 1864 based on a translation from Donders' Dutch manuscript. It had an immediate impact and was widely praised for its clarity and insight, and for its application of experimental results to clinical practice. It has been described as "an epochal work, one of the few pivotal books that can be said to have established a scientific basis for ophthalmic practice."[5] It provided a comprehensive review of refractive errors and accommodation, with coverage of topics such as the dioptric system of the eye, the mechanism of accommodation, use and optics of spectacles, and the analysis and treatment of refractive and accommodative conditions.

The first use of a graph for presenting accommodation and convergence data appears to have been in the 1858 doctoral dissertation of Donders' student MacGillavry. The first formal publication of accommodation and convergence graphs was in Donders' book. MacGillavry and Donders plotted convergence on the x-axis and accommodation on the y-axis. The units diopters and prism diopters had not yet been invented, so they used degrees and minutes for convergence and reciprocal Parisian inches for accommodation. Ranges of accommodation were plotted at various amounts of convergence.[6]

Donders published on a wide variety of other topics in ophthalmology and physiology. Hirschberg[7] observed that Donders "influenced the entire scientific world, not only by his publications, but also orally in the lecture hall and in the laboratory." Donders was recognized by various ophthalmological awards, a statue in Utrecht, and his likeness on a Dutch postage stamp.

## GLENN ANSEL FRY (1908-1996)

Glenn Fry was born in Wellford, South Carolina. He received an A.B. degree

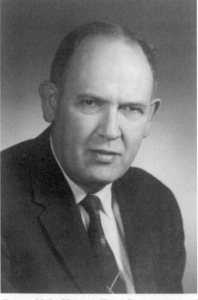

from Davidson College in North Carolina in 1929. This was followed by an M.S. degree in psychology and physiology in 1931 from Duke University and a Ph.D. in psychology in 1933 also from Duke.[8] In 1935, he became the director of the optometry school at The Ohio State University. The school was at that time known as the Applied Optics program and was operated within the Department of Physics.[9] In 1937, it became the School of Optometry. Fry continued as its director until 1966. Fry was responsible for starting the first graduate program in physiological optics associated with an optometry school, with the first M.S. degrees being awarded in 1938 and the first Ph.D. in 1942.[10]

Fry published more than 250 papers on a variety of topics in optometry and vision science, including color vision, space perception, visual ergonomics, accommodation and convergence, geometrical

*Figure 19.3. Glenn A. Fry (photo courtesy of International Library, Archives, and Museum of Optometry, St. Louis).*

optics, ophthalmic optics, and ocular optics.[11] He was well known for the intricate instrumentation he designed and built for vision experiments and his ability to integrate theoretical concepts from various fields with clinical principles.[12]

Fry published a number of papers on accommodation and convergence starting in the late 1930s and continuing into the 1950s.

Hofstetter[13] observed that the first suggestion that an accommodation and convergence graph be used for routine clinical purposes was made by Lesser in 1933, but that Lesser's uniquely designed graph "suffered from inadequate explanation." In about 1938, Fry introduced a graph form for analysis of patient accommodation and convergence findings at Ohio State.[13] In 1943, he published a paper detailing the elements of the clinical accommodation and convergence graph essentially as it is used today.[14]

As a consequence of his research, administrative work, and service in numerous commissions, committees, and professional organizations, Fry received many awards, including the Tillyer Medal of the Optical Society of America, the Distinguished Service Award of the American Optometric Association, the Gold Medal of the Illuminating Engineering Society, the Prentice Medal of the American Academy of Optometry, and six honorary degrees.[12] Former graduate students, many of whom have gone on to distinguished careers in optometry and vision science, speak admiringly of Fry's energy and intellectual abilities. Fry continued to be active in research and optometric activities well past his retirement, publishing his last paper just months before his death at 87 years of age.

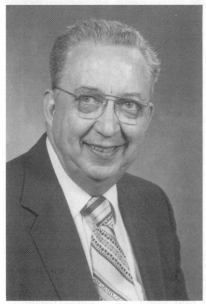

Figure 19.4. Harold M. Haynes (photo courtesy of Pacific University).

## HAROLD M. HAYNES (1926-1997)

Harold M. Haynes was born in Pittsburgh and was raised in Point Pleasant, West Virginia.[15] He completed optometry school at the Northern Illinois College of Optometry in 1946. He joined the faculty of Pacific University College of Optometry in Forest Grove, Oregon, in 1948, and remained a faculty member there until his retirement from full-time teaching in 1992. Most of his teaching responsibility was in courses in case analysis, theoretical optometry, vision training, and strabismus. Various authors[16-19] have credited him with the development of MEM dynamic retinoscopy. A paper Haynes published in 1960 details the dynamic retinoscopy procedure involving estimation of the motion of the retinoscopic reflex with lenses "interposed only momentarily to check the examiner's estimates."[20] Haynes was the first to report a study on accommodation in infants.[21]

Haynes was heavily involved in local government activities, helping to found Forest Grove's Committee for Citizen Involvement and helping to write the charter for the city of Forest Grove in the 1970s.[15,22]

## HENRY W HOFSTETTER (1914-2002)

Henry Hofstetter was born at Windsor Hills, Ohio, of Swiss and German immigrant parents. Raised on the family farm in northeastern Ohio, the crippling of his left hand by polio at the age of sixteen may have led him away from farming as a career.[23] After attending Western Reserve University and Kent State University, he taught all eight grades in a one-room school in Middlefield, Ohio, for three years. A brother-in-law, who was a jeweler and who fitted spectacles, encouraged Hofstetter to study optometry. Hofstetter entered The Ohio State University, and in 1939, completed the B.S. degree in optometry, at that time the terminal professional degree at Ohio State. He then completed M.S. and Ph.D. degrees in physiological optics in 1940 and 1942.

Hofstetter's Ph.D. was the first awarded in a physiological optics program associated with an optometry school.[10] His dissertation research, under the guidance of Glenn Fry, was a haploscopic study of accommodation and convergence

235

relationships. Hofstetter's most comprehensive publication on accommodation and convergence was his two-part paper on the zone of clear single binocular vision.[24] It was followed by several other papers on accommodation and convergence, many of them showing applications of a graph for clinical data analysis.[13] Hofstetter did much to popularize the use of the accommodation and convergence graph through his publications and lectures.

After completion of his Ph.D. degree, Hofstetter served on the Ohio State faculty for six years. From January, 1949 to July, 1952, he was Dean of the Los Angeles College of Optometry. From 1952 to 1970, he was the Director of the optometry school at Indiana University.[25] From 1970 to his retirement in 1980, he was a faculty member at Indiana University,

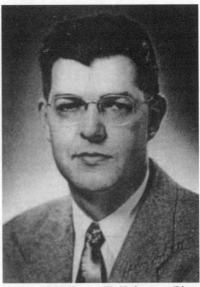

*Figure 19.5. Henry W Hofstetter. (Photo courtesy of Indiana University)*

being named Rudy Professor of Optometry in 1974. Hofstetter authored four textbooks and over 500 articles. Perhaps his best known book is *Optometry: Professional, Legal, and Economic Aspects*, published in 1948 and reprinted in 1964. He also co-edited five editions of the *Dictionary of Visual Science*. In addition to papers on accommodation and binocular vision, Hofstetter also published on optometry history, refractive errors, optometric education, international optometry, color vision, ocular optics, presbyopia, occupational vision, visual acuity, and other topics.

Hofstetter served in dozens of commissions, committees, organizations, and consulting positions, and was well known for his organizational and administrative skills. He was the first full-time educator to become the president of the American Optometric Association.[26] He was president of the Association of the Schools and Colleges of Optometry and was founding president of the Optometric Historical Society. He also assumed leadership positions in numerous committees and local organizations.[22] Hofstetter received many awards, including International Optometrist of the Year from the International Optometric and Optical League, Prentice Medal from the American Academy of Optometry, Apollo Award and Distinguished Service Award from the American Optometric Association, Orion Award from the Armed Forces Optometric Society, Distinguished Service Award from the World Council of Optometry, and five honorary degrees.[27] Many former students and colleagues remember Hofstetter's deliberate and carefully considered answers to questions, and they speak highly of his positive influence, kind manner, and helpful mentoring.[28]

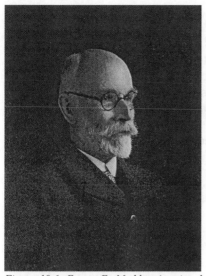

# ERNEST EDMUND MADDOX (1863-1933)

Ernest E. Maddox was a distinguished British ophthalmologist. Maddox attended the University of Edinburgh, where he graduated with an M.B. degree in 1882 and received the M.D. in 1889. In 1894, he became F.R.C.S.E.[29] He practiced for about ten years in Edinburgh and then in Bournemouth until his retirement. He published extensively, particularly in refraction and binocular vision, and experimented on the relation of accommodation and convergence.[30,31] His books were *The Clinical Use of Prisms and the Decentering of Lenses*, published in 1889, with a second edition in 1893, and a third edition in 1907; *Tests and Studies of the Ocular Muscles*, published in 1898, followed by a second edition in 1907; and *Golden Rules of Refraction*, published in 1902.

*Figure 19.6. Ernest E. Maddox (reprinted with permission from Duke-Elder S, Wybar K. Ocular Motility and Strabismus, vol. 6 in: Duke-Elder S, ed. System of Ophthalmology. St. Louis: Mosby, 1973:246. ©1973)*

In his early description of what have now come to be known as the Maddox components of convergence, Maddox listed three factors: initial convergence, accommodative convergence, and fusion supplement.[30,31] In the second edition of his book, *The Clinical Use of Prisms and the Decentering of Lenses*, published in 1893, Maddox noted that Edmund Hansen Grut had observed that the usual parallelism of the lines of sight in the initial convergence was due to a "tonic element."[32] Grut[33] suggested that the eyes were brought from the anatomical position of rest to the functional position of rest by tonus in the extraocular muscles. It was in his 1893 book that Maddox presented the four components as we recognize them today: "...there are four elements of convergence, though the first and third are perhaps closely related. The four are: (1) Tonic; (2) Accommodative; (3) Convergence due to 'knowledge of nearness,' or in other words, 'Voluntary convergence,' for we cannot, without special practice, converge the eyes voluntarily, under ordinary conditions, without doing so by thinking of a near object; (4) Fusion convergence. Of these four elements I have included the second and third under the one name of 'accommodative convergence,' to simplify practical work. On looking at a near object, the voluntary and accommodative elements of convergence bear very different proportions to each other in different individuals."[34]

Several tests were devised by Maddox and have subsequently been associated with his name. Maddox first described the principle of the Maddox rod in 1890.[35] Maddox described the Maddox rod as "a short glass rod" which produces "a streak of light, by acting as a strong cylindrical lens."[36] In the second edition of *The Clinical Use of Prisms*, Maddox described two methods by which the rod could be used to measure convergence posture. One of them, which Maddox called the glass rod test, involved the use of a prism to align the streak and the light. In Maddox's words, "On looking at a distant flame with this before one eye, it appears converted into a long streak of light, which there is no desire to regard as a false image of the flame, from its dissimilarity, especially if red glass be used. If the streak pass through the flame, equilibrium is perfect, but if otherwise, its distance indicates the amount of latent deviation. The prism that is able to bring the line and the flame together is the measure of it."[36] This procedure is what we refer to today as the Maddox rod test.

Another method proposed by Maddox using the glass rod to measure convergence posture involved the use of a "tangent scale." A flame was held at the zero point on the scale and numbers on either side of zero were calibrated to give a measurement of convergence for a specified distance. The patient was to report the number through which the streak of light from the glass rod passed. Maddox[37] noted that similar tangent scales were suggested before his by Landolt and Hirschberg in about 1875. Maddox's tangent scale differed in that the numbers were legible to the patient and it was used with the Maddox rod. Maddox[38] described the use of the Maddox rod together with a scale in 1890. This test is generally referred to today as the modified Thorington test. I have examined several editions of Thorington's book *Refraction and How to Refract*, and to date I have not found a discussion of what has come to be known as the modified Thorington test. Thorington did describe a test with a numbered scale, but the scale is doubled with a dissociating prism, and the number on the doubled scale to which an arrow on the first scale points is the measure of the phoria. The earliest references I have been able to find which have used the terms Thorington test or modified Thorington test were papers by Scobee and Green[39] and by Hirsch[39,40] in the late 1940s.

Duke-Elder and Wybar[42] described Maddox as "a wholly delightful and very modest person," whose publications were "characterized by clear and original thinking, punctilious exactitude and lucid expression." They also note of Maddox that "Practical originality was one of his most striking attributes, a faculty which led him to introduce many inventive but always simple devices…"

## MEREDITH WALTER MORGAN, JR. (1912-1999)
Meredith W. Morgan was born in Kingman, Arizona, and at an early age moved to Richmond, California, near Berkeley. Morgan's father was a certified railroad watchmaker, and after completing an education in optometry in 1918 from Benson's College of Optometry and Ophthalmology, established a practice in Richmond.[43]

Morgan entered the University of California Berkeley in 1930. He was one of twelve students who graduated from Berkeley in 1934 in physics/optometry. At that time, the optometry program at the University of California was conducted within the physics department.[44] In 1934, he entered optometry practice with his father, while also pursuing graduate studies in physiology at University of

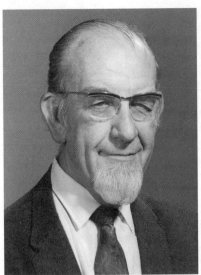

California Berkeley. He received an M.A. degree in physiology in 1939 and the Ph.D. in 1941. His Ph.D. research investigated neural control of ocular accommodation.[44] This was followed by a number of papers he published in the 1940s on physiological and clinical aspects of accommodation and convergence in *American Journal of Physiology* and in *American Journal of Optometry and Archives of the American Academy of Optometry*. He continued to contribute articles on accommodation and convergence to the literature for many years thereafter.

Morgan became a member of the optometry faculty at Berkeley in 1942. He was Dean of the optometry school at Berkeley from 1960 to 1973. By 1988, his published papers numbered more than 68, and he had supervised the research of more physiolog-

*Figure 19.7. Meredith W. Morgan (photo courtesy of International Library, Archives, and Museum of Optometry, St. Louis).*

ical optics graduate students than any other member of the Berkeley faculty.[43] His books include *The Optics of Ophthalmic Lenses* (1978), *The Optics of Ophthalmic Lenses: Problem Sets* (1982), *Vision and Aging* edited by Alfred A. Rosenbloom and Morgan (1986, 1993), and *Principles and Practice of Pediatric Optometry* edited by Rosenbloom and Morgan (1990).

Morgan's teaching, research, administrative work, and service on many committees and commissions were rewarded by the Prentice Medal of the American Academy of Optometry, the Apollo Award of the American Optometric Association, the Berkeley Citation for exceptional service to the university, and four honorary degrees.[44] Morgan has been depicted as "a kind and gentle man" who "represented the finest qualities of our profession and science."[44] He was well known for his laugh, which has been variously described as "infectious,"[43] "exuberant...distinctive,"[44] and "booming."[45]

## IVAN S. NOTT (1892-1969)

Ivan Nott was a Canadian optometrist, as were his brothers Herbert and William. Early in his career he held various positions, including practice with his brother Herbert in Winnipeg and working in the instrument division of the former Consolidated Optical Company in Toronto. He lectured widely in Canada on optometric techniques and instrumentation. In 1921 and 1922, he taught at the Central Technical School in Ophthalmic Optics.[46] In the 1920s, he joined the Toronto practice of noted Canadian optometrist Wellington G. Maybee and later took over the practice. In 1969, Fisher wrote that "Nott's practice was one of the best. He rendered a high quality of optometrical services even by today's standards."[46]

In 1925, Nott described a method of dynamic retinoscopy which he called the observation behind fixation method[47] and which we now call Nott retinoscopy. Nott contributed other papers on accommodation, convergence, and refraction to the literature, including two in the *American Journal of Optometry*.[48,49] He assembled a 60-page booklet for the American Optical Company entitled *The Stereoscopic Development of the Fusion Faculty* (1926), which discussed vergence disorders and vision therapy for them, with emphasis on training methods using stereoscopes and loose prisms. Nott also wrote a home study document on subjective refraction for the American Optometric Association.[46] Nott was editor of the *Canadian Optometrist* journal from 1929 to 1937.

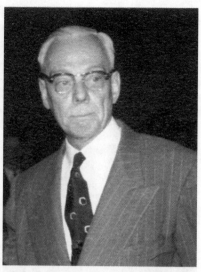

Figure 19.8. Ivan S. Nott (photo courtesy of University of Waterloo School of Optometry Library).

## KENNETH NEIL OGLE (1902-1968)

Kenneth Ogle was born in Colorado, and graduated from Colorado College in 1925. From 1925 to 1930, except for a year as a teaching fellow in physics at the University of Minnesota, he studied physiological optics at Dartmouth College with Adelbert Ames.[50] Ogle's 1930 Ph.D. thesis was entitled *The Resolving Power of the Human Eye*. Ogle conducted research at the Dartmouth Eye Institute at Dartmouth College from 1930 until it closed in 1947. The Dartmouth Eye Institute featured a remarkable collaboration of ophthalmologists, optometrists, and basic scientists in investigations of binocular vision.[51] From 1947 to 1967, he worked in the Section of Biophysics of the Mayo Clinic and the Mayo Graduate School of Medicine at the University of Minnesota as a research consultant and professor.

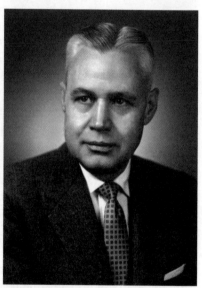

Figure 19.9. Kenneth N. Ogle (used by permission of Mayo Historical Unit, Mayo Clinic, Rochester, Minnesota).

Ogle made extensive research contributions to binocular vision, with studies of aniseikonia, horopters, space perception, stereopsis, fixation disparity, and other areas. For many years, as observed by Duke-Elder and Wybar,[52] "he made the subject of fixation disparity essentially his own." He published books which were highly respected: *Researches in Binocular Vision* (1950),

*Optics: An Introduction for Ophthalmologists* (1961, 1968), and *Oculomotor Imbalance in Binocular Vision and Fixation Disparity*, by Ogle, Martens, and Dyer (1967). Ogle received the Proctor Medal from the Association for Research in Vision and Ophthalmology, the Tillyer Medal from the Optical Society of America, and two honorary degrees. Glenn Fry characterized him as "a friendly and ever-helpful person," qualities which "endeared him to his many friends."[53]

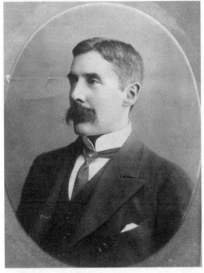

## ARCHIBALD STANLEY PERCIVAL (1862-1935)

A.S. Percival was a British ophthalmologist who was known for his work in optics and in accommodation and convergence studies. He received B.A. and M.A. degrees from Cambridge. His clinical training was at St. George's Hospital in London. His medical credentials included M.R.C.S. (Membership of the Royal College of Surgeons), M.B. (Bachelor of Medicine), and B.Ch. (Bachelor of Surgery).[54]

Percival had interest and ability in mathematics,[54,55] as is evident in his publications. One of his contributions in optics was the design of what he called "periscopic lenses" developed to reduce the periph-

*Figure 19.10. Archibald S. Percival (photo courtesy of Piers Percival).*

eral aberrations of spectacles.[56] Some of his formulas were used in 1949 by Harold Ridley in constructing the first intraocular lens implant.[55] The respect with which Percival was held in the area of optical calculations can be demonstrated by a statement by Duke-Elder in the preface to the first edition of his *Practice of Refraction*: "the mathematical problems involved in the theory of spectacles will be found in Percival's 'Prescribing of Spectacles'…from which I have quoted largely."[57]

Percival freely shared his knowledge with both the optometrists of his day and with ophthalmologists, a characteristic which was not common in his time.[55] He wrote several books on optics, mathematics, and spectacle prescribing: *Optics, A Manual for Students* (1899), *Practical Integration for the Use of Engineers, Etc.* (1907, 1909), *The Prescribing of Spectacles* (1910, 1912, 1928), *Geometrical Optics* (1913), *Perspective, The Old and The New Method* (1921), and *Mathematical Facts and Formulae* (1933).

In an 1892 paper, Percival put forward his idea of an "area of comfort" within the zone of clear single binocular vision,[58] the concept which has led to what is commonly called Percival's criterion. In that paper, he presented case reports of the prescription of prism for the alleviation of asthenopia and related it to the area of comfort on corresponding graphs. Percival also elaborated on the area of comfort in his book *The Prescribing of Spectacles*.[59]

## CHARLES F. PRENTICE (1854-1946)

Charles Prentice was the only child of James Prentice (1812-1888), a leading New York optician and instrument maker, to survive infancy. James Prentice was born and apprenticed in London, and came to the United States in 1842.[60] James insisted that Charles get a better education in optics than he thought available in the United States at the time and sent him to Germany to study for three years at the Royal Polytechnicum at Karlsruhe.[61] His studies emphasized engineering, physics, and mathematics.

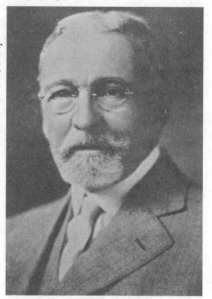

When Prentice returned to the United States, he worked for a few years as a mechanical engineer and draftsman in various jobs until he started work with his father, taking over the business after his father died. At the time Charles Prentice

*Figure 19.11. Charles F. Prentice (photo courtesy of International Library, Archives, and Museum of Optometry, St. Louis).*

started practicing optometry, practitioners in the field usually called themselves opticians, and the term optometrist did not become popular until the early twentieth century. Prentice favored the word opticist over optometrist. In 1886, he copyrighted the term opticist and wrote in favor of its uniform adoption.[62]

Hirsch and Wick[63] described Prentice as an idealist who refused to compromise and had an "intense desire to excel." When a challenge came from an ophthalmologist in 1892 that his charging for an examination constituted the practice of medicine without a license, Prentice responded by launching a crusade for licensure laws in optometry.[64-67] As a result of the efforts of Prentice and others, the first optometry licensure law was passed in Minnesota in 1901. Prentice became the first president of the New York State Board of Optometry in 1908, when the optometry licensure law was established there.[68]

Prentice published several booklets and papers on ophthalmic optics and refraction. His book *Ophthalmic Lenses* appeared in 1886, followed by *Dioptric Formulae for Combined Cylindrical Lenses* in 1888. Those two publications and a number of his journal articles were published in a collection entitled *Ophthalmic Lenses, Dioptric Formulae for Combined Cylindrical Lenses, The Prism Dioptry, and Other Optical Papers* (1900, 1907).

In an 1890 paper,[69] Prentice devised the term and concept of prism dioptry, which we now know as the prism diopter. In a revision of that paper published in the book collecting some of his works, he noted that soon after the publication of the original paper in 1890, he devised a "simple apparatus (phorometric chart) for estimating the deviation of the visual axes."[70] Prentice's "phorometric chart" was similar to Maddox's tangent scale or the modified Thorington test. Prentice used a +12 D cylindrical lens instead of Maddox rod, and a blackboard "having on its surface eight vertically and eight horizontally arranged dots, which are separated by 6 centimeter distances, so that each interval of space between the dots represents 1Δ at 6 meters from the eye. A light is placed behind a piece of red glass in a circular opening in the center of the board."[70] Unlike Maddox's tangent scale test, there were no numbers so the patient had to count to the dot the line intersected. Prentice is also known for Prentice's rule, the formula by which the prismatic effect of the decentration of lenses is calculated.

Borish[71] credited Prentice (or Thorington) with a phoria test in which a horizontal row of letters and numbers is doubled with a base-up prism over the left eye. In the center of the row of letters and numbers is an arrow pointing downward. The magnitude and direction of the phoria is indicated by the letter or number to the arrow in the upper row points in the lower row.

From 1912 to 1921, Prentice contributed several articles on ophthalmic lenses and prisms and optical terms to the *American Encyclopedia of Ophthalmology*. Prentice and Andrew Jay Cross helped draw up the curriculum for the optometry school at Columbia University, which in 1910 became the first university to offer optometry studies.[72] Prentice is often referred to as "The Father of Optometry" for his campaigning for the professionalization of optometry.[61,65]

## CHARLES SHEARD (1883-1963)

Charles Sheard was born in Dolgeville, New York. His academic degrees were all in physics, A.B. from St. Lawrence University in 1903, M.A. from Dartmouth in 1907, and Ph.D. from Princeton in 1912. He was on the faculty at The Ohio State University from 1907 to 1919. Starting in 1914, he was the founding Director of the Applied Optics program, as the optometry school was then known, at Ohio State. That started a long association with optometry in which he frequently spoke at optometry meetings and actively contributed to numerous optometric committees and organizations, including helping to found the American Academy of Optometry[73] and working to develop educational standards.[74] From 1919 to 1924, he was in charge of scientific work at the American Optical Company in Southbridge, Massachusetts.[75] It was during that time that he

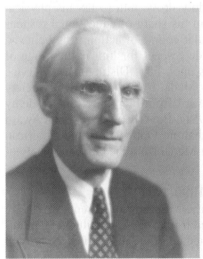

*Figure 19.12. Charles Sheard (photo courtesy of International Library, Archives, and Museum of Optometry, St. Louis).*

founded and was editor of the *American Journal of Physiological Optics*.[76] From 1924 to 1949, he was Professor of Biophysics at the University of Minnesota and Director of the Division of Physics and Biophysics at the Mayo Clinic. He then served as Distinguished Lecturer in Physiological Optics at Tulane University and in 1952-53 was interim Dean of the Los Angeles College of Optometry.

Sheard wrote extensively about accommodation, convergence, dynamic retinoscopy, and clinical testing procedures in both journal articles and monographs. His name is associated with a guideline for assessing strain on fusional vergence, now known as Sheard's criterion. In his book, *Dynamic Ocular Tests*, first published in 1917, he listed 18 numbered tests as a routine battery of tests in a clinical vision examination.[77] It appears that Sheard's 18 tests were modified to form the "21 point examination" emphasized throughout most of the twentieth century by the Optometric Extension Program (OEP).[78,79] The set of 21 numbered tests in the OEP exam (see Table 17.1) is similar to Sheard's 18 numbered tests.

Along with his work on accommodation and convergence, some of the other topics Sheard wrote about were ophthalmic optics, dark adaptation, effects of radiant energy on plant and animal tissues, applications of spectrophotometry to biology and medicine, and the physiology of temperature regulation. Books he wrote include: *Dynamic Ocular Tests* (1917), *Physiological Optics* (1918), *Ocular Accommodation* (1920), *Dynamic Skiametry and Methods of Testing the Accommodation and Convergence of the Eyes* (1920), *Transmission of Radiant Energy by Ophthalmic Glasses* (1921), and *Life-Giving Light* (1933). Some of his most noted writings were collected in *The Sheard Volume: Selected Writings in Visual and Ophthalmic Optics* (1957).

It was said of Sheard that "his sense of duty drove him to tax his physical capacity to the utmost. He took more than his share of educational responsibility and was never afraid of an unpopular course of action if he believed it to be right."[73] An indication of the wide respect for him is the range of professional groups that conferred awards upon him: Distinguished Service Medal in Optometry (1930), Ward Burdick Medal from the American Society of Clinical Pathologists (1947), Honor Award from the American Academy of Ophthalmology and Otolaryngology (1951), Beverly Myers Nelson Award of the Foundation for Education in Ophthalmic Optics from the American Board of Opticianry (1951), and the Tillyer Medal from the Optical Society of America (1957).[80]

## ARTHUR MARTEN SKEFFINGTON (1890-1976)

A.M. Skeffington was born in Kansas City, Missouri, of parents originally from England and Denmark.[81] He graduated from Needles Institute of Optometry in Kansas City in 1917, and then opened an office in Kearney, Nebraska. In about 1926, Skeffington closed his office when he formed an association with E.B. Alexander of Oklahoma to provide educational opportunities for practicing optometrists.[81,82] In 1928, Skeffington and Alexander founded the

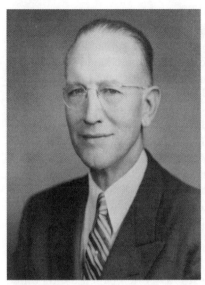

Optometric Extension Program (OEP). Because the quality of the educational background of the practicing optometrists of that time varied widely, OEP sought to upgrade the profession by presenting educational programs and literature and by emphasizing a comprehensive examination – a 21 point examination. Skeffington and colleagues emphasized that an important outcome of the analysis of the results of the 21 point exam is the prescription of lenses to relieve the visual stress associated with nearpoint activities. They designed a case analysis system, often called OEP analysis (discussed in chapter 17), to evaluate the findings in the 21 point exam.[83,84]

*Figure 19.13. A.M. Skeffington (photo courtesy of International Library, Archives, and Museum of Optometry, St. Louis).*

In his role as OEP Director of Education, Skeffington traveled extensively to lecture and confer with optometrists at various conferences and study group meetings.[81] He also met with numerous investigators in fields such as psychology, neurosciences, physiology, and education from whom he could glean information to incorporate into his broad concept of vision. One of Skeffington's major contributions was emphasizing that vision care did more than relieve eyestrain and improve visual acuity because vision is the dominant sense for acquiring information and for directing movement. Further he emphasized that providing vision care involved more than care for the eyes, because in the visual process, ocular function is integrated with activity in other sensory and neural structures and with cognitive function. He came down firmly on the nurture side of the nature versus nurture debate at a time when nature often seemed to be the dominant concept. Because his concepts have influenced the thinking of many practitioners, he is often referred to as the Father of Behavioral Optometry.[81,85,86]

Books published by Skeffington were *Procedure in Ocular Examination* (1928) and *Differential Diagnosis in Ocular Examination* (1931). In addition, OEP published several collected volumes of his serial publications for its membership, including *Analytical Optometry* (1938-1951), *Practical Applied Optometry* (1951-1958), *Introduction to Clinical Optometry* (1964), *Clinical Optometry in Theory and Practice* (1973), and *The Best of Skeffington* (1975-1976). Skeffington's zeal can be demonstrated by an observation that he did "impose upon optometry the sense of urgency in the upgrading of the practice patterns of the profession. Skeffington's sheer force, and his appeal to his audiences, marked him as a natural leader."[87] Skeffington received the Apollo Award of the American Optometric Association in 1961.

# JAMES THORINGTON (1858-1944)

James Thorington was a native of Davenport, Iowa.[88] He graduated from Jefferson Medical College in Philadelphia in 1881. He served as surgeon for the Panama Railroad until 1889. He then established practice in Philadelphia where he worked for fifty years.[88] For many years he was an ophthalmology professor at the Philadelphia Polyclinic Hospital. Thorington wrote several books, some of them continuing into many editions: *Retinoscopy* (1897, 1898, 1899, 1901, 1906, 1911), *Refraction and How to Refract* (1900, 1902, 1904, 1909, 1910), *The Ophthalmoscope and How to Use it* (1906), *Prisms, Their Use and Equivalents* (1913), and *Refraction of the Human Eye and Methods of Estimating the Refraction* (1916, 1930, 1939). Thorington's son, James Monroe Thorington (1894-1989), also an ophthalmologist in Philadelphia, revised and edited Thorington's book *Refraction of the Human Eye and Methods of Estimating the Refraction* for its third edition in 1939.

Thorington devoted significant space in some of his books to the characteristics of prisms and to dissociated phoria testing procedures. Thorington's name is associated with the dissociated phoria test today often called the modified Thorington test. As discussed earlier, that test may actually have originated with Maddox. Thorington's description of the test is as follows: "This tangent scale of Prentice with a central light as a fixing object and a Maddox rod before the left eye furnished an ideal test as the record of the amount of the deviation can be stated by the patient. Each line of displacement of the streak is equivalent to one centrad or prism-diopter."[89] The Prentice tangent scale as portrayed by Thorington was a numbered grid. Maddox's description of the test appeared earlier than Thorington's. Furthermore, it does not appear to have been Thorington's habit to deflect credit for his own contributions, because while he did claim credit in his books for some of his contributions, such as a schematic eye,[90] a "pointed line test" for subjective astigmatism testing,[91] a double prism designed to facilitate hyperphoria testing,[92] and equipment for retinoscopy,[90] he did not claim credit for the phoria test now known as the modified Thorington. Therefore, it appears that priority goes to Maddox, and it might be more properly called the Maddox tangent scale test instead of the modified Thorington test.

As mentioned earlier in the discussion of Prentice's contributions, Borish[71] attributed another dissociated phoria test to Thorington or Prentice. A description of that test by Thorington appears as follows in one of his books: "Another method for testing lateral insufficiency at the reading distance of 13 in. is to have a card about 6 in. square, and on this card to draw a heavy black line about 4 in. long; this line to be placed exactly horizontal. At the middle of the horizontal line draw a heavy black line, ½ in. long extending vertically from the horizontal line, this short vertical line to be capped with an arrow point. The horizontal line is divided off into equal spaces, each 3 1/3 mm. apart and numbered from 1 to 15 each side of the arrow; those to the left of the arrow are marked 'esophoria,' and those to the right of the arrow are marked 'exophoria.' To use this method, a prism of 8 centrads is placed base down before the right eye; this doubles the scale vertically; the upper scale belongs to the right eye. The number and the word in the upper scale to which the arrow in the lower scale points is the approximation in centrads of the amount of the esophoria or exophoria."[93] Here again, Thorington does not claim to have originated the test. And an earlier description of the test appears in one of Maddox's books.[94] A few paragraphs after his description of the test, Thorington refers to the line scale as a "Maddox scale."[93]

Thorington's books are characterized by clear descriptions of testing procedures. Their popularity is indicated by the fact that some of the books went through several additional printings after the appearance of each new edition. Thorington received an honorary A.M. degree from Ursinus College.[88]

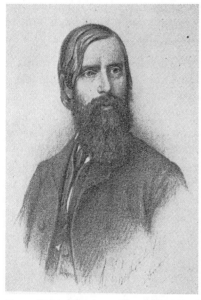

Figure 19.14. Albrecht von Graefe (Reprinted by permission from Duke-Elder S, Ashton N, Smith RJH, Lederman M. The Foundations of Ophthalmology: Heredity, Pathology, Diagnosis, and Therapeutics, vol. 7 in: Duke-Elder S, ed. System of Ophthalmology. St. Louis: Mosby, 1962:232 ©1962).

## ALBRECHT VON GRAEFE (1828-1870)

Albrecht von Graefe was born in Berlin. His father was a famous German surgeon, Carl Ferdinand von Graefe (1787-1840). When he entered the University of Berlin in 1843, Albrecht von Graefe was the youngest student on record there.[95] He graduated from medical school in 1847, after which he spent three years studying with noted ophthalmologists across Europe, among them being von Arlt in Prague, Sichel and Desmarres in Paris, Bowman in London, and the Jaegers (father and son) and von Brücke in Vienna.[95,96] Donders was also in London when von Graefe was and they formed a friendship that continued for many years.[97]

In 1850, von Graefe returned to Berlin and started practicing ophthalmology. It is said that von Graefe worked exceedingly long hours in patient care, writing, and lecturing.[97,98] The combination of long-standing frail health and an arduous work schedule led to von Graefe's early demise from tuberculosis at 42 years of age.[97] Historians of ophthalmology are effusive in their praise for von Graefe. Ullman[99] proclaimed him "the greatest ophthalmologist of the 19th century." Albert and Henkind[100] called "his contributions vast, his influence remarkable" and noted that his "classic articles are milestones...cornerstones of enduring worth..." Shastid[97] said that he "was a very charitable and kindly man. All his patients, rich and poor, high and low, were alike welcome." In 1969, Duke-Elder and Jay[95] went even farther in calling von Graefe "undoubtedly the greatest ophthalmologist who ever existed."

In 1854, von Graefe founded the journal *Archiv für Ophthalmologie*. The first issue, published in January, 1854, consisted of 480 pages, of which von Graefe authored 400 pages himself.[101] He served as editor, with Donders and von Arlt joining him as co-editors soon after the beginning of the journal. That journal continues today as *Graefe's Archive for Clinical and Experimental Ophthalmology*, an international journal produced in Heidelberg and published in English.[102] von Graefe was president of the Berlin Medical Society for over 18 years, and he helped to found the German Ophthalmological Society.[102]

Von Graefe wrote about conditions ranging across the whole field of eye care. His contributions included theory as well as testing methods, diagnosis, and surgical procedures.[101] After Helmholtz announced construction of an ophthalmoscope in 1851, von Graefe was one of the first to use it and describe the observations made with it.[97,103] Authors writing about von Graefe note in particular his contributions in glaucoma, cataract, and strabismus.[97,101,103,104]

The prism diplopia phoria test commonly known as the von Graefe test was described in 1861 by von Graefe.[101] The test target used by von Graefe for lateral phorias was a dot with a vertical line passing through it.[105]

Postage stamps honoring von Graefe were issued by both West Germany and East Germany in 1978 on the 150th anniversary of his birth.[104,106,107] A monument with a statue of von Graefe was unveiled in 1882 in Berlin.[108] An award medal presented by the Ophthalmological Society of Heidelberg every ten years bears a likeness of Albrecht von Graefe on one side.[109] An ophthalmology encyclopedia, *Handbuch der gesamten Augenheilkunde*, was dedicated to von Graefe after his death.[110] It was edited by Alfred Graefe (1830-1899, Albrecht's cousin) and Theodor Saemisch (1833-1909) and was published in seven volumes from 1874 to 1880. A second edition appeared in fifteen volumes from 1899 to 1933.

## REEFERENCES

1. Arrington EE. *History of Optometry. Chicago: White, 1929:113-116.*

2. Gregg JR. *American Optometric Association – A History. St. Louis: American Optometric Association, 1972:11-15.*

3. ter Laage RJChV. *Franciscus Cornelis Donders. In: Gillispie CC, ed. Dictionary of Scientific Biography. New York: Charles Scribner's Sons, 1971;4:162-164.*

4. Duke-Elder S, Abrams D. *Ophthalmic Optics and Refraction, vol. 5 in: Duke-Elder S, ed. System of Ophthalmology. St. Louis: Mosby, 1970:255.*

5. Albert DM, Henkind P. *Men of Vision: Lives of Notable Figures in Ophthalmology. Philadelphia: Saunders, 1993:142.*

6. Donders FC. *On the Anomalies of Accommodation and Refraction of the Eye - With a Preliminary Essay on Physiological Dioptrics. London: New Sydenham Society, 1864:111-114.*

7. Hirschberg J. *The History of Ophthalmology, vol. 10. Transl. by Blodi FC. Bonn: Wayenborgh, 1991:19.*

8. Sheedy JE. *The enduring legacy of Glenn Fry, Ph.D. J Am Optom Assoc 1996;67:375-376.*

9. Hebbard FW. *A brief biography of Glenn A. Fry. Am J Optom Physiol Opt 1976;53:339.*

10. Goss DA. *A history of M.S. and Ph.D. programs offered by schools and colleges of optometry in North America. Optom Vis Sci 1993;70:616-621.*

11. Publications of Glenn A. Fry. *Optom Vis Sci 1990;67:574-576.*

12. Augsburger A. *A celebration of the life of Glenn Ansel Fry September 10, 1908-January 5, 1996.* Optom Vis Sci 1996;73:223-224.

13. Hofstetter HW. Graphical analysis. In: Schor CM, Ciuffreda KJ, eds. *Vergence Eye Movements: Basic and Clinical Aspects.* Boston: Butterworths, 1983:439-464.

14. Fry GA. Fundamental variables in the relationship between accommodation and convergence. Optom Weekly 1943;34:153-155, 183-185.

15. Colby RN. *Professor, activist Harold M. Haynes dies.* The Oregonian (Portland, OR). March 25, 1997; B6.

16. Greenspan SB. M.E.M. retinoscopy. Refraction Letter December, 1974;(16).

17. Rouse MW, Hutter RF, Shiftlett R. *A normative study of the accommodative lag in elementary school children.* Am J Optom Physiol Opt 1984;61:693-697.

18. Valenti CA. *The Full Scope of Retinoscopy, rev. ed.* Santa Ana, CA: Optometric Extension Porgram, 1990:8.

19. Birnbaum MH. *Optometric Management of Nearpoint Vision Disorders.* Boston: Butterworth-Heinemann, 1993:169.

20. Haynes HM. *Clinical observations with dynamic retinoscopy.* Optom Weekly 1960;51:2243-2246, 2306-2309.

21. Haynes H, White BL, Held R. *Visual accommodation in human infants.* Science 1965;148:528-530.

22. http://www.co.washington.or.us/deptmts/cao/geninfo/haynes.htm. *Accessed Auguest 17, 2007.*

23. Morgan MW. *A biographical sketch of Henry Hofstetter.* Optom Vis Sci 1993;70:612-613.

24. Hofstetter HW. *The zone of clear single binocular vision.* Am J Optom Arch Am Acad Optom 1945;22:301-333, 361-384.

25. Goss DA. *History of the Indiana University Division of Optometry.* Indiana J Optom 2003;6:28-74.

26. Heath GG. *Henry W Hofstetter.* In: In Honor of Retiring Faculty, Indiana University, April, 1980.

27. Goss DA. *Henry W Hofstetter, OD, PhD, FAAO 1914-2002.* Optom Vis Sci 2002;79:467-468.

28. Baldwin WR, Bailey NJ, Penisten DK, Woo GC, Marshall EC, Goss DA. *Henry W Hofstetter (1914-2002): Tributes and reminiscences.* Indiana J Optom 2002;5:18-25.

29. Cooper JB. *Obituary – Dr. Ernest E. Maddox.* Br J Ophthalmol 1934;18:55-58.

30. Maddox EE. *Investigations in the relation between convergence and accommodation of the eyes.* J Anat Physiol 1886;20:475-508, 565-584; 1887;21:21-42.

31. Maddox EE. *Investigations in the relation between convergence and accommodation of the eyes.* Ophthal Rev 1886;5:341-353.

32. Maddox EE. *The Clinical Use of Prisms and the Decentering of Lenses, 2nd ed.* Bristol: John Wright, 1893:90.

33. Grut EH. *A contribution to the pathogeny of concomitant squinting (convergent and divergent); being the Bowman lecture.* Trans Ophthalmol Soc UK 1890;10:1-41.

34. Maddox EE. *The Clinical Use of Prisms and the Decentering of Lenses, 2nd ed.* Bristol: John Wright, 1893:106.

35. Maddox EE. *A new test for heterophoria.* Ophthal Rev 1890; 9:129-133.

36. Maddox EE. *The Clinical Use of Prisms and the Decentering of Lenses, 2nd ed.* Bristol: John Wright, 1893:126-127.

37. Maddox EE. *Tests and Studies of the Ocular Muscles, 3rd ed.* Philadelphia: Keystone, 1907:224.

38. Maddox EE. *The investigation by the rod-test of pareses and paralyses of the ocular muscles.* Ophthal Rev 1890;9:287-290.

39. Scobee RG, Green EL. *Tests for heterophoria – reliability of tests, comparisons between tests, and effect of changing testing conditions.* Am J Ophthalmol 1947;30:436-451.

40. Hirsch MJ, Bing LB. *The effect of testing method on values obtained for phoria at forty centimeters.* Am J Optom Arch Am Acad Optom 1948;25:407-416.

41. Hirsch MJ. *Clinical investigation of a method of testing phoria at forty centimeters.* Am J Optom Arch Am Acad Optom 1948;25:492-495.

42. Duke-Elder S, Wybar K. Ocular Motility and Strabismus, vol. 6 in: Duke-Elder S, ed. System of Ophthalmology. St. Louis: Mosby, 1973:245.

43. Peters HB, Enoch JM, Sarver MD. Meredith Walter Morgan – A salute. Am J Optom Physiol Opt 1988;65:322-324.

44. Carter D, Enoch JM, Goodlaw E, Westheimer G. Meredith W. Morgan, 1912-1999, Professor of Physiological Optics and Optometry, Dean of the School of Optometry, University of California at Berkeley. Ophthal Physiol Opt 1999;20:169-171.

45. Adams AJ. Meredith W. Morgan, OD, PhD, FAAO (1912-1999). Optom Vis Sci 2000;77:6-7.

46. Fisher EJ. Tribute to Ivan S. Nott, 1892-1969. Can J Optom 1969;30:105.

47. Nott IS. Dynamic skiametry, accommodation and convergence. Am J Physiol Opt 1925;6:490-503.

48. Nott IS. Accommodative astigmatism. Am J Optom 1928;5:268-273.

49. Nott IS. Convergence, accommodation and fusion. Am J Optom 1929;6:19-29.

50. Boeder P. Obituary: Kenneth N. Ogle. Invest Ophthalmol 1968;7:234-235.

51. Bisno DC. Eyes in the Storm – President Hopkins's Dilemma: The Dartmouth Eye Institute. Norwich, VT: Norwich Press, 1994.

52. Duke-Elder S, Wybar K. Ocular Motility and Strabismus, vol. 6 in: Duke-Elder S, ed. System of Ophthalmology. St. Louis: Mosby, 1973:517-518.

53. Fry GA. Eulogy: Kenneth N. Ogle. J Am Optom Assoc 1968;39:570.

54. Anonymous. Obituary: A.S. Percival. Br J Ophthalmol 1936;20:123-124.

55. Percival SPB. Letter to Richard Keeler, July 13, 2005.

56. Percival AS. Periscopic lenses. Br J Ophthalmol 1926;10:369-379.

57. Duke-Elder S. The Practice of Refraction, 5th ed. St. Louis: Mosby, 1949:vi.

58. Percival AS. The relation of convergence to accommodation and its practical bearing. Ophthal Rev 1892;11:313-328.

59. Percival AS. The Prescribing of Spectacles, 3rd ed. Bristol, England: John Wright & Sons, 1928:119-136.

60. Prentice CF. Legalized Optometry and the Memoirs of its Founder. Seattle: Casperin Fletcher, 1926:197-198.

61. Hirsch MJ, Wick RE. The Optometric Profession. Philadelphia: Chilton, 1968:129.

62. Hofstetter HW. Optometry: Professional, Economic, and Legal Aspects. St. Louis: Mosby, 1948:90.

63. Hirsch MJ, Wick RE. The Optometric Profession. Philadelphia: Chilton, 1968:131.

64. Prentice CF. Legalized Optometry and the Memoirs of its Founder. Seattle: Casperin Fletcher, 1926.

65. Hofstetter HW. Optometry: Professional, Economic, and Legal Aspects. St. Louis: Mosby, 1948:32-33.

66. Gregg JR. The Story of Optometry. New York: Ronald Press, 1965:190-195.

67. Hirsch MJ, Wick RE. The Optometric Profession. Philadelphia: Chilton, 1968:131-139.

68. Christensen J. Chronology of Charles Prentice's life. Hindsight: Newsletter Optom Hist Soc 2000;31:2-5.

69. Prentice CF. A metric system of numbering and measuring prisms. Arch Ophthalmol 1890;19(1). In: Prentice CF. Ophthalmic Lenses, Dioptric Formulae for Combined Cylindrical Lenses, The Prism Dioptry, and Other Optical Papers, 2nd ed. Philadelphia: Keystone, 1907:105-124.

70. Prentice CF. Ophthalmic Lenses, Dioptric Formulae for Combined Cylindrical Lenses, The Prism Dioptry, and Other Optical Papers, 2nd ed. Philadelphia: Keystone, 1907:121.

71. Borish IM. Clinical Refraction, 3rd ed. New York: Professional Press, 1970:816-817.

72. Hirsch MJ, Wick RE. The Optometric Profession. Philadelphia: Chilton, 1968:163.

73. Koch CC. Minnesota honors Charles Sheard. Am J Optom Arch Am Acad Optom 1963;40:102-105.

74. Hofstetter HW. Optometry: Professional, Economic, and Legal Aspects. St. Louis: Mosby, 1948:295-312.

75. Koch CC. Charles Sheard 1883-1963. Am J Optom Arch Am Acad Optom 1963;40:757-758.

76. Richards OW. Charles Sheard, Edgar D. Tillyer Medalist for 1957. J Opt Soc Am 1958;48:205-214.

77. Sheard C. The Sheard Volume: Selected Writings in Visual and Ophthalmic Optics. Philadelphia; Chilton, 1957:43.

78. Borish IM. 21 points. Newsletter Optom Hist Soc 1987;18:23-24.

79. Hendrickson H. 21 points and more. Newsletter Optom Hist Soc 1987;18:55-56.

80. Sheard C. The Sheard Volume: Selected Writings in Visual and Ophthalmic Optics. Philadelphia; Chilton, 1957:436.

81. Cox JL. A.M. Skeffington, O.D. – the Man. J Behav Optom 1997;8:3-6.

82. Hoare AE. The Skeffington saga – Part 2, Skeffington, the mission. Optom World 1966;53(7):8, 10,14,16,18,22,24.

83. Birnbaum MH. Optometric Management of Nearpoint Vision Disorders. Boston: Butterworth-Heinemann, 1993:121-160.

84. Schmitt EP. The Skeffington Perspective of the Behavioral Model of Optometric Data Analysis and Vision Care. Bloomington, IN: Authorhouse, 2006.

85. Birnbaum MH. Behavioral optometry: a historical perspective. J Am Optom Assoc 1994;65:255-264.

86. Maples WC. A.M. Skeffington: the father of behavioral optometry – his contributions. Proc SPIE 1998;3579:17-23.

87. Hoare AE. The Skeffington saga – Part 2, Skeffington, the man. Optom World 1966;53(5):9,12, 15,16,18.

88. Anonymous. Dr. J. Thorington is dead at 86. The Evening Bulletin (Philadelphia). October 20, 1944; 5.

89. Thorington J. Prisms, Their Use and Equivalents. Philadelphia: Blakiston, 1913: 98-99.

90. Thorington J. Retinoscopy (Or Shadow Test) in the Determination of Refraction at one meter Distance with the Plane Mirror, 6th ed. Philadelphia: Blakiston, 1911: 3, 63-65.

91. Thorington J. Refraction and How to Refract Including Sections on Optics, Retinoscopy, the Fitting of Spectacles and Eye-glasses, etc. Philadelphia: Blakiston, 1900:139.

92. Thorington J. Prisms, Their Use and Equivalents. Philadelphia: Blakiston, 1913: 90-93.

93. Thorington J. Refraction of the Human Eye and Methods of Estimating the Refraction. Philadelphia: Blakiston, 1916: 267-269.

94. Maddox EE. The Clinical Use of Prisms and the Decentering of Lenses. Bristol: John Wright, 1889: 86-87.

95. Duke-Elder S, Jay B. Diseases of the Lens and Vitreous; Glaucoma and Hypotony, vol. 11 in: Duke-Elder S, ed. System of Ophthalmology. St. Louis: Mosby, 1969: 613-615.

96. Hirschberg J. The History of Ophthalmology, vol.11 (part 1-a). Trans. by Blodi FC. Bonn: Wayenborgh, 1992: 214-254.

97. Shastid TH. Albrecht von Graefe. In: Wood CA, ed. The American Encyclopedia and Dictionary of Ophthalmology. Chicago: Cleveland Press, 1915: 5621-5624.

98. Tower P. Albrecht von Graefe: a survey of his correspondence. Arch Ophthalmol 1964;71: 619-624.

99. Ullman EV. Albrecht von Graefe: the man in his time. Am J Ophthalmol 1954;38: 525-543, 695-711, 791-809.

100. Albert DM, Henkind P. Men of Vision: Lives of Notable Figures in Ophthalmology. Philadelphia: Saunders, 1993: 361-369.

101. Remky H. Albrecht von Graefe: facets of his work on the occasion of the 125th anniversary of his death (20 July 1870). Graefe's Arch Clin Exp Ophthalmol 1995;233: 537-548.

102. Foerster MH. Graefe's Archive: 150 years. Graefe's Arch Clin Exp Ophthalmol 2004;242: 451-452.

103. Duke-Elder S, Ashton N, Smith RJH, Lederman M. The Foundations of Ophthalmology: Heredity, Pathology, Diagnosis, and Therapeutics, vol. 7 in: Duke-Elder S, ed. System of Ophthalmology. St. Louis: Mosby, 1962: 233-234.

104. Tan SY, Zia JK. Medicine in stamps: Albrecht von Graefe (1828-1870): founder of scientific ophthalmology. Singapore Med J 2007;48: 797-798.

105. von Graefe A. Uber die musculare Asthenopie. Archiv für Ophthalmol 1861;8:314-367.

106. Blodi FC. Ophthalmology and philately: I. Ophthalmologists on stamps. – Albrecht von Graefe (1828-1870). Arch Ophthalmol 1979;97: 1653.

107. Haas LF. Albrecht von Graefe (1828-70). J Neurol Neurosurg Psychiatry 1998;64: 504.

108. Duke-Elder S, Jay B. Diseases of the Lens and Vitreous; Glaucoma and Hypotony, vol. 11 in: Duke-Elder S, ed. System of Ophthalmology. St. Louis: Mosby, 1969: 378-379.

109. Galst JM. Ophthalmological numismatics: a look at the past. Arch Ophthalmol 2000;118: 1589.

110. Hirschberg J. The History of Ophthalmology, vol.11 (part 1-a). Trans. by Blodi FC. Bonn: Wayenborgh, 1992: 6, 246.

# Appendix A
# Answers to Selected Practice Problems

## Chapter 1

1. (a) 1.82 D

   (b) 1.22 D

   (c) 1.00 D

   (d) 4.50 D

   (e) 2.78 D

   (f) 1.53 D

   (g) 2.00 D

2. (a) 19 Δ

   (b) 11.8 Δ

   (c) 6.1 Δ

   (d) 25.7 Δ

# Chapter 2

Patient AK:

Calculated ACA = [15 − (-2) + (-2)] / 2.50 = 6 Δ/D

Patient ED:

Calculated ACA = [15 − (-1) + (-3)] / 2.50 = 5.2 Δ/D

Gradient ACA = [(-3) − (-7)] / 1 = 4 Δ/D

Patient DB:

Calculated ACA = [15 − 0 + 8] / 2.50 = 9.2 Δ/D

Gradient ACA = [8 − 1] / 1 = 7 Δ/D

Patient SR:

Calculated ACA = [15 − 0 + (-10)] / 2.50 = 2 Δ/D

Gradient ACA = [(-10) − (-11)] / 1 = 1 Δ/D

Patient LP:

Calculated ACA = [16.7 − (-1) + (-2)] / 3 = 5.2 Δ/D

Patient TC:

Calculated ACA = [14.8 − (-2) + (-6)] / 2.50 = 4.3 Δ/D

Gradient ACA = [(-6) − (-9)] / 1 = 3 Δ/D

Patient BE:

Calculated ACA = [15.7 -2 + 4] / 2.50 = 7.1 Δ/D

Gradient ACA = [4 − (-1)] / 1 = 5 Δ/D

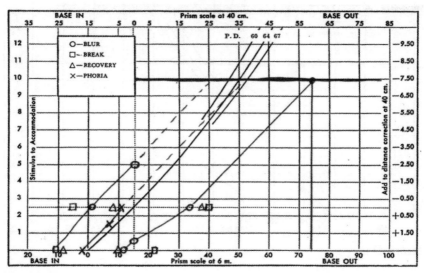

# Chapter 3

## Patient AR

Calculated ACA = [15 – (-2) + (-4)] / 2.50 = 5.2 Δ/D
Gradient ACA = 4 Δ/D

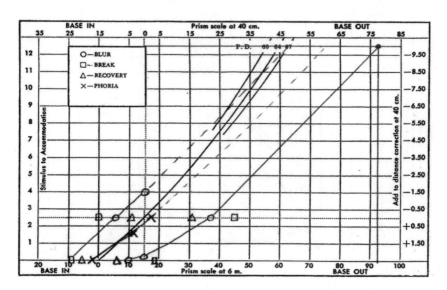

## Patient BP

Calculated ACA = [14.5 – (-2) + (-2)] / 2.50 = 7.4 Δ/D
Gradient ACA = 5 Δ/D

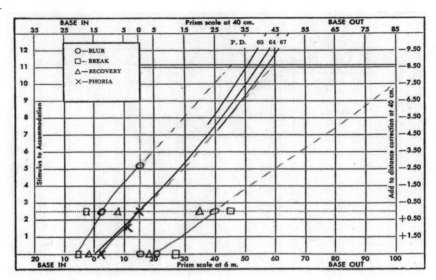

## Patient DT
Calculated ACA = [15 − (2) + (0)] / 2.50 = 5.2 Δ/D
Gradient ACA = 4 Δ/D

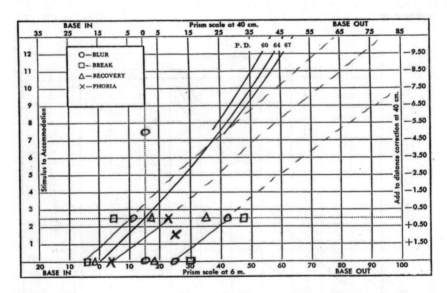

## Patient GL
Calculated ACA = [14.1 − 3 + 8] / 2.50 = 7.6 Δ/D

It appears that the +1.00 D gradient phoria and the PRA are not consistent with other test findings. An answer for the gradient ACA is not given because the higher esophoria with the plus add than with the BVA may be due to procedural or measurement error.

256

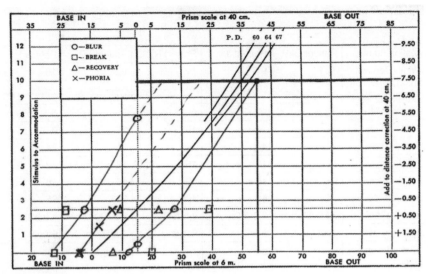

## Patient DK

Calculated ACA = [15 − (−4) + (−8)] / 2.50 = 4.4 Δ/D
Gradient ACA = 4 Δ/D

2.  (a) (100/10) + (+2.00 − 0) = 12.0 D

    (b) (100/8) + (−2.50 − (−1.00)) = 11.0 D

# Chapter 5

|         | Problem 1 | Problem 2 | Problem 3 |
|---------|-----------|-----------|-----------|
| NRV     | 17        | 5         | 12        |
| PRV     | 12        | 24        | 15        |
| NFV     | 9         | 8         | 10        |
| PFV     | 20        | 21        | 17        |
| Demand  | 8         | 3         | 2         |
| Reserve | 12        | 5         | 15        |

# Chapter 6

| Question number | Patient GH | Patient JK | Patient RP | Patient LP | Patient MS |
|---|---|---|---|---|---|
| 1. width Percival comfort zone, 40 cm | 12.7 | 9.3 | 11.3 | 9.3 | 10 |
| 2. demand, 40 cm | 2 | 12 | 5 | 8 | 6 |
| 3. NRV, 40 cm | 14 | 24 | 10 | 20 | 6 |
| 3. PRV, 40 cm | 24 | 4 | 24 | 8 | 24 |
| 3. NFV, 40 cm | 12 | 12 | 15 | 12 | 12 |
| 3. PFV, 40 cm | 26 | 16 | 19 | 16 | 18 |
| 4. reserve, 40 cm | 24 | 4 | 10 | 8 | 6 |
| 5. calc. ACA | 5.9 Δ/D | 2.8 Δ/D | 8.1 Δ/D | 2.2 Δ/D | 6.9 Δ/D |
| 5. gradient ACA | 3 Δ/D | 2 Δ/D | 9 Δ/D | 2 Δ/D | 5 Δ/D |
| 6. Sheard's crit., distance | yes | no 1.3Δ BI | Yes | yes | yes |
| 6. Sheard's crit., 40 cm | yes | no 6.7Δ BI | Yes | no 2.7Δ BI | no 2Δ BO |
| 7. Percival's crit., distance | yes | no 2.7Δ BI | no 0.7Δ BO | yes | yes |
| 7. Percival's crit., 40 cm | yes | no 5.3Δ BI | no 1.3Δ BO | no 1.3Δ BI | no 4Δ BO |
| 8. 1:1 rule, distance | NA | NA | NA | yes | no 1ΔBO |
| 8. 1:1 rule, 40 cm | NA | NA | no 1Δ BO | NA | no 1.5Δ BO |

NA = not applicable

# Chapter 7

1. b, c, e, f
2. Patient PB: 40 cm BO blur, break, and recovery

   Patient RL: distance BI break and recovery; 40 cm blur and break

   Patient LM: distance BI recovery; 40 cm BI recovery

   Patient LE: distance BO blur, break and recovery; 40 cm BO blur and recovery

# Chapter 8

1. Patient MR: normal accommodative facility

   Patient LG: accommodative disorder

   Patient TB: vergence disorder

2.

| Amplitude | Test distance | Lens powers | Failure criterion |
|-----------|---------------|-------------|-------------------|
| 7.0 D | 32.0 cm | ±1.00 D | <10 cpm |
| 8.0 D | 28.0 cm | ±1.25 D | <10 cpm |
| 9.0 D | 24.5 cm | ±1.50 D | <10 cpm |

# Chapter 10

1.

| Dissociated phoria | Associated phoria | Mallett classification |
|--------------------|-------------------|------------------------|
| 8 Δ exo | 0 | Compensated exophoria |
| 3 Δ eso | 0 | Compensated esophoria |
| 9 Δ exo | 3ΔBI | Uncompensated exophoria |
| 6 Δ eso | 2ΔBO | Uncompensated esophoria |
| 6 Δ exo | 2ΔBO | Paradoxical fixation disparity |

4. curve type, slope, x-intercept, y-intercept, Sheedy's criterion

5.

| Clinical FDC parameter | Patient PM | Patient CR | Patient JB | Patient RM | Patient BP |
|------------------------|-----------|-----------|-----------|-----------|-----------|
| Curve type | I | II | III | I | I |
| Slope | -1 min/Δ | -0.7 min/Δ | -0.7 min/Δ | 0 | -1.3 min/Δ |
| y-intercept | 4 min eso | 2 min eso | 4 min exo | 0 | 4 min exo |
| x-intercept | 9Δ BO | 3Δ BO | 6Δ BI | 0 | 9Δ BI |
| Sheedy's criterion | 3Δ BO | 3Δ BO | 6Δ BI | 0 | 3Δ BI |

# Chapter 11

|  | Patient RP | Patient DE | Patient AT | Patient BC |
|---|---|---|---|---|
| b. calc. ACA | 2.0 Δ/D | 8.7 Δ/D | 3.4 Δ/D | 8.4 Δ/D |
| c. gradient ACA | 1 Δ/D | 8 Δ/D | 3 Δ/D | 7 Δ/D |
| d. Sheard's crit., dist. | met | met | not met 2.7Δ BO | not met 3.7Δ BI |
| d. Sheard's crit., 40 cm | not met 4Δ BI | not met 2Δ BO | met | met |
| e. Percival's crit., dist. | met | met | not met 4. 7Δ BO | met |
| e. Percival's crit., 40 cm | not met 0.3Δ BI | not met 3Δ BO | met | met |
| f. 1:1 rule, distance | NA | NA | not met 3Δ BO | NA |
| f. 1:1 rule, 40 cm | NA | not met 1.5Δ BO | NA | NA |
| g. case type | Convergence insufficiency | Convergence excess | Divergence insufficiency | Divergence excess |
| h. Mallett class., dist. | --- | --- | Uncompensated esophoria | Uncompensated exophoria |
| h. Mallett class., 40 cm | Uncompensated exophoria | Uncompensated esophoria | --- | Compensated exophoria |

|  | Patient DW | Patient HH | Patient SM | Patient NE |
|---|---|---|---|---|
| b. calc. ACA | 4.0 Δ/D | 6.4 Δ/D | 5.2 Δ/D | 1.8 Δ/D |
| c. gradient ACA | 3 Δ/D | 5 Δ/D | 4 Δ/D | 1 Δ/D |
| d. Sheard's crit., dist. | not met 3Δ BI | not met 3. 7Δ BO | met | met |
| d. Sheard's crit., 40 cm | not met 4. 7Δ BI | not met 3.3Δ BO | met | not met 3.3Δ BI |
| e. Percival's crit., dist. | not met 0. 7Δ BI | not met 4Δ BO | met | met |
| e. Percival's crit., 40 cm | not met 0. 7Δ BI | not met 4Δ BO | met | met |
| f. 1:1 rule, distance | NA | not met 3.5Δ BO | NA | NA |
| f. 1:1 rule, 40 cm | NA | not met 3Δ BO | NA | NA |
| g. case type | Basic exophoria | Basic esophoria | Fusional vergence dysfunction | Pseudo convergence insufficiency |
| h. Mallett class., dist. | Uncompensated exophoria | Uncompensated esophoria | --- | --- |
| h. Mallett class., 40 cm | Uncompensated exophoria | Uncompensated esophoria | Compensated exophoria | Uncompensated exophoria |

NA = not applicable

# Chapter 12

1. $2.50 - (1.50 / 2) = +1.75$ D
2. $3.00 - (2.50 / 2) = +1.75$ D
3. $+1.00$ D
4. $+1.25$ D

# Chapter 13

1. Min. expected amplitude $= 15 - (0.25)(20) = 10$ D;

   7.0 D is lower than minimum expected;

   Accommodative insufficiency;

   Plus adds and/or vision therapy

2. Patient SN: AR $= 2.00$ D; lag $= 0.50$ D

   Patient CD: AR $= 2.17$ D; lag $= 0.43$ D

   Patient GI: AR $= 1.47$ D; lag $= 1.03$ D

   Patient PC: AR $= 1.79$ D; lag $= 0.71$ D

3. lag $= 1.25$ D; high; yes, accommodative insufficiency

4. Patient CA:

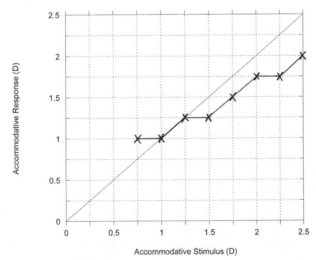

MEM $= 0.50$ D lag
Low neutral $= +1.25$ D add

Patient AT:

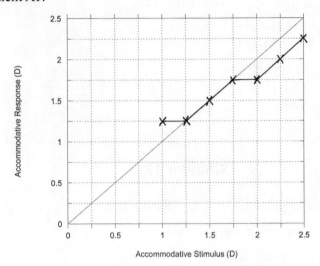

MEM = 0.25 D lag
Low neutral = +0.75 D add

Patient BP:

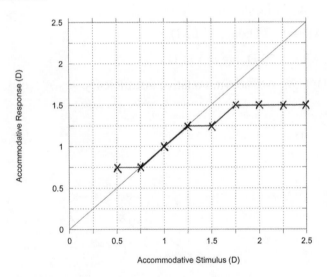

MEM = 1.00 D lag
Low neutral = +1.25 D add

Patient OC:

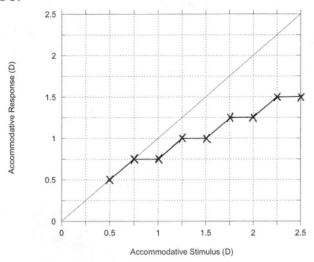

MEM = 1.00 D lag
Low neutral = +1.75 D add

Patient FL:

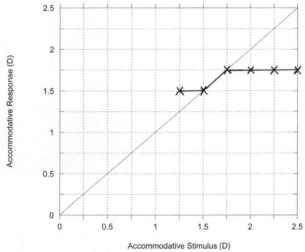

MEM = 0.75 D lag
Low neutral = +0.75 D add

# Chapter 16

1. CAC = 0.50 D / 6Δ = 0.08 D/Δ

2. CAC = 0.25 D / 6Δ = 0.04 D/Δ

3. PCT = 4.7 – 3 = 1.7 Δ/D

4. calculated ACA = [15 – (-2) + (-4)] / 2.50 = 5.2 Δ/D

   Gradient ACA = 4 Δ/D

   PCT = 5.2 – 4 = 1.2 Δ/D

5. PCT = [(15 + (-14) – (-2)] / 2.50 = 1.2 Δ/D

# Appendix B
# Equipment Sources

Bernell
4016 N. Home Street
Mishiwaka, IN 46545
(800) 348-2225
www.bernell.com

i.O.O. Sales Limited
56-62 Newington Causeway
London SE1 6DS
United Kingdom
admin@ioosales.co.uk
www.ioosales.co.uk

Keystone View
Nevada Capital Group, Inc.
2200 Dickerson Road
Reno, Neveda 89503
(866) 574-6360
sales@keystoneview.com
www.keystoneview.com

Optego Vision Inc.
341 Deloraine Avenue
Toronto, Ontario M5M 2B7
Canada
orders@optego.com
www.optego.com/index.htm

Optometric Extension Program
1921 E. Carnegie Avenue, Suite 3-L
Santa Ana, CA 92705-5510
(949) 250-8070
www.oepf.org

Stereo Optical, Inc.
3539 N. Kenton Avenue
Chicago, IL 60641
(800) 344-9500
sales@stereooptical.com
www.stereooptical.com

# Appendix C
# Glossary and Acronyms

**ACA ratio (or AC/A ratio)** – the ratio of accommodative convergence to accommodation; the amount of accommodative convergence, usually in prism diopters, that occurs with one diopter of accommodation.

**Accommodative convergence** – convergence due to the neurological link of accommodation and convergence and occurring as a result of the stimulation of accommodation.

**Accommodative excess** – an accommodative disorder characterized by a lead of accommodation and which can also show a low NRA, minus on the BCC, and slowness on the plus side of the monocular and binocular lens rock.

**Accommodative facility tests** – tests which determine how quickly patients can clear letters as accommodative stimulus is alternated between two levels, measured in cycles per minute, one cycle being a start on the lower stimulus level to clarity with a change to the higher stimulus and back to clarity on the lower stimulus level; also known as accommodative rock because accommodative stimulus is rocked back and forth between two levels.

**Accommodative infacility** – an accommodative disorder characterized by slowness on monocular and binocular facility testing, generally on both plus and minus sides of the lens rock, and which can also show low NRA and PRA findings.

**Accommodative insufficiency** – an accommodative disorder characterized by a high lag of accommodation and/or a low amplitude of accommodation and which can also show a low PRA, high plus on the BCC, and slowness on the minus side of the monocular and binocular lens rock.

**Accommodative response** – the amount of increase in optical power of the eye due to a change in the accommodative apparatus of the eye, the dioptric amount of which can be measured with dynamic retinoscopy or an optometer.

**Accommodative stimulus** – the magnitude of accommodation that would be necessary to focus the object of regard on the retina, the dioptric amount of which is determined by subtracting the amount of any plus add from the reciprocal of the viewing distance in meters or by adding the amount of any minus add to the reciprocal of the viewing distance in meters.

**Amplitude of accommodation** – the maximum amount of accommodation that an individual can exert, usually determined using the near point of accommodation on a push-up test.

**AR** – accommodative response.

**AS** – accommodative stimulus.

**Associated phoria** – amount of prism required to reduce fixation disparity to zero.

**Base-in limit** – the blur finding on base-in fusional vergence range testing, or the break if no blur is reported; equal to the NRV.

**Base-out limit** – the blur finding on base-out fusional vergence range testing, or the break if no blur is reported; equal to the PRV.

**Basic esophoria** – a vergence disorder characterized by esophoria at distance and near, normal ACA ratio, low base-in vergence ranges at distance and near, low PRA, and reduced ability on the minus side of the binocular lens rock.

**Basic exophoria** – a vergence disorder characterized by high exophoria at distance and near, normal ACA ratio, low base-out vergence ranges at distance and near, low NRA, and reduced ability on the plus side of the binocular lens rock.

**BCC** – binocular cross cylinder test.

**BD** – base-down prism.

**BI** – base-in prism.

**Binocular cross cylinder test** – a test in which a cross cylinder creates an astigmatic interval and the patient views a cross grid pattern with lines parallel to the principal meridians of the cross cylinder; the spherical lens add with which the patient reports the cross grid lines being equally dark is the add which makes the dioptric accommodative response equal to the dioptric accommodative stimulus.

**BO** – base-out prism.

**Brock string** – a training procedure in which a string with beads for fixation is used in vision therapy to improve vergence function.

**BU** – base-up prism.

**BVA** – acronym for maximum plus binocular subjective refraction to best visual acuity.

**CAC ratio** – ratio of the amount of convergence accommodation occurring with a change in convergence, usually expressed in diopters per prism diopter.

**Calculated ACA ratio** – the ratio of accommodative convergence to accommodation determined by taking one dissociated phoria at distance through the BVA and another dissociated phoria at near through the BVA.

**Chiastopic fusion** – fusion in free space of two similar laterally separated targets, with fusion achieved by a crossing of the lines of sight of the two eyes inside the plane of the targets, such that the left eye views the right target and the right eye views the left target.

**Convergence excess** – a vergence disorder characterized by normal distance phoria, esophoria at near, high ACA ratio, low base-in vergence ranges at near, low PRA, and reduced ability on the minus side of the binocular lens rock.

**Convergence insufficiency** – a vergence disorder characterized by normal distance phoria, high exophoria at near, low ACA ratio, low base-out vergence ranges at near, and a receded NPC.

**Demand** – amount of fusional vergence required to maintain binocular vision; equal to the magnitude of the dissociated phoria.

**Dissociated phoria** – the amount by which the lines of sight of the two eyes, with fusion disrupted, differ from the position the lines of sight would assume if they intersected at the object of regard, usually measured in prism diopters.

**Distance rock** – an accommodative facility procedure in which dioptric accommodative stimulus is changed by changes in viewing distance; also used as a training procedure in vision therapy to improve the latency and velocity of accommodative responses.

**Divergence excess** – a vergence disorder characterized by high exophoria at distance, normal nearpoint phoria, high ACA ratio, and low base-out vergence ranges at distance.

**Divergence insufficiency** – a vergence disorder characterized by esophoria at distance, normal nearpoint phoria, low ACA ratio, and low base-in ranges at distance.

**FDC** – fixation disparity curve.

**Fixation disparity** – a slight vergence misalignment during binocular fixation, the overconvergence (eso fixation disparity) or the undercovergence (exo fixation disparity) being small enough that binocular fusion is present.

**Fixation disparity curve** – a plot of the amount of fixation disparity as a function of the prism through which the patient views.

**Fixation disparity curve parameters** – numerical values which can be used to describe the configuration and placement of the fixation disparity curve on the graph designed for it; they are curve type, slope, y-intercept, x-intercept, and center of symmetry; for clinical purposes, Sheedy's criterion can be used to replace the center of symmetry.

**Fusional convergence** – convergence occurring in response to retinal disparity in order to maintain binocular fusion (synonyms, fusional vergence, disparity vergence).

**Fusional vergence dysfunction** – a vergence disorder characterized by normal phorias and ACA ratio, low fusional vergence ranges, low NRA and PRA, and reduced vergence facility.

**Fusional vergence ranges** – tests to determine the powers of base-in or base-out (or vertical) prism that can be added until the patient reports target letters blurring, breaking into two, and recovering back into one.

**Gradient ACA ratio** – the ratio of accommodative convergence to accommodation determined by taking two dissociated phorias at the same near viewing distance through two different lens powers.

**Lag of accommodation** – a condition in which accommodative response is less than accommodative stimulus; quantified by subtracting the dioptric accommodative response from the dioptric accommodative stimulus; when a lag of accommodation is present, the retina is conjugate with a point farther from the patient than the object being viewed.

**Lead of accommodation** – a condition in which accommodative response is greater than accommodative stimulus; quantified by subtracting the dioptric accommodative stimulus from the dioptric accommodative response; when a lead of accommodation is present, the retina is conjugate with a point closer to the patient than the object being viewed.

**Lens rock** – an accommodative facility testing procedure in which dioptric accommodative stimulus is changed with lenses; also used as a training procedure in vision therapy to improve the latency and velocity of accommodative responses.

**Low neutral dynamic retinoscopy** – a retinoscopy procedure in which the patient views a nearpoint target and the examiner adds spherical lenses until neutrality is observed, providing a measure of the add power that makes the dioptric accommodative response equal to the dioptric accommodative stimulus.

**MEM dynamic retinoscopy** – monocular estimation method dynamic retinoscopy, a retinoscopy procedure in which the patient views a nearpoint target and the examiner estimates how far accommodation is from conjugacy with the target by judging the speed, width, and brightness of the retinoscopic reflex, that estimate of dioptric distance from neutrality being a measure of the lag (or lead) of accommodation.

**MEM-LN retinoscopy** – a dynamic retinoscopy procedure combining principles of MEM and low neutral dynamic retinoscopy to obtain accommodative response measurements at several accommodative stimulus levels.

**Minus add** – minus lens power added to the BVA; e.g., a -1.00 D add refers to a lens that is 1.00 D more minus than the BVA.

**Morgan's norms** – means, standard deviations, and normal ranges derived by Morgan for dissociated phorias, fusional vergence ranges, relative accommodation, and gradient ACA ratio.

**Negative fusional vergence (NFV)** – amount of fusional divergence that can be exerted starting from an amount of prism equal to the dissociated phoria, determined by the addition of base-in prism (synonym, negative fusional convergence, NFC).

**Negative relative accommodation (NRA) test** – test finding the amount of plus added binocularly to the first sustained blur at near; also known as the plus to blur test.

**Negative relative vergence (NRV)** – amount of fusional divergence that can be exerted starting from zero prism, determined by the addition of base-in prism (synonym, negative relative convergence, NRC).

**NFC** – negative fusional convergence; see negative fusional vergence, NFV.

**NFV** – negative fusional vergence.

**Nott dynamic retinoscopy** – a dynamic retinoscopy procedure in which the patient views a nearpoint target and the examiner moves the retinoscope away farther from the patient and farther behind the target until neutrality is observed; the difference between the reciprocal of the distance in meters from the spectacle plane to the target (accommodative stimulus) and the reciprocal of the distance from the spectacle plane to the retinoscope (accommodative response) is the lag of accommodation.

**NPC** – near point of convergence; the point at which a patient reports diplopia or the examiner first notes binocular convergence has ceased as a near point object is brought closer to the eyes.

**NRA** – negative relative accommodation.

**NRC** – negative relative convergence; see negative relative vergence, NRV.

**NRV** – negative relative vergence.

**1:1 rule** – a guideline used to assess strain on fusional vergence in esophoria; it states that the base-in recovery should be at least the amount of the esophoria.

**Orthopic fusion** – fusion in free space of two similar laterally separated targets, with fusion achieved by a crossing of the lines of sight of the two eyes behind the plane of the targets, such that the left eye views the left target and the right eye views the right target.

**PCT ratio** – ratio of change in proximal convergence occurring with a change in test distance, usually expressed in prism diopters per diopter.

**PD** – interpupillary distance.

**Percival's criterion** – a guideline used to assess strain on fusional vergence; it compares the base-in blur (or break if no blur reported) and the base-out blur (or break if no blur reported) and states that the lesser of those two limits should be at least half of the greater.

**PFC** – positive fusional convergence; see positive fusional vergence, PFV.

**PFV** – positive fusional vergence.

**Phoria** – term used as a synonym for dissociated phoria, and not to be confused with associated phoria in which case the words associated and phoria are always used together (see definitions of dissociated phoria and associated phoria).

**Phoria line** – the line which connects the dissociated phoria points on an accommodation and convergence graph.

**Plus add** – plus lens power added to the BVA; e.g., a +1.00 D add refers to a lens that is 1.00 D more plus than the BVA.

**Positive fusional vergence (PFV)** – amount of fusional convergence that can be exerted starting from an amount of prism equal to the dissociated phoria, determined by addition of base-out prism (synonym, positive fusional convergence, PFC).

**Positive relative accommodation (PRA) test** – test finding the amount of minus added binocularly to the first sustained blur at near; also known as the minus to blur test.

**Positive relative vergence (PRV)** – amount of fusional convergence that can be exerted starting from zero prism, determined by addition of base-out prism (synonym, positive relative convergence, PRC).

**PRA** – positive relative accommodation.

**PRC** – positive relative convergence; see positive relative vergence, PRV.

**Presbyopia** – the normal reduction in amplitude of accommodation which occurs with age and which results in the necessity of a plus lens add for satisfactory clarity of nearpoint vision.

**Prism adaptation** – an increase in tonic vergence (resulting in an eso shift in dissociated phoria) after use of positive fusional vergence, or a decrease in tonic vergence (resulting in an exo shift in dissociated phoria) after use of negative fusional vergence; also known as vergence adaptation or fusional aftereffects.

**Prism rock** – a testing or training procedure in which a patient views alternately through some amount of base-in prism and some amount of base-out prism, used as a test to evaluate the quickness of fusional vergence responses or used in vision therapy to improve vergence function.

**Proximal convergence** – convergence due to an awareness of nearness.

**PRV** – positive relative vergence.

**Pseudo convergence insufficiency** – a vergence disorder secondary to accommodative insufficiency, characterized by high exophoria at near, low base-out vergence ranges at near, high lag of accommodation, and receded NPC which improves with a plus add.

**Reserve** – amount of fusional vergence left over after binocular fusion has been achieved; equal to the NRV in esophoria and equal to the PRV in exophoria.

**Response ACA ratio** – the ratio of accommodative convergence to the change in accommodative response.

**Sheard's criterion** – a guideline used to assess strain on fusional vergence; it states that the fusional vergence reserve should be at least twice the amount of the demand on fusional vergence.

**Sheedy's criterion** – on a fixation disparity curve, the minimum amount of prism (x-axis value) on the flattest segment of the curve.

**Stimulus ACA ratio** – the ratio of accommodative convergence to the change in accommodative stimulus.

**Tonic convergence** – vergence at the physiological position of rest of the eyes; vergence position during distance fixation under unfused conditions and with no accommodation occurring.

**Tranaglyph** – a training device consisting of paired red and green targets on plastic sheets viewed through red and green filters, used in vision therapy to improve vergence function.

**Vectogram** – a training device consisting of paired polarized targets on plastic sheets viewed through Polaroid filters, used in vision therapy to improve vergence function.

**Vergence facility tests** – tests which determine how quickly patients can fuse a target when convergence stimulus is alternated between two stimulus levels, measured in cycles per minute.

**ZCSBV** – zone of clear single binocular vision; the area on a graph of accommodation and convergence representing the dimensions of distance, lens power, and prism power within which a patient has clear single binocular vision.

# Appendix D
# Phorometry Test Procedures

The following tables summarize phoropter procedures and examples of instructions given for von Graefe dissociated phorias, rotary prism fusional vergence ranges, relative accommodation, and binocular cross cylinder tests. Additional information concerning the performance of these tests can be found in chapters 2 (phorias), 3 (fusional vergence ranges and relative accommodation), and 13 (binocular cross cylinder). Some practitioners substitute the modified Thorington or another dissociated phoria test for the von Graefe test. They may also substitute prism bar vergence ranges outside the phoropter for rotary prism vergence ranges performed in the phoropter. Procedures for the modified Thorington test and for prism bar vergences are discussed in chapters 2 and 3. Work done by Drs. Jaimie Kruger and Rana Zargar in the Special Projects course at Indiana University School of Optometry served as a first draft for the development of these tables.

| Test | Phoropter and target set-up to start the test | Instructions and adjustment of phoropter during test | Results and recordings |
|---|---|---|---|
| **Distance Lateral Phoria** | -BVA lenses<br>-Distance PD<br>-Single letter one line larger than best visual acuity (or vertical line of letters)<br>-12 BI OD (measuring prism), 6 BU OS (dissociating prism) | "How many letters do you see?"<br>"Is the upper letter to the right or left?"<br>"Watch the lower letter and keep it clear."<br>"I will be moving the upper letter. Say 'now' when the top letter is directly above the bottom one in a straight line." (reduce BI)<br>"Say 'now' again when the two letters are aligned one above the other." (reduce BO or increase BI) | -Average of the two if they are within 3 prism diopters of each other.<br><br>-If not within 3 prism diopters then repeat measurements and average two closest |
| **Distance Vertical Phoria** | -BVA lenses<br>-Distance PD<br>-Single letter one line larger than best visual acuity (or horizontal line of letters)<br>-12 BI OD (dissociating prism) 6 BU OS (measuring prism) | "How many letters do you see?"<br>"Is the upper letter to the right or left?"<br>"Watch the upper letter."<br>"I will make the lower target move; say now when the two letters are lined up side by side at the same height." (reduce BU)<br>"I will be moving the letters back in the other direction say 'now' when they align side by side again" (reduce BD) | -Average of two if they are within 2 prism diopters of each other.<br><br>-If not within 2 prism diopters then repeat measurements and average two closest. |

| | | | |
|---|---|---|---|
| **Distance Vertical Vergences** | -BVA lenses<br>-Distance PD<br>-Risley prisms with 0 pointed sideways before both eyes<br>-Single letter one line larger than BVA (or horizontal line of letters) | "How many letters (or lines) do you see?" (should see one).<br>"When it breaks into two say 'two.' When it goes back into one again say 'one'." (increase BD over one eye; then increase BU over that same eye) | -Record Break/ Recovery<br><br>(BD is supra-vergence; BU is infravergence) |
| **Distance BI Vergences** | -BVA lenses<br>-Distance PD<br>-Risley prisms with 0 pointed up before both eyes<br>-Single letter one line larger than BVA (or vertical line of letters) | "How many letters (or lines) do you see?" (should see one).<br>"Look at the letter and try to keep it clear."<br>"Say 'blur' if the letter blurs or 'two' if it breaks into two." (increase BI over both eyes)<br>"Say 'one' when it goes back into one again." (decrease BI over both eyes) | -Record:<br> Blur/Break/ Recovery<br><br>-Record X for the blur if no blur reported |
| **Distance BO Vergences** | -BVA lenses<br>-Distance PD<br>-Risley prisms with 0 pointed up in front of both eyes<br>-Single letter one line larger than BVA (or vertical line of letters) | "Say 'blur' if the letter blurs or 'two' if it breaks into two." (increase BO over both eyes)<br>"Say 'one' when it goes back into one again." (decrease BO over both eyes) | -Record:<br> Blur/Break/ Recovery<br><br>-Record X for the blur if no blur reported |
| **Near Lateral Phoria** | -BVA lenses or tenta-tive add for presby-opes<br>-Near PD<br>-block or vertical line of approx. 20/30 letters<br>-12 BI OD (measuring prism), 6 BU OS (dissociating prism) | "How many sets of letters do you see?"<br>"Is the upper set to the right or left?"<br>"Watch the lower letters and keep them clear."<br>"I will be moving the upper letters. Say 'now' when the top chart is directly above the bottom one in a straight line." (reduce BI)<br>"Say 'now' again when the two charts are aligned one above the other." (reduce BO or increase BI) | -Average of the two if they are within 3 prism diopters of each other.<br><br>-If not within 3 prism diopters than repeat measurements and average two closest |

| | | | |
|---|---|---|---|
| **Gradient Phoria** | -Near PD<br>- block or vertical line of approx. 20/30 letters<br>-12 BI OD (measuring prism), 6 BU OS (dissociating prism)<br>-Add +1.00 D to BVA lenses or can add -1.00 D if above 6 exo at near | "How many sets of letters do you see?"<br>"Is the upper set to the right or left?"<br>"Watch the lower letters and keep them clear."<br>"I will be moving the upper letters. Say 'now' when the top chart is directly above the bottom one in a straight line." (reduce BI)<br>"Say 'now' again when the two charts are aligned one above the other." (reduce BO or increase BI) | -Average of the two if they are within 3 prism diopters of each other.<br><br>-If not within 3 prism diopters than repeat measurements and average two closest |
| **Near Vertical Phoria** | -BVA lenses or tentative add for presbyopes<br>-Near PD<br>-block or horizontal line of approx. 20/30 letters)<br>-12 BI OD (dissociating prism)<br>- 6 BU OS (measuring prism) | "How many charts do you see?"<br>"Is the upper letter to the right or left?"<br>"Watch the upper letters."<br>"I will make the lower target move and say now when the two charts are lined side by side at the same height." (reduce BU)<br>"I will be moving the letters back in the other direction say 'now' when they align side by side again" (reduce BD) | -Average of two if they are within 2 prism diopters of each other.<br><br>-If not within 2 prism diopters then repeat measurements and average two closest. |
| **Near Vertical Vergences** | -BVA lenses or tentative add for presbyopes<br>-Near PD<br>-Risley prisms with 0 pointed sideways before both eyes<br>-block or horizontal line of approx. 20/30 letters | "How many charts do you see?" (should see one).<br>"When the letters break into two say 'two,' when they go back into one again say 'one'." (increase BD over one eye; then increase BU over that same eye) | -Record Break/ Recovery<br><br>(BD is supravergence; BU is infravergence) |
| **Near BI Vergences** | -BVA lenses or tentative add for presbyopes<br>-Near PD<br>-Risley prisms with 0 pointed up before both eyes<br>-block or vertical line of approx. 20/30 letters | "How many charts do you see?" (should see one).<br>"Look at the letters and try to keep them clear."<br>"If the letters begin to blur say 'blur,' when the chart breaks into two say 'two'. (increase BI over both eyes) When it goes back to one again say 'one'." (decrease BI over both eyes) | -Record: Blur/Break/Recovery<br><br>Record X for the blur if no blur reported |
| **Near BO Vergences** | -BVA lenses or tentative add for presbyopes<br>-Near PD<br>-Risley prisms with 0 pointed up before both eyes<br>- block or vertical line of approx. 20/30 letters | "If the letters begin to blur say 'blur', when the chart breaks into two say 'two'. (increase BO over both eyes) When it goes back into one again say 'one'." (decrease BO over both eyes) | -Record: Blur/Break/Recovery<br><br>Record X for the blur if no blur reported |

| | | | |
|---|---|---|---|
| **Binocular Cross Cylinder (BCC)** | -Near PD<br>-Set auxiliary to +/-0.50 cross cylinder<br>-Use cross cylinder grid target<br>-Dim illumination<br>-Plus add (approx. +1.75 D for non-presbyopes; more plus as presbyopia advances; or can start at NRA endpoint) | "Which lines are blacker and more distinct—the lines going up & down or the lines going across" (vertical expected, add plus if horizontal) If the vertical lines are darker, say "Tell me when the two sets of lines are equally distinct or when the lines going across are darker" (reduce plus in 0.25 D steps binocularly) | -Reduce plus until patient reports equal or, if no equal, horizontal lines are darker<br><br>-Record the difference from BVA or tentative add |
| **NRA (plus to blur)** | -BVA lenses or, if presbyope, use the tentative add<br>-Near PD<br>-Near Snellen chart with 20/20 line target at 40 cm | "Can you read the bottom line?" "Try to keep that line of letters clear". "Tell me when these letters become blurred but you can still read them." (increase plus binocularly in 0.25 D steps) | -Binocularly add plus until patient reports sustained blur but can still read the line<br><br>-Record the difference from BVA or tentative add |
| **PRA (minus to blur)** | -BVA lenses or if presbyope, use the tentative add<br>-Near PD<br>-Near Snellen chart with 20/20 line target at 40 cm | "Can you read the bottom line?" "Try to keep that line of letters clear". "Tell me when these letters become blurred but you can still read them." (increase minus binocularly in 0.25 D steps) | -Binocularly add minus until patient reports sustained blur but can still read the line<br><br>-Record the difference from BVA or tentative add |

# Index

## A

absolute presbyopia, 138–39
ACA ratio
average, 61–62
CAC ratio compared to, 224–25
calculated, 17, 36, 37, 61–62, 196, 205
categories of, 16
defined, 42
drug effects on, 195–96
gradient (*see* gradient ACA ratio)
inverse of, 205
norms for, 65–66
PCT ratio calculation, use in, 196, 198
plotting, 223
response ACA ratio, 16, 36, 37
stimulus ACA ratio, 16, 17–19, 36, 37
in vergence disorders, 51, 111, 120, 122, 124, 198–99
accommodation
amplitude of (*see* amplitude of accommodation)
change in, 15
drug effects on, 195
improving, 38, 121
lag of (*see* lag of accommodation)
lead of, 152, 158–59
myopia relationship to, 208, 209
near point of (*see* near point of accommodation)
accommodation and convergence graph
alternative forms of, 205–6
first use of, 233
Fry, G. use of, 234
fusional vergence, plotting on, 25, 44–45
Hoffstetter, H.M. use of, 236
overview of, 2–5
relative accommodation, plotting, 25–26
tests plotted on, 7, 24
accommodation-convergence relationship, 193–94, 204, 237
accommodation tests, 1, 25, 151–55, 156–57, 163–64, 204. *See also under specific test, e.g.:* negative relative accommodation (NRA) test
accommodation-vergence relationship, 199
accommodative adaptation, 224
accommodative convergence
change in, 107, 144, 193–94, 196

defined, 15, 42
fusion, maintaining through, 143, 158–59
inducing, 16
plotting, 223
recognition of, 237
as vergence response factor, 200
accommodative disorders
accommodative fatigue, 157
asymptomatic, 164
case studies, 164–65
classification of, 73, 74
excess, 157, 158
exophoria, high secondary to, 37–38
infacility, 157, 165
insufficiency, 120, 157, 158, 162, 165
nonpresbyopic, 151–65
oculomotor dysfunction symptoms similar to, 228
prevalence of, 1, 7
terminology for, 157
accommodative facility
exercises, 165, 173
interpretation of, 4
tests, 70–77, 78, 156, 157
accommodative posture, 221
accommodative ranges, 140–41, 221
accommodative response
accommodative stimulus and, 36, 153, 154, 159–62
factors determining, 199
Haynes normative data for, 221
testing, 152, 153
vision therapy effect on, 176
accommodative rock, 158
accommodative stimulus
in accommodative facility tests, 70, 72
accommodative response and, 36, 153, 154, 159–62
calculating, 5
change in, 151, 152
lens and prism effects on, 5, 6–7
overview of, 1
for selected distances, 3t
tonic convergence relationship to, 42
in vision therapy, 172, 175, 176, 180–81, 183
accommodative vergence, 49
adaptation difficulties, avoiding, 141
adaptations, negative, 217

adaptive vision disorder, 164
Alexander, E.B., 244–45
Alpern, M., 195
American Optical (AO) vectographic slide, 88f, 89, 91, 189
American Optometric Association, 232, 236, 240
ametropia, 1, 17, 26, 36
amplitude of accommodation, 140, 151
    in accommodative insufficiency, 158
    improving, 171
    plotting, 4, 7, 29
    in presbyopia, 138–39, 141, 143, 144, 147
    testing, 24, 26–27, 30, 156, 157
anatomic resting position of eyes, 42
aniseikonia, 120
anti-cholingergic drugs, 195
AR. See accommodative response
AS. See accommodative stimulus
associated phoria
    definition and overview of, 83–84
    dissociated phoria coexisting with, 91
    esphoria, uncompensated, 119
    measuring, 55, 88, 89–91, 93, 189
    in presbyopia, 146
    prescription for, 91, 93, 122
    target of, 88, 90
    vision therapy for, 143
    zone of zero (ZZAP), 208
asthenopia
    accommodative and binocular impairment without, 164
    in basic esophoria, 118
    in exophoria, 142, 143
    in fixation disparity, 96
    fusional vergence strain associated with, 49, 82
    in reading and near work, 120
    sources, potential of, 201
    treatment for, 241
    vergence facility, reduced in, 78
B
base-in associated phoria, 91
base-in fusional vergence range, 7, 24
base-in prisms
    convergence stimulus, effect on, 6, 7
    for exophoria, 11, 50, 143
    in fixation disparity, 90, 93, 94–95, 99
    in fusional vergence range testing, 24
    near vision, improving through, 146
    prescribing, 224
    SILO effect and, 39
    in testing, 12

in vergence disorder treatment, 115, 118
base-in testing, 7
base-in to blur, break and recovery, 7, 25, 26, 31, 65, 144
base-out associated phoria, 93
base-out fusional vergence range, 7
base-out prisms
    convergence stimulus, effect on, 6, 7
    for esophoria, 11, 51, 52–53
    in fixation disparity, 85, 93, 94–95
    in fusional vergence range testing, 24
    SILO effect and, 39
    in vergence disorder treatment, 113–14, 123
base-out testing, 7
base-out to blur, break and recovery, 7, 25, 28, 31, 65, 144
basic esophoria, 107, 118–19, 198, 199
basic exophoria, 107, 116–18, 198, 199
basic orthophoria with restricted zone (term), 120
BCC. See binocular cross cylinder (BCC) test
bell retinoscopy, 156
Bernell lantern farpoint target, 89–90
Bernell near-point target, 95
best visual acuity (BVA), 3, 5, 11, 24
BI. See base-in prisms
binocular cross cylinder (BCC) test, 154–55
    lag of accommodation assessed through, 152
    plotting, 223
    in presbyopia, 140, 142
    tests, other compared to, 156, 157
binocular dysfunction, 74
binocular fusion, 39
binocular lens rock, 173, 180
binocular vision syndromes, 18, 19
binocular vision zone. See zone of clear single binocular vision (ZCSBV)
Birnbaum, M.H., 162, 164, 201
blurred vision, 118, 158, 164
BO. See base-out prisms
Borish, I.M., 187, 190, 216, 243, 246
Borish card, 95, 189
Borish nearpoint chart, 91
Brock string, 172, 180, 182, 183
C
CAC ratio, 192–93, 223, 224–25
caffeine, 196
calculated ACA ratio, 17, 36, 37, 61–62, 196, 205

278

Carter, D.B., 121
centering, 219
chiastopic fusion, 174
childhood myopia, 207, 208
cholingergic drugs, 195
compensated esophoria, 93
compensated exophoria, 91
computer-related vision problems, 142, 201
convergence
  amplitude testing, 4, 24, 27–28
  change in, 194
  in lens rock testing, 72
  near point of, 7, 27, 28
  types of, 15–16
convergence accommodation, 192–94, 199, 223
convergence-accommodation relationship, 193–94, 204, 237
convergence excess, 19, 107, 111–13, 118, 124, 198, 199
convergence insufficiency, 19, 107, 108. See also pseudoconvergence insufficiency
  classification of, 199
  identifying, 165
  prevalence of, 108, 117, 198
  treatment for, 110–11
  vision therapy for, 179, 180
convergence stimulus
  calculating, 3, 5, 6
  lens and prism effects on, 5, 6, 7
  overview of, 1–2
  for selected distances, 4
  in vision therapy, 172, 174–75, 180, 181, 182, 183
cover test, 10, 122, 187, 202
Cross, A.J., 153, 232–33, 243
Cross dynamic retinoscopy, 153
crystalline lens, aging effect on, 147
D
dark focus, 192, 197–98
dark vergence, 198
Daum, K.M., 176, 177, 178, 193, 202, 224, 225
defocus theory, 209
Delgadillo, H.M., 77
demand line, 5, 18
depth of focus, 203–4
Developmental Eye Movement (DEM) Test, 230
diplopia, 10, 81, 86, 117, 118, 142
direct observation eye movement testing method, 229

disparity-induced vergence (term), 192
disparity vergence (term), 192
Disparometer, 81, 82, 92, 93–94, 100, 189
displacement, testing for, 10
dissociated phoria
  associated phoria and, 83–84, 91
  asymptomatic, 190
  defined, 10
  esophoria, 118
  fixation disparity correlation to, 82
  fusional vergence associated with, 49
  norms for, 61, 62, 64, 65–66, 219, 223
  oculomotor imbalance diagnosis, role in, 88
  plotting, 4, 7, 223
  proximal convergence effect on, 39
  in pseudoconvergence insufficiency, 107
  testing and measuring, 7, 10–15, 16, 36–37, 39, 42, 43, 45, 85, 108, 142, 187, 188–89, 201–2, 246–47
  vergence posture relationship to, 70
dissociated (term), 10
distance blur, 164
distance fixation, 24
distance phoria
  in binocular vision syndromes, 19
  dark vergence, relationship to, 198
  lateral, testing for, 12, 13, 14
  testing, 36
  through subjective refraction, 42
  as tonic convergence measure, 15
  as tonic vergence measure, 198
distance rock
  defined, 70
  test, 71, 76–77, 151, 156–57
  in vision therapy, 173, 181, 183
distortion in testing, 10
divergence excess, 19, 107, 114–16
divergence insufficiency, 19, 107, 113–14
Donders, F.C., 3, 138, 233, 247, 248
Duane's binocular vision syndromes, 18, 19
dynamic retinoscopy
  development of, 232
  MEM (see MEM dynamic retinoscopy)
  MEM-LN, 160–62
  nearpoint plus ads indicated by, 228
  norms, 155–56
  Nott (see Nott dynamic retinoscopy)
  plotting, 4
  tests, other combined with, 157
  types of, 152–54

E
electronic eye movement testing techniques, 229, 230
emmetropia, 17
equilibrium findings, 219
Eskridge, J.B., 189
eso dissociated phoria, 93
eso fixation disparity, 83, 84, 86, 91, 93, 95, 98
esophoria
    basic, 107, 118–19, 198, 199
    compensated, 93
    defined, 10
    fixation disparity in, 96, 100
    fusional convergence in, 44, 49
    lags of accommodation in, 194
    negative relative vergence (NRV) relationship to, 49
    plotting, 46
    plus add effect on, 143
    ranges and norms for, 66, 122
    stimulus ACA ratio, effect on, 17
    tests for patients with, 43, 52, 55, 72
    treatment for, 50–51, 219
    uncompensated, 93, 119
    vision therapy in, 50, 107
ethyl alcohol, 195–96
exclusion in testing, 10
exodeviations, 176, 177
exo dissociated phoria, 84, 85, 91
exo fixation disparity, 81, 83, 84, 86, 90, 91, 95, 98, 143
exophoria
    accommodative lead in, 158–59
    accommodative problems as cause of high, 37–38, 162
    basic, 107, 116–18, 198, 199
    compensated, 91
    defined, 10
    fixation disparity in, 100
    fusional convergence in, 44, 49
    plotting, 46
    plus adds as factor contributing to, 89, 143
    positive relative vergence (PRV) relationship to, 49
    in presbyopia, 142–43
    ranges and norms for, 66, 122
    reducing, 115
    stimulus ACA ratio, effect on, 17
    tests for patients with, 44f, 54–55, 72
    treatment for, 11, 50, 55, 219
    uncompensated, 91, 93
    vertical alignment in, 11
    vision therapy in, 50, 107
extraocular muscles, range of motion for, 229
eye movements
    minimum, 187
    overview and types of, 228
    reading and, 201, 228–29, 230
    testing, 229–30
eyestrain
    in accommodative disorders, 158
    in basic exophoria, 117
    causes of, 42
    fusional vergence disorder associated with, 49, 54
    in vergence disorders, 125, 216

F
false convergence insufficiency. See pseudo convergence insufficiency
fixation disparity, 4, 81–86, 88–100, 122, 240
fixation disparity curve (FDC), 84–86, 88, 89, 93–99, 122, 189, 197
focus, depth of, 203–4
free-posture test, 7
free space fusion exercises, 174–75, 182, 183
Fry, G., 3, 193, 234–35, 241
fusional aftereffects, 84, 195
fusional convergence, 15, 42–46, 91, 194, 196, 201, 237
fusional vergence
    accommodation associated with, 192
    binocular lens rock performance limited by, 173
    demand on, 216
    plotting, 25, 44–45, 223
    prism adaptation caused by, 199–200
    slow, 195
    stress on, 49–55, 82
    tests, 7, 43, 77, 202–3
    treatment for, 107, 118
    vision therapy for, 143, 146, 159, 183
fusional vergence dysfunction, 107, 119–20
fusional vergence range
    norms for, 61, 64, 66
    oculomotor imbalance diagnosis, role in, 88
    proximal convergence effect on, 39
    results, displaying, 4, 7
    testing, 24–25

G
García, A., 73–75
Gilmartin, B., 198

Godio, L.P., 208
Goss, D.A., 63, 156
gradient ACA ratio, 36
  definition and overview of, 17–18
  norms for, 62, 63, 65
  PCT ratio, calculating with aid of, 196
  plus add, determining with aid of, 111–12
graphical display of clinical data, 204–5. See also accommodation and convergence graph
  accommodation, 2–5
  alternative forms of graph, 205–6
  convergence, 2–5
  dissociated phorias, plotting, 14–15, 16
  scales, 6–7
  strabismus, 206–8
Griffin, J.R., 77, 97, 119–20, 121, 122–23
Grisham, J.D., 77, 97, 108, 110, 119–20, 121, 122–23, 176, 178, 180
Groffman Visual Tracing test, 230
Grut, E.H., 237
H
Hall, P., 156
Haynes, H.M., 76, 156, 160, 161, 162, 235
Haynes' normative analysis, 220–23
headaches, 117, 125, 158
heterophoria, 91
Hirsch, M.J., 242
Hofstetter, H., 3, 138, 139, 204, 205, 234, 235–36
Hogan, R.E., 198
horizontal fixation disparity curve (FDC), 189
horizontal imbalances, 187
Howell phoria card, 202
hyperopia, 115, 141
hyperopic refractive error, 118
I
ill-sustained accommodation (term), 157
inhibitory test, 7
integrative analysis, 216
intraocular lens transplant, first, 241
J
Jackson, T.W., 63, 156
jump vergences, 182, 183
K
King-Devick Test, 229
L
lag of accommodation, 36–38
  in accommodative insufficiency, 158
  in esophoria, 194
  estimating, 159
  myopia relationship to, 209

testing, 151, 152–55, 156
lateral fixation disparity, 83
lateral phoria, 10, 12, 14
lead of accommodation, 152, 158–59
Leibowitz, H.W., 198
lens adds
  presbyopic, 139–40, 141
  vergence disorder treatment with, 49, 55, 107, 108
lens capsule, aging effect on, 147
lenses
  accommodative and convergence stimuli, effects on, 5, 7
  adaptation to, 142
  fixation disparity change with, 86
  plus lenses, 217
  prescription of, 204, 216
  for vergence disorder, 124–25
lens powers, categories of, 5
lens rock testing, 70–71, 72, 73–74, 151, 156–57
lens rock training, 173, 174
lines of sight
  in association disphoria, 93
  in fixation disparity, 81, 93
  positions of, 42–43, 44
Locke, L.C., 156
low neutral dynamic retinoscopy, 152, 153, 154, 155, 156, 157, 159–60
M
Maddox, E.E., 237–38, 246, 247
Maddox classification of convergence, 15, 42, 49, 201, 237
Maddox rod, 13, 14, 246
Maddox rod test
  overview of, 10, 187, 237–38
  Prentice, C.F. test compared to, 243
  prism use in, 11
  repeatability of, 202
Maddox wing test, 10, 11
Mallett, R.F.J., 91, 93
Mallett far-point testing unit, 89, 90, 91
Mallett near-point testing unit, 90, 95, 120
MEM dynamic retinoscopy
  development of, 235
  lag of accommodation assessed through, 120, 152–53, 158, 159
  norms for, 155, 156, 162
  tests, other combined with, 157, 160
MEM-LN retinoscopy, 160–62
minimum eye movement, 187
minus adds, 5

minus to blur test, 7, 25–26, 151. See also positive relative accommodation (PRA) test
monocular estimation method (MEM). See MEM dynamic retinoscopy
monocular estimation method (MEM)-low neutral (LN) retinoscopy, 160–62
monocular lens rock, 173, 180–81
Morgan, M., 61, 219, 238–39
Morgan's test norms and clinical analysis, 61–62, 63, 110, 123, 218
   development of, 215, 219–20
   for distance base-in break and recovery, 65, 66
   exophoria, 118
   fusional vergence ranges, 190
   vergence disorders, 108
Muscle Imbalance Measure cards, 13
myopia, 115, 141, 164, 207, 208–9

**N**

Narayan, B., 224
near phoria
   accommodation lag effect on, 37
   in binocular vision syndromes, 19
   lateral, testing for, 12, 13, 14
   in presbyopia, 142
   testing, 36
   vertical, 13
nearpoint fixation, 24
near point of accommodation, 26, 138, 139
nearpoint of convergence (NPC), 7, 27, 28, 108, 111
nearpoint phoria, 15–16
near vision, blurred, 138, 146
near work
   avoidance of, 217
   difficulties with, 158, 216–17, 218
   prescription for, 143
negative fusional vergence (NFV), 43, 45
negative relative accommodation (NRA) test, 46, 47, 64, 139, 151, 156, 157, 163–64. See also plus to blur test
negative relative vergence (NRV), 43, 44–45, 49
night myopia, 198
nonfusable (independent) objects, 10
non-strabismic binocular disorders, 1, 7
normative analysis, 215–16
Nott, I.S., 153, 239–40
Nott dynamic retinoscopy
   CAC ratio, determining with, 224
   development of, 240
   lag of accommodation, measuring through, 152, 153, 158

ranges, 155, 156, 157
NPC, 7, 27, 28, 108, 111
NSUCO Oculomotor Test, 229

**O**

oculomotor dysfunction, 228–30
oculomotor imbalance, 88
oculomotor symptoms, relieving, 120
office-based vision therapy, 180
Ogle, K.N., 240–41
one-to-one rule, 52–53, 54, 55, 119, 122, 123
ophthalmoscope, 248
optical reflex accommodation, 197, 199
Optometric Extension Program, 245
Optometric Extension Program analysis, 215, 216–19, 244
orthophoria, 124
orthopic fusion, 174, 175
orthoptics, 204
Owens, D.A., 198

**P**

paradoxical fixation disparity, 84
paralysis of accommodation (term), 157
parasympatholytic (anti-cholingergic) drugs, 195
parasympathomimetic (cholingergic) drugs, 195
Payne, C.R., 121
PCT ratio, 192, 196–97, 198
pencil pushups, 180
Percival, A.S., 241–42
Percival's criterion, 53–54, 215, 241–42
performance tests, 203
phoria line
   accommodation lag effect on, 37
   defined, 14–15
   plotting, 18, 36, 37
   in proximal convergence, 39
   as stimulus ACA ratio factor, 18–19
phorias. See associated phoria; dissociated phoria; distance phoria; near phoria
phorometric chart, 243
phorometry test, 273–76
phoropter, 90, 94
Pierce Saccade Test, 229
placebo vision therapy, 180
plus adds
   accommodative convergence, effect on, 144
   accommodative function, improving through, 38, 143, 158, 224
   defined, 5
   fixation disparity treatment with, 93, 111, 113

nearpoint, 228
testing through, 142
vergence disorder treatment with, 115, 120, 121, 123, 216
plus to blur test, 7, 25–26, 47, 151
Polaroid testing goggles, 90, 94
positive fusional vergence (PFV), 43, 45
positive relative accommodation (PRA) test, 25, 46, 47, 64, 151, 156, 157, 163–64
positive relative vergence (PRV), 43, 44, 49
Pratt system, 223–24
Prentice, C.F., 242–43, 246
Prentice's rule, 243
presbyopia, 26, 89, 138–47
prescription, checking, 203
prism adaptation, 84–85, 195, 199–200, 224
prism bar, 24, 65
prism diopters (PDs), 1–2, 4t, 5, 242
prism flippers, 77, 78
prism rock, 174, 182
prisms
    for accommodative convergence errors, 224
    for asthenopia, 241
    dissociated phoria testing, use in, 11, 12
    drawbacks of, 216
    effects on accommodative and convergence stimuli, 5–6
    fixation disparity, prescription for, 89, 97, 99
    fusional vergence range testing, use in, 24
    prescription of, 204
    vergence disorder, prescription for, 49, 55, 107, 108, 110, 121, 122, 123
proximal accommodation, 196, 197, 199
proximal convergence, 15–16, 31, 36, 38–39, 42, 196, 197
proximal vergence, 49, 197, 200
pseudoconvergence insufficiency, 37–38, 107, 120–21, 162–63, 165
pursuits, 228, 229
push-away training, 172
push-up test, 151
push-up training, 171–72, 180
R
Rainey, B.B., 195
reading
    ability, visual skills associated with, 201
    asthenopic symptoms associated with, 120
    difficulty in, 138, 146–47, 158, 217, 228
    eye movements associated with, 201, 228–29, 230
    headaches after, 164
reading glasses, 124–25, 142, 147
reading segments, base-in prisms for, 143
reduced fusional vergence (term), 119
refractive disorders, 1, 120, 201
refractive error, 141, 217
relative accommodation
    norms for, 61, 66, 219
    plotting, 4, 7, 223
    testing, 7, 24, 25, 151
relative vergence, 46
response ACA ratio, 16, 36, 37
resting position of eyes, 42
restricted zone cases (term), 119
retinal correspondence, 208
retinal disparity, 194, 199
retinoscopy, 198. See also type of retinoscopy, e.g.: dynamic retinoscopy
Ridley, H., 241
Rosenfield, M., 195, 197
rotary prism, 11, 12
Rouse, M.W., 155
Rutstein, R.P., 189, 208
S
saccades, 228, 229
Saladin, J.J., 49, 52, 63, 88, 96
Saladin Card, 81, 93, 94, 100, 189
Scheiman, M., 179, 180, 188, 215–16
Schor, C.M., 88, 96, 194, 195, 224
Sheard, C., 36, 153, 243–44
Sheard's criterion, 49–52, 54, 55, 110, 111, 113, 116, 118, 119, 120, 122, 123, 125, 215
Sheedy, J.E., 49, 52, 63, 88, 94, 143
Sheedy Disparometer, 81, 82, 92, 93–94
Sheedy's criterion, 96, 97, 98, 99, 110, 122
SILO response, 39, 196
Skeffington, A.M., 216–17, 244–45
slow fusional vergence (term), 195
smooth vergences, 183
Snellen card, 140
Sohrab-Jam, G., 228
Somers, W., 156
spherical lens adds, 49, 224
step stimulus, 182
stereoscope, 122, 187
stimulatory test, 7
stimulus ACA ratio, 16, 17–19, 36, 37

strabismus, 115, 206–8
subjective refraction
    to best visual acuity (BVA), 3, 5, 11
    defined, 26
    distance phoria through, 42
    test findings taken through, 30, 38, 39
suppression, 120, 171–72

**T**

tentative add, 142
Thorington, J., 243, 246–47
Thorington test, modified
    development of, 246–47
    equipment used in, 13
    norms for, 63, 64, 65
    overview of, 10, 238
    Prentice, C.F. test compared to, 243
    procedures for, 13–14
    repeatability of, 202
    scale use in, 11
    von Graef test in addition to, 122, 187
tonic convergence, 15, 42, 43, 237
tonic vergence, 49, 196, 198–99, 200
tranaglyphs, 172–73, 180, 182
triad convergence (term), 193
tropia line, 206–7

**U**

uncompensated esophoria, 93, 119
uncompensated exophoria, 91, 93

**V**

vectograms and tranaglyphs, 172–73, 180,
    182
vergence, 42, 196, 208–9. *See also* fusional
    vergence
vergence adaptation (term), 84, 195
vergence disorders. *See also vergence
    disorder type, e.g.:* convergence insuf-
    ficiency
    analysis of, 108–21, 216
    asymptomatic, 164
    case studies, 124–25
    case types, 31, 107, 109, 123, 198–99,
    218–19
    diagnosis of, 66, 91
    fixation disparity use in, 89
    lens rock rates in, 73
    oculomotor dysfunction symptoms
    similar to, 228
    prevalence of, 7
    treatment for, 49, 55, 107
    vision therapy for (*see* vision therapy:
    for vergence disorders)
vergence facility, 77–78
vergence posture, 70
vergence ranges, 65, 219

vergence response, 200
vergence stimulus, 107
vergence tests
    comprehensive, 215
    facility, 77–78
    normative values for, 1
    in presbyopia, 142
    reliability of, 202–3
vergence training, 107
version eye movements, 228
vertical deviations, uncorrected, 120
vertical distance phoria, 14
vertical fixation disparity curve (FDC),
    189
vertical imbalances, 187–90, 201
vertical phoria, 13, 187, 188–89, 190
vertical prism, 187, 188–89, 190
Visagraph, 230
vision therapy
    for accommodative disorders, 38, 97,
    158–59, 165, 171, 173, 175–76, 177,
    178, 179, 181
    for esophoria, 50, 107
    for exophoria, 50, 107
    for fixation disparity, 96, 97, 99
    for fusional vergence, 53, 114, 146
    for oculomotor dysfunction, 230
    for presbyopia, 143
    procedures, sequence of, 183
    results, graphical representation of,
    183
    for vergence disorders, 49, 55, 107,
    108, 110, 111, 115, 117, 118, 120, 123,
    125, 158–59, 171–73, 174–77, 178–79,
    180, 181, 199, 216
    for vertical imbalances, 187, 188
visual-verbal naming tests, 229–30
voluntary convergence, 237
von Graefe, A., 247–48
von Graefe prism dissociation technique
    applications of, 190
    development of, 248
    overview of, 10
    plotting results of, 188
    procedures for, 11–13
    repeatability of, 202
    tests, other combined with, 122, 187

**W**

Wesson Fixation Disparity Card, 81, 92, 94,
    100
Wick, B., 94–95, 96, 156, 188, 197, 215–
    16, 242

**Y**

Young, F., 209

# Z

zone of clear single binocular vision
(ZCSBV), 24
accommodation tests and, 163–64
depth of focus effects on, 203–4
graphical analysis of, 27, 28–31, 36, 37,
39, 44–45, 46, 62, 205
Percival's criterion, 53, 241–42
in presbyopia, 143–44
proximal convergence and, 38
publications on, 236
in strabismus, 206, 207
vergence adaptation and, 195
vergence disorders, assessing with aid
of, 108, 110–11, 112, 114, 118, 119,
120, 121, 123, 124, 125, 165
zone of zero associated phoria (ZZAP)
compared to, 208
zone of zero associated phoria (ZZAP),
208

# ABOUT THE AUTHOR

**D**avid A. Goss holds a B.A. degree from Illinois Wesleyan University, B.S. and O.D. degrees from Pacific University, and a Ph.D. in physiological optics from Indiana University. Between optometry school and Ph.D. studies, he practiced optometry in the office of Drs. Allen Lande and Donovan Crouch in Storm Lake, Iowa. He is a Fellow of the American Academy of Optometry (FAAO) and an Academic Fellow of the College of Optometrists in Vision Development (FCOVD-A). He was on the faculty of the College of Optometry at Northeastern State University in Tahlequah, Oklahoma from 1980 to 1992. While at Northeastern State University, he was an optometry staff member at the W.W. Hastings Indian Health Service Hospital, Tahlequah, Oklahoma. He has been on the faculty of the Indiana University School of Optometry since 1992.

Teaching responsibilities have included courses in binocular vision testing procedures and case analysis, ocular motility, ocular optics, refractive development, and vision development. Most of his research papers have been in the areas of myopia and other refractive errors, accommodation and binocular vision testing procedures, and optometry history. In addition to the previous editions of this book, his published books include *Eye and Vision Conditions in the American Indian*, 1990 (with Linda L. Edmondson as co-editor); *Clinical Management of Myopia*, 1999 (with Theodore Grosvenor); and *Introduction to the Optics of the Eye*, 2002 (with Roger W. West). He is the editor of *Hindsight: Journal of Optometry History* and the *Indiana Journal of Optometry*. Service on journal review boards includes boards for the *Journal of the American Optometric Association*, *Optometry and Vision Development*, and the *Journal of Behavioral Optometry*.